Philosophical and Theoretical Perspectives for Advanced Nursing Practice

FOURTH EDITION

Edited by

William K. Cody, RN, PhD, FAAN
Director
Presbyterian School of Nursing
Queens University of Charlotte
Charlotte, North Carolina

Previous Editions Edited by the Late Janet W. Kenney, RN, PhD

JONES AND BARTLETT PUBLISHERS
Sudbury, Massachusetts
BOSTON   TORONTO   LONDON   SINGAPORE

World Headquarters
Jones and Bartlett Publishers
40 Tall Pine Drive
Sudbury, MA 01776
978-443-5000
info@jbpub.com
www.jbpub.com

Jones and Bartlett Publishers Canada
6339 Ormindale Way
Mississauga, Ontario L5V 1J2
CANADA

Jones and Bartlett Publishers International
Barb House, Barb Mews
London W6 7PA
UK

Jones and Bartlett's books and products are available through most bookstores and online booksellers. To contact Jones and Bartlett Publishers directly, call 800-832-0034, fax 978-443-8000, or visit our website, www.jbpub.com.

Substantial discounts on bulk quantities of Jones and Bartlett's publications are available to corporations, professional associations, and other qualified organizations. For details and specific discount information, contact the special sales department at Jones and Bartlett via the above contact information or send an email to specialsales@jbpub.com.

Production Credits

Acquisitions Editor: Kevin Sullivan
Associate Editor: Amy Sibley
Production Director: Amy Rose
Associate Production Editor: Kate Hennessy
Marketing Manager: Emily Ekle
Composition: Jason Miranda, Spoke & Wheel

Manufacturing and Inventory Coordinator: Amy Bacus
Cover Design: Timothy Dziewit
Cover Image: © Photos.com
Printing and Binding: Malloy, Inc.
Cover Printing: Malloy, Inc.

Library of Congress Cataloging-in-Publication Data
Philosophical and theoretical perspectives for advanced nursing practice / [edited by] William K. Cody and Janet W. Kenney.-- 4th ed.
    p. ; cm.
  Includes bibliographical references index.
  ISBN-13: 978-0-7637-4030-6
  ISBN-10: 0-7637-4030-6
  1. Nursing--Philosophy. 2. Nursing models.
  [DNLM: 1. Nursing Theory. 2. Nursing--trends. 3. Nursing Research. 4. Philosophy, Nursing. WY 86 P569 2006] I. Cody, William K. II. Kenney, Janet W.
  RT84.5.P53 2006
  610.73'01--dc22

                            2006000742

Printed in the United States of America
10 09 08 07 06   10 9 8 7 6 5 4 3 2 1

Contents

Acknowledgments

This book came into being through the efforts of the late Dr. Janet Kenney, who nurtured it through its first three editions. It has long been well received, and it has come to occupy a special place in graduate nursing programs. In this light, it has been a very special privilege for me to attempt to follow on the heels of Dr. Kenney's original authorship and editorship. This book would not have been possible without the heroic efforts of Kevin Sullivan, Amy Sibley, Kate Hennessy, and their associates at Jones and Bartlett, who have been more than generous in working with me to complete the manuscript. I wish also to acknowledge the incomparable support and tremendous inspiration I receive every day from my beloved life partner, Timothy Koch.

Preface

The practice of nursing at an advanced level requires a deep understanding of theory and the ability to apply theory effectively in providing healthcare services to people. Indeed, if such understanding and ability is not found within a given nurse, in any specialty whatsoever, his or her practice *cannot* be considered to be advanced at all. This text, therefore, was originally edited by the late Janet Kenney and has been further revised by William Cody to meet the needs of students in graduate programs in nursing to establish a reflective dialogue with a variety of contemporary perspectives of nursing practice, to develop their own perspectives of nursing practice, and to grow in their abilities to apply theories effectively.

The place of theory in nursing *practice* has, in reality, long been considered somewhat vague and tenuous. A situation persists today that has been referred to as the "theory-practice gap," in which theory and practice are perceived as interacting imperfectly, infrequently, and sometimes insignificantly. What nurses on a trajectory to enter into advanced practice must understand is that it is *vital* for advanced practice nurses of all stripes to possess deep understandings of knowledge that can only be learned through the formal study of nursing—which means precisely philosophical and theoretical perspectives of nursing—and to master the skills of using that knowledge in service to humankind. This value for specialized knowledge is at the core of any and every discipline.

All formalized and regulated professional practice is guided by some kind of knowledge. Such knowledge is developed, traditionally, in and between and around disciplines. Although the topographic map of disciplines across academe has shifted and morphed appreciably in the past several decades, it is still the case that disciplines exist to serve humankind through astute stewardship of knowledge within a circumscribed area. Advanced practitioners and scholars within a discipline continually push the boundaries of knowledge within that discipline and are generally the only persons sanctioned by society to do so. It would be irresponsible of any discipline to elevate persons within it to positions of authority and influence who have not demonstrated a reasonable mastery of the disciplinary knowledge.

Knowing is a process. Knowledge itself is process. It is not any one thing permanently. The volume of information available to persons of means in the developed areas of the globe has roughly doubled every *18 months* since the beginning of the information age toward the end of the previous millennium, and this process continues. Memorization of facts, data, and techniques is an entirely outmoded way of preparing professionals for practice in the new millennium. Rather, it is the *process* of coming to know, the *values* that provide the reasons for wanting to know, and the *evidence* that is adduced to establish a warrant for believing anything that require deep reflection, analysis, and open-ended dialogue. This book is designed to facilitate such reflective and dialogical processes.

William K. Cody, RN, PhD, FAAN

Authors

Marion Allen, RN, PhD

Ellen Clark Birx, RN, PhD

Geertje Boschma, RN, PhD

Anne Boykin, PhD

Sandra Schmidt Bunkers, RN, PhD, FAAN

Patricia G. Butterfield, RN, MS

Barbara A. Carper, RN, EdD

William K. Cody, RN, PhD, FAAN

W. Richard Cowling, III, RN, PhD

Susan M. Duncan, RN, PhD

Lynne M. Dunphy, PhD, FNP, CNS

Nancy Edgecombe, RN, PhD(c), MN

Joyce J. Fitzpatrick, PhD, FAAN

Jacqueline Fawcett, RN, PhD, FAAN

Sally Gadow, RN, PhD

Louise A. Jensen, RN, PhD

Joy L. Johnson, RN, PhD

Janet W. Kenney, RN, PhD

Shaké Ketefian, RN, EdD, FAAN

Dorothy Kleffel, RN, MPH, DNSc

Nicole Letourneau, RN, PhD, MN, BN

Kim Lutzen, RN, PhD

Patricia Marck, RN, PhD

Brendan McCormack, DPHIL, BScNsg, PGCEA, RGN, RMN

Gail J. Mitchell, RN, MScN

Elizabeth J. Monti, MSN, CRNA

Betty Neuman, PhD, FAAN

Rosemarie Rizzo Parse, RN, PhD, FAAN

Nola J. Pender, RN, PhD, FAAN

John R. Phillips, RN, PhD

Diane Pelletier Raymond

Richard W. Redman, RN, PhD

Pamela G. Reed, RN, PhD, FAAN

Donna M. Romyn, RN, PhD

Janet C. Ross-Kerr, PhD, RN

Mahvash Salsali, PhD

Savina Schoenhofer, PhD

Rozella M. Schlotfeldt, RN, PhD, FAAN

Mary Cipriano Silva, RN, PhD, FAAN

Martha S. Tingen, PhD, RN, ANP, CS

Ann E. Tourangeau, RN, PhD

Patricia Hinton Walker, PhD, FAAN

Fay Warnock, RN, PhD

Jean Watson, PhD, FAAN

Jill E. Winland-Brown, EdD, MSN, FNP-c

Judith Wuest, RN, MN

Part One

THE NURSING DISCIPLINE AND THE DEVELOPMENT OF NURSING KNOWLEDGE

Florence Nightingale is hailed throughout the English-speaking world as the founder of modern nursing. As she was a woman of action and a great advocate for improvements in health care in the 19th century British Empire, it is often forgotten that Florence Nightingale was primarily a *writer*. Her great and lasting influence in healthcare came about through the power of her *ideas* laid out in prose and circulated in official reports, essays, and books.

Nightingale is sometimes thought of as the first nurse theorist (Tomey & Alligood, 2002) although it is doubtful that she would have understood what the term meant, had she heard it in the 1850s. Focusing largely on hygiene, nutrition, and rest, Nightingale (1859/1969) created a system for delivering effective care to patients in the context of her time. She created schools for the training of women called to do this work, and she recorded her ideas in writing for preservation and dissemination. Formal schools modeled more-or-less on the Nightingale model grew up rapidly in the late 19th century. The trend spread to America, where it proliferated. Although its progenitor was unquestionably an intellectual giant of her time, nursing was not viewed by many, over the ensuing decades, as a highly intellectual pursuit. The Anglo-American tradition of nursing, from Nightingale's time until very recently, was construed largely as vocational rather than professional, as applied rather than basic science, and as a subordinate category of labor, rather than a distinct and learned discipline.

Nursing history reflects a number of important events in the first century after Nightingale opened her schools, such as the emergence of formalized public health nursing and university education for nurses. The creation of new models of nursing and the dissemination of eloquent discourse about concepts and principles of nursing were hardly expected during that era, however, and developments in nursing philosophy and

theory were few and far between. It was not until the publication of Hildegarde Peplau's *Interpersonal Relations in Nursing* in 1952 that a work of scholarship named as *a theory of nursing* by its author was published. Slowly, additions the literature on philosophy and theory in nursing began to appear.

Considerable nursing theoretical literature in the 1950s and 1960s focused on simply naming what many nurses believed to be present in the content and context of the best nursing (e.g., Henderson, 1966). A feature of the evolving literature was the borrowing and application of theories and concepts from other disciplines, which can be detected to some extent in most of the various frameworks put forth (see Tomey & Alligood, 2002). The whole interesting project of the creation of theory to guide nursing practice became a popular topic in the scholarly nursing literature. Such endeavors came to be viewed as extremely important to nursing's future among nurse scholars who laid the groundwork for the nursing theory-based practice movement that continues in force today.

Perhaps the most salient feature of the nursing theoretical literature that arose in the 1960s was the notion that *the whole person* and *health in all its dimensions*, taken together, comprise the proper focus of nursing care. When this idea first arose, it was taken for granted that the proper approaches for study or care-planning would be to merely alternate or combine extant biological, psychological, sociological, and spiritual concepts and methods. In 1970, Martha Rogers put forward a radically different vision of nursing science as a new emergent in human history with a new and unique single focus: *the unitary human being*, more than and different from the sum of parts, and knowable only as unitary, not through particulate approaches. Thus, a new paradigm of nursing was born.

The 1970s and 1980s were an exciting time in the evolution of nursing philosophy and theory. During those decades at least 20 significant nursing frameworks intended to guide practice were published; the notion that a nurse, a nursing unit, and a nursing school should have an explicit theoretical framework for practice was popularized; research to test and expand the extant frameworks became more common and proliferated in doctoral programs in nursing; and thus, discourse about philosophy and theory in nursing became a permanent and indispensable constituent of nursing scholarship. Through the early 1990s, the literature was rife with spirited dialogue and debate around issues of nursing philosophy and theory.

In the last decade, much of the scholarly dialogue and debate in nursing centered around issues of practice and research in which the preceding discourses about philosophy and theory seemingly played little part. Master's programs in nursing increasingly turned into practitioner programs largely teaching medical knowledge, and schools with doctoral programs in nursing increasingly focused on research that would bring in government funding, which was rarely framed in a context of nursing's disciplinary knowledge. Nevertheless, there is today a sense that a critical mass has been achieved, a corner has been turned, a milestone has been passed. Now, rooted precisely in the philosophy and theory of nursing, there are very real reasons that a talented person might choose to become a nurse rather than a physician, a psychologist, or a social worker. Further, there are intriguing ideas in nursing philosophy and theory that can be explored more thoroughly through nursing scholarship than through any other means. There are also challenges to human betterment that nursing may well be the discipline best suited philosophically to meet. Whether or not nurse scholars make extensive use of nursing's extant theories or fervently embrace nursing's stated paradigms, most nurse scholars today

would agree with these assertions. The distinctiveness of nursing's disciplinary knowledge base is a reality that cannot be ignored.

In Part One of this book, five scholars explore questions that are fundamental to understanding the knowledge base of the discipline. In Chapter 1, I seek to bring clarity to the evidence-based practice movement through a discussion of fundamental assumptions underlying *evidence-based care* and *values-based practice*. I propose a new way of looking at evidence and values which, hopefully, then can be used in turn to shed light and spark discussion of the remainder of the book. In Chapter 2, Schlotfeldt discusses considerations in determining what constitutes the knowledge base of the discipline of nursing, and then identifies five areas for systematic inquiry to grow the knowledge base of nursing. In Chapter 3, a much-cited article, Carper discusses fundamental patterns of knowing in nursing, which she groups into four: empirics, esthetics, personal knowledge, and moral knowledge. In Chapter 4, Monti and Tingen explore the multiple paradigms identified in nursing science and offer a non-partisan overview of the debates. In Chapter 5, Phillips asks and answers the question: What constitutes nursing science? In sum, in this section, readers are invited to consider in several different ways the questions that are fundamental to generate knowledge to guide advanced practice in nursing.

References

Henderson, V. (1966). *The nature of nursing: A definition and its implications for practice, research, and education.* New York: Macmillan.

Nightingale, F. (1969). *Notes on nursing: What it is and what it is not.* New York: Dover. (Original published in 1859).

Peplau, H. E. (1952). *Interpersonal relations in nursing.* New York: G. P. Putnam's Sons.

Rogers, M. E. (1970). *An introduction to the theoretical basis of nursing.* Philadelphia: F. A. Davis.

Tomey, A. M., & Alligood, M. R. (Eds.). (2002). *Nursing theorists and their work* (5th ed.). St. Louis, MO: Mosby.

Chapter 1

Values-Based Practice and Evidence-Based Care: Pursuing Fundamental Questions in Nursing Philosophy and Theory

William K. Cody, RN, PhD, FAAN

Possibly the single most important philosophical question to be posed within a practice discipline is "*what guides practice?*" In nursing, historically, a long list of traditions and rules from a variety of sources served to guide practice before (and since) the advent of nursing theories. In science, traditionally, the short answer to the question "what guides practice?" usually has been rendered as *theory*, and nursing has developed a strong body of theories; however, many powerful and subtle forces influence choices in practice. By reflecting on the manifold influences on one's choices in practice, the practitioner can construct a personal answer to the fundamental question "what guides my practice?"

A clear understanding of what guides practice helps the practitioner to pursue useful knowledge more efficiently, to represent one's disciplinary perspective more articulately, and to communicate more effectively with clients and the multidisciplinary team. This book is concerned with philosophical and theoretical perspectives to guide nursing practice. It is important to note that nursing could not take its place in the academic sun and be recognized as the distinct discipline that it is today until it could point to a domain of human knowledge specific to the discipline, *knowable* only through the formal study of nursing (Coyne, 1981). This domain was mapped through the creative, deliberative construction of nursing theories over the past 50 years.

Value-Laden Theory and the Fallacy of Value-Free Science

A theory's power is proportionate to the breadth of situations and events it can encompass. There are a number of frameworks in nursing that are capable of guiding nursing practice across a range of situations and events, which reflects the maturity of nursing's knowledge base. Some nurse scholars have expressed doubt that these frameworks can guide practice broadly because they are abstract or because they are humanistic in orientation or because they include nonobjective dimensions or because many have not been extensively tested under controlled conditions. Grounding of a theoretical framework in an underlying philosophy, however, *strengthens* the theory as a guide to practice by making explicit the assumptions and values that form its underpinnings. Many nursing frameworks have explicitly incorporated values such as caring, profound respect for all persons, and attentive presence into their conceptualizations and propositions. Learning these frameworks has profoundly changed the lives of many advanced practice nurses.

In the mid twentieth century, a movement for "value-free" science rooted in the philosophies of science known as positivism, logical positivism, and logical empiricism wielded pervasive influence. This movement in its various guises sought essentially to purge science of all thought not arising from either *empirical observation or strict rules of logic*. Its influence on the sciences has lingered despite subsequent developments in philosophy of science that weakened or refuted most of its claims (Proctor, 1991). The fact that scientists are human means that science cannot be value free. Values are fundamental constituents of the human lifeworld. Indeed, there is warrant to say even that *science itself is a value*. That nursing's body of theory is heavily and explicitly value laden can today be seen as a *strength*, not a weakness, of our body of knowledge.

The hopes and expectations that grew strong in the 1980s, that nurses, nursing units, and nursing schools would adopt, use, support, and grow nursing's own theories have today been somewhat diminished by the influences of other forces converging upon the practice of nursing. These forces are multifarious and include the advent of prospective payment systems, shortened hospital lengths of stay, digitization of healthcare documentation, higher education of influential nurses in nonnursing disciplines, and the persistent need for two-year nursing programs to meet workforce demands. Along with all of these factors, the attenuated growth of the nursing theory movement can also be attributed to the failure of many members of our own discipline to recognize the uniqueness and value of our own body of knowledge and to face down criticisms from other quarters courageously.

The Clarion Call for Evidence-Based Practice

In contemporary nursing, there is a persistent clarion call to adopt *evidence-based practice*, implement it, teach it, study it, and standardize it (Melnyk & Fineout-Overholt, 2004). Many nurse leaders holding advanced degrees would answer the question "what guides nursing practice?" today by saying without hesitation, "Evidence." *Evidence-based practice* refers, in the main, to the use of rigorously derived empirical findings preferentially as the basis for intervention and nonintervention. It is not unique to nursing. The nomenclature for this movement varies, and one sees literature referring to evidence-based *practice* and literature referring to evidence-based *care*. In this chapter, a basis for differentiating the two will be proposed.

The evidence-based practice movement, although centered on the findings of empirical research and the findings of integrative reviews of empirical research, includes proponents of various different kinds of evidence, including ethical considerations and other dimensions of life (Goodman, 2003). The movement is not without its internal controversies and divergent views (e.g., Franks, 2004; Timmermans & Berg, 2003; Welsh & Lyons, 2001). Still, for the most part, the movement and the vast majority of the related literature focus on the use rigorous and replicable research findings to inform, or even determine, questions of intervention and nonintervention in healthcare.

Standards of care can be said to approximate the state of the art in evidence-based practice. Note here the difference in terminology (standards of *care*), which is significant. A set of standards of care is typically based on multiple research studies accumulated over time. It is constructed by large panels of experts to provide practitioners with a well-thought out synthesis of the available evidence for intervention and nonintervention. These standards of care adhere predominantly to the medical model in their approach, but they are commonly used by nurses, health educators, and others. Some sets of standards achieve such familiarity among practitioners across disciplines that they are known chiefly by brief acronyms such as "JNC-7," which is the *Seventh Report of the Joint National Committee on Prevention, Detection, Evaluation and Treatment of High Blood Pressure* (U.S. Department of Health and Human Services, 2004). Equivalent sets of guidelines exist for many diseases and conditions. It would be difficult to argue against such standards of care within the parameters for which they are designed because they represent feats of combined intellectual achievement that no one person could conceivably match. They help to ensure the availability of the consensus of best reasoned options for care to millions of people.

The evidence base for many of the conventions of tradition-laden and routinized healthcare, however, the truth be told, can be rather weak. Also, for any number of possible *unique* acts of intervention or caregiving, there may be no research evidence at all. Does this mean, then, that we have no guide for practice in human situations in which there is insufficient research to support recommendations? Or does it mean that knowledge resources other than strongly conclusive research must be brought to bear on situations as guides to practice? Good-

man (2003) proposes dealing with uncertainty (as to treatment) in medicine through "management, acknowledgement, and reduction [of the uncertainty]" (p. 131). Interestingly, Goodman does not turn to values for guidance in the absence of convincing evidence one way or another. One aim of the evidence-based practice movement is to minimize *bias*, and attention to the values of the practitioner can be read as an open invitation to allow bias to rule. Such an interpretation of the dynamics of personal and professional values in practice ignores the fact that many or most healthcare practitioners in fact have a *value* (i.e., a bias) for objective evidence of efficacy and for the use of good evidence in planning care. With or without evidence, it is the practitioner's values that drive her or his performance in providing care.

In reality, no formal guide to practice or any body of knowledge in any discipline can be both broad and specific enough to guide *all* actions in every situation. Practitioners are human, and life is complex, ever-changing, and unpredictable. Historically, this philosophical problem has been discussed in the discourse concerned with *praxis*.

Understanding Praxis

The discourse on evidence-based practice in nursing could benefit from an exploration of the literature on *praxis*, a concept that has been well examined from ancient times to the present. In demurring from engagement with the literature on *praxis*, the proponents of evidence-based practice limit discussion of considerations other than evidence that have a strong bearing on practice.

Praxis has been defined and described in several different ways. Aristotle related *praxis* to human situations requiring practical reasoning to inform action. Habermas (1973), Freire (1993), and Bernstein (1999), in the 20th century, have contributed to our contemporary understandings of *praxis*, which always unfolds embedded in human situations replete with the complications of multidimensional human interactions, the uncertain, and the unknowable. Persons pursue reasoning related to their peculiar situations based on an understanding of what is good and what contributes to human well-being. *Praxis* and practical reasoning always unfold in a context that is profoundly interpersonal and relatively unpredictable. The end is not predetermined, and as possible *ends* evolve situationally, possible *means* evolve as well. Thus, *praxis* is creative and dialogical. In political and pedagogical discourse, praxis has even been explicated as the practice of freedom.

Practice as *Praxis*

If practice is examined in the light of this voluminous literature of over 2,000 years, it must be viewed as driven by far more than scientific evidence alone. Even the most diehard logical positivist would concede, at a minimum, the need for a *code of ethics* to provide parameters of conduct for science-based practice. Many considerations other than scientific evidence can be identified as reasons for action and as knowledge to guide practice.

The *practice* of nursing is intentional and deliberate action, guided by nursing science and other sources of knowledge, performed by nurses, and intended for the benefit of persons and society. In this regard, it is comparable to other professional practices. The moment-to-moment acts of nursing practice are chosen from a wide variety of options by each individual nurse in the ever-unfolding and unpredictable context of interrelationships with persons, families and communities, their meanings to the persons involved, and the values that are interwoven among the meanings. The animus underlying nursing practice is the intention to benefit people. However, the actions, behaviors, and words that provide the benefits change from moment to moment with the situation.

Each nurse is responsible for her or his own practice in a fundamental and inescapable way. The actions entailed in professional nursing practice are also the responsibility of, and occur under the stewardship of, the nursing profession itself, by way of its regulatory bodies and professional associations. These bodies determine the expectations of all the nurses within their spheres of influence, and these expectations are laid out in accord with conventions such as the nursing process and standards of ethics. In short, practice is predominantly driven by the personal and professional *values* of the nurse. It is owned and controlled by the individual nurse to a great extent although governed by certain bodies representing the profession and the state.

Care

Human care is a recognizable and structured interaction in human societies through which persons give and receive assistance with basic human needs, in wellness and in illness, across the lifespan, before birth, throughout life, and beyond death. Specialized care of various kinds is delivered by professionals and is largely deemed to be deliverable only by such professionals. In contemporary society, human care, hereinafter *care*, should be and is largely consumer driven. Care delivery is governed, at the individual level, largely by the recipient of care or the guardian or designee of the recipient, who has the right to accept or refuse whatever care is offered.

It is axiomatic across healthcare disciplines that clients have a right to be *offered* care based on the best evidence available. It is not for the practitioner to decide ultimately what intervention, if any, the client will receive; rather, this decision rests with the client, who has the right to be well-informed about the evidence and to make a choice. What evidence is most valued by the practitioner varies from one practitioner to the other, but all are expected to adduce evidence to justify their recommendations and offerings to clients. It is important to note that from the practitioner perspective care is *offered* and, within the bounds of ethics, not ordered, required, or forced, for care, in a fundamental sense, belongs to the consumer. It is the consumer's to request, accept, or reject in accord with personal values. It is the professional's responsibility to offer that for which there is best evidence. As demonstrated above, this expectation is exemplified in the standards of care that delineate the best knowledge that the health sciences have to offer at a given time.

Differentiating Practice and Care

The discourse on evidence-based practice does not differentiate clearly between *practice* and *care*. This conflation of what should be two distinct concepts is especially troubling in nursing, wherein scholars have emphasized nursing's special commitment to care and caring for generations. Upon reflection, however, one can discern a fundamental difference between the nature and structure of professional practice on the one hand and the care that is delivered by professionals on the other. In **Table 1–1**, four ways of differentiating practice and care are specified.

Practice belongs to the practitioner and is driven by values. Only the actor has the agency to initiate

and cease deliberate actions. The practitioner is assumed to have control over her or his own actions and to be responsible for them. Nothing can remove the onus of individual responsibility from any professional practitioner, neither haste in service to one's charges, nor pressure from one's hierarchical superiors, nor lack of key information. This responsibility and relative autonomy is further emphasized at the societal level by assigning control and governance of the profession largely to the members of the profession itself. Professional practice is governed by the individual practitioner, her or his discipline, the governments of states and countries, laws, and societal norms. Professional practice is relatively discipline specific in that education and licensure to perform complex and sophisticated tasks to benefit others, for pay, is typically regulated in a context of disciplinary knowledge, expertise, socialization, and customary expectations.

Practice is necessarily and profoundly practitioner driven. The knowledge base and decision-making capacity of the practitioner are among the very defining factors of professional practice. Practice, as stated before, is highly contextual and situational. Many factors impinge on moment-to-moment decision-making in practice. No external resource for decision-making can be absorbed by the practitioner thoroughly and rapidly enough to inform all action or inaction in situation to an extent equal to individual

Table 1–1 Differentiating Practice and Care

Practice	Care
Belongs to the practitioner	Belongs to the consumer
Controlled by the practitioner, by the profession, and by society	Controlled by the consumer, by rules/laws, and by society
More discipline-specific, since it is more practitioner-driven	More interdisciplinary, since it is more consumer-driven
Values-based	Evidence-based

knowledge and experience. This immediacy of intention and action is in the nature of all multidimensional, deliberative interactions among human beings.

That which most fundamentally drives one's practice is one's *values*. Values are by definition the cherished beliefs that prompt and inspire choices and actions over time. Making similar choices repeatedly and performing similar actions repeatedly over time confirms the value as an abiding cherished belief within one's world of meaning (Parse, 1998). The way a nurse practices and the way she or he provides care to persons reflects her or his personal and professional values (Woodbridge & Fulford, 2003). Spending time with clients may reflect a value for offering attentive presence. Frequently urging clients to make changes in health maintenance routines may reflect the values of norms or problem solving. One's values are constituents of *who one is* and thus are reflected in all that one does.

Care is the prerogative of the consumer and is structured by evidence. Only the consumer/client (or her/his legitimate designee) has the right to accept or reject care, even though typically care is designed and prescribed or recommended by others (i.e., professionals). This assertion is an outgrowth of the ongoing paradigm shift toward person-centered care, attending to the whole person, and respect for individual and cultural differences. The professional caregiver's responsibility is to see that the consumer's choice of care is informed and that the delivery of care is carried out competently. Legal protections and social sanctions exist to ensure that the consumer's rights to be well-informed and to receive competent care are protected.

As described above, standards of care represent something close to the consensus state of the art of evidence-based care. All clients of healthcare professionals have the right to expect that care will be offered that is structured to the extent possible in accord with broadly recognized standards of care.

Values-Based Practice and Evidence-Based Care

We live our values. The strongest confirmation of a value is to act on it repeatedly, which also describes rather precisely how we construe professional practice. The practitioner chooses how to practice based on personal values. The client chooses what care to receive based on personal values. The practitioner offers care to address the client's needs and desires, care that is structured based on the best evidence available.

As the philosopher Raz (2003) has pointed out in his book *The Practice of Value,* "Concepts of false values cannot have instances" (p. 24). This is another way of saying essentially that we live our values. To frame this proposition more colloquially, *if you don't live it, it's not your value.* In contrast, there can be false evidence. Indeed, the history of science is replete with instances of evidence misinterpreted and misunderstood. Evidence is a phenomenon that emerges only as evidence of something. The answer is already halfway there when the question is posed.

Standards of care are rewritten periodically based on newly emergent evidence, and it is not unusual for standards to seesaw back and forth between yea and nay to certain procedures between one edition of guidelines and the next. Surely something more substantial, lasting, and meaningful to both nurse and client must underpin nursing practice. To this author's way of thinking, that underpinning is found in the interface of personal meanings and values with the meanings and values structured in a theoretical framework for nursing practice. Readers are invited to use this text to assist them in identifying the values and meanings that inform and inspire their practice.

Suggestions for Further Reflection

In this chapter, I have sought to inspire and facilitate reflection on the question "what guides practice?" Many of the readings throughout the rest of this book put forward ideas about philosophy and theory in nursing that will prompt further reflection, and hopefully dialogue and debate, about the question. In Chapter 3, Carper provides a schema for organizing the knowledge necessary for nursing practice, categorized as empirics, esthetic knowing, ethical knowing, and personal knowing. How do values and evidence relate to Carper's ways of knowing? Are values and evidence equally relevant to all types of knowing, or is evidence more pertinent to one type and are values more pertinent to another? In Chapter 4, Monti and Tingen present multiple paradigms of nursing science, in which vastly different worldviews underpin theory development and practice. Does this then mean that different values underpin practice and evidence is considered differently from different perspectives?

In Chapter 8, Parse describes how adopting an explicitly values-based theoretical perspective transforms practice. In Chapter 9, Bunkers puts forward 16 tenets for framing nursing knowledge for the 21st century, all of which are explicitly value laden. Evidence is scarcely mentioned at all. Does this mean that a philosophy that is explicitly values driven does not value evidence? Or does it mean that evidence accrues when one abides with the 16 value-laden tenets? In Chapter 10, Wuest discusses the contrast between traditional values of professionalism and the values of caring and justice reflected in the feminist literature. In Chapter 11, Ketefian and Redman propose that the process of knowledge development itself is embedded in systems of cultural values and perspectives and question whether it

is appropriate for Western values by their dominance in science and the professions to shape knowledge development in non-Western societies. One might well ask, "How can one accurately perceive evidence if one is using the wrong cultural lens to seek it?"

In Johnson's examination of nursing art in Chapter 15, it is easy to see that values are threaded throughout the five conceptualizations of nursing art that she puts forth, but perhaps not so easy to ferret out the role of evidence in the performance of nursing art. Cowling, in Chapter 17, and Gadow, in Chapter 18, explicitly connect with a values-laden ontology in describing an appreciative practice methodology and describing an ethos of relational narrative, respectively. In Chapter 19, Butterfield points out that in many cases, the evidence one seeks in order to understand health concerns may be found not at the individual level but at the societal level. How counterproductive, and arguably inhumane, for example, to press for behavior change at the individual level to resolve a difficulty that stems fundamentally from societal neglect?

In Chapter 21, Boykin and Schoenhofer reconceptualize outcomes in a way that challenges the hegemony within the outcomes literature of strict adherence to objective and quantifiable outcomes. In the theory of nursing as caring, rather, enhancing personhood is conceptualized as the central desired outcome. Chapters 23, 24, and 25 reflect three different attitudes toward the place of human values, meanings, hopes, and dreams in relation to science, reflecting three divergent ways of organizing constructs of science, values, and evidence. In Chapter 26, Carper's categories of knowing are revisited and the meaning of evidence in each way of knowing is specified. Chapters 27 and 28 explicitly focus on issues surrounding the use of evidence from two competing perspectives.

The interplay of values and evidence in determining how to practice and what kind of care to deliver occurs at the very core of healthcare decision-making. The contemporary advanced practice nurse is challenged to develop the ability to appreciate and understand a wide variety of human values in a rapidly changing multicultural society. She or he is equally challenged to develop the ability to discern strong and weak evidence and how to structure healthcare services based on the preponderance of the evidence. Both abilities are cultivated best within the context of a broad and deep appreciation of theoretical and philosophical perspectives of nursing offered in this text.

References

Bernstein, R. J. (1999). *Praxis and action: Contemporary philosophies of human activity*. Philadelphia: University of Pennsylvania Press.

Coyne, A. B. (1981). Prologue. In R. R. Parse, *Man-living-health: A theory of nursing* (pp. vii–xii). New York: John Wiley.

Franks, V. (2004). Evidence-based uncertainty in mental health nursing. *Journal of Psychiatric and Mental Health Nursing, 11*, 99–105.

Freire, P. (1993). *Pedagogy of the oppressed* (M. B. Ramos, Trans.). New York: Continuum.

Goodman, K. W. (2003). *Ethics and evidence-based medicine: Fallibility and responsibility in clinical science*. Cambridge, UK: Cambridge University Press.

Habermas, J. (1973). *Theory and practice* (J. Viertel, Trans.). Boston, MA: Beacon.

Melnyk, B. M., & Fineout-Overholt, E. (2004). *Evidence-based practice in nursing and healthcare: A guide to best practice*. Philadelphia: Lippincott Williams & Wilkins.

Parse, R. R. (1998). *The human becoming school of thought: A perspective for nurses and other health professionals*. Thousand Oaks, CA: Sage.

Proctor, R. (1991). *Value-free science? Purity and power in modern knowledge*. Cambridge, MA: Harvard University Press.

Raz, J. (2003). *The practice of value*. Oxford, UK: Oxford University Press.

Timmermans, S., & Berg, M. (2003). *The gold standard: The challenge of evidence-based medicine and standardization in health care*. Philadelphia: Temple University Press.

U.S. Department of Health and Human Services. (2004). *Seventh Report of the Joint National Committee on Prevention, Detection, Evaluation and Treatment of High Blood Pressure*. Rockville, MD: Author.

Welsh, I., & Lyons, C. M. (2001). Evidence-based care and the case for intuition and tacit knowledge in clinical assessment and decision making in mental health nursing practice: An empirical contribution to the debate. *Journal of Psychiatric and Mental Health Nursing, 8*, 299–305.

Woodbridge, K., & Fulford B. (2003). Good practice? Values-based practice in mental health. *Mental Health Practice, 7*(2), 30–34.

Chapter 2

Structuring Nursing Knowledge: A Priority for Creating Nursing's Future

Rozella M. Schlotfeldt, RN, PhD, FAAN

Nursing's future will be created only as the discipline underlying nursing practices is identified, structured, and continuously updated by systematic inquiry. The kinds of knowledge contained within the discipline are identified and an approach to its structure is proposed.

There can be little doubt that one of the highest priorities for creating an appropriate future for nursing is that of identifying, structuring, and continuously advancing the knowledge that underlies the practices of professionals in the field. That statement can be made because a consensus has not yet been attained concerning the subject matter that must be mastered by those who seek to practice general and specialized nursing. Surely by the beginning of the twenty-first century, nursing's body of knowledge will be identified, selected, verified, and agreed upon by qualified professionals in the field, effectively structured, and continuously updated to reflect newly discovered knowledge. Also, knowledge judged to be erroneous, inadequate, and outdated should be deleted. This knowledge will be derived from basic and clinical scientific nursing research, both quantitative and qualitative, from philosophic and historical inquiries, and from

Source: Schlotfeldt, R. (1989). Structuring nursing knowledge: A priority for creating nursing's future. *Nursing Science Quarterly, 1*(1): 35–38. Reprinted by permission of and copyright © 2002 Sage Publications, Inc.

evaluation research designed to establish valid criterion measures, devices, and approaches to establishing the efficacy and value of nursing's caring functions as they are relevant to the health, function, comfort, well-being, productivity, self-fulfillment, and happiness of human beings.

The thesis of this chapter is that only qualified professionals in the field, including general and specialist practitioners, educators, administrators, investigators, historians, philosophers, and theorists, should be given responsibility by the profession (however that is defined) to identify, verify, structure, and continuously update the extant content or subject matter that, at the minimum, should be included in the intellectual armamentaria of all professional nurses. This responsibility of the profession is essential to four functions: (a) the creation of comparable programs of study at the first professional degree level; (b) control of the profession's goals, mission, and accomplishments; (c) a valid procedure for licensing (not registering) all who quality as professionals in the field; and (d) certification of bona fide nursing specialists.

Nursing as a Profession

Two major criteria must be fulfilled by any occupational group whose members earn and achieve the status of a profession, or more appropriately for nursing, a learned helping profession. First, a profession must have an institutionalized goal or social mission. Learned professions are valued by the societies whose members give them positive sanction for two major reasons: (a) the services learned professionals render are judged to be essential and beneficial for all members of society during particular times in their lives, and (b) members of each learned profession have identified and come to a consensus about the knowledge that practitioners must master and use selectively, creatively, humanely, effectively, and ethically in providing those essential services. As a second criterion, each profession must support a cadre of investigators whose role is to advance its knowledge continuously with a view toward improving its practices.

The traditional learned professions have included the clergy, lawyers, and physicians. The clergy have been valued and supported because they are expected to be knowledgeable and skillful in providing spiritual comfort and well-being for all those who consult them. Lawyers are expected to master coded law and to apply their discipline fairly and skillfully in fulfilling the goal of preserving social harmony and justice. Physicians have been valued because knowledge of human ills and disabilities and their causes and knowledge of the means to eliminate, attenuate, or manage them and alleviate their noxious consequences are considered essential to the well-being of society. Are the caring functions and mission of nurses, namely, appraising and optimizing the health, function, comfort, independence, and potential of human beings, any less valued than spiritual comfort and well-being? Are they any less desirable than social harmony and justice? Are they any less

important than finding causes for, diagnosing, and treating human ills?

Unfortunately, the caring functions typically provided by nurses were for too long considered to be mere extensions of the duties and obligations of wives and mothers, for which large amounts of professional knowledge were not considered essential (Reverby, 1987). Lay members of societies have typically not recognized and nurses themselves have been remarkably tardy in identifying and organizing the several kinds of professional knowledge that are fundamental to executing the caring functions that nurses typically provide.

The essential and often crucial nature of nurses' caring functions in promoting the health and well-being of all human beings is finally being recognized by thinking people, including scholarly nurses. There is now general agreement (at least verbal agreement) that nursing's social mission is to appraise and assist human beings in their quest to optimize their health status, health assets, and health potential (Fawcett, 1983). Furthermore, general agreement exists that there is or should be a body of structured knowledge that professionals in the field agree represents the discipline that is fundamental to general and specialty nursing practices.

Nursing scholars have discussed, described, and characterized the discipline (Donaldson & Crowley, 1978), and in the recent past, the American Association of Colleges of Nursing (1986) has reported findings from a "national effort to define the essential knowledge, practice, and values that the baccalaureate nurse should possess" (p. 1). Panel members expressed the belief that the essentials so delineated can be achieved within the traditional baccalaureate degree program in nursing and that the baccalaureate represents first-level professional preparation in nursing.

The efforts that have been made toward establishing the discipline represent significant steps toward achieving the goal of identifying, organizing, and achieving a consensus concerning the specific body of extant knowledge that underlies nursing practices. It must be noted, however, that there has not yet been a concerted effort to identify and obtain agreement about the currently available knowledge that is fundamental to nursing's growing number of declared specialties or even to obtain a consensus about the requisite knowledge and skills that define what nursing's specialties are. It must be recognized also that the subject matter that constitutes the discipline has not yet been identified and structured, and agreement has not been reached concerning appropriate and needed inclusions from qualified professionals in the field. This paper presents an approach to organizing the several kinds of knowledge contained within the discipline, a possible next step toward having qualified professionals select and structure the specific extant subject matter of the discipline about which agreement is needed.

Knowledge of the Discipline

Figure 2–1 shows the kinds of professional knowledge contained within the discipline, which is depicted as a large sphere having a permeable and expandable membrane (represented by the second sphere) to permit the continuous addition of newly discovered knowledge and the deletion of that found through systematic inquiry to be erroneous, inadequate, or irrelevant.

The largest segment of the sphere (**Figure 2–1a**) represents nursing's scientific subject matter. Therein belongs all of nursing science (i.e., the verified facts, principles, and laws that have been discovered through scientific inquiry to be valid, relevant, and useful for nursing practice); included also are extant scientific theories that guide scientific investigations in nursing and those that have been proposed by scholarly

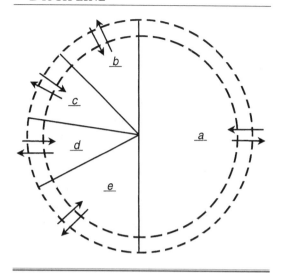

Figure 2–1 THE NURSING DISCIPLINE

nurses as promising explanations of phenomena that are of particular concern to nurses.

To date, much of nursing science has been discovered by basic scientists and subsequently found through empirical evidence and systematic study to be relevant. Nurse investigators have also been adding to nursing's scientific knowledge by testing the relevance and utility of theories generated by basic scientists in clinical nursing situations (Chinn, 1984). Few investigations have yet been reported that test scientific theories regarding human phenomena that are of particular concern to nurses but 'not to basic scientists (Silva, 1986). A plausible reason is that there is little agreement among nurses concerning the human phenomena that are of concern to nurses and how they should be characterized and classified and how knowledge of them should be advanced.

In general, nurses accept the notion that human beings are biopsychosocial beings (Engel, 1977). It is proposed here that the subjects that nurses serve also exemplify assets of the human spirit of which relevant knowledge is inadequate.

Those assets surely include human spirituality and other qualities of the human spirit, such as determination, verve, courage, beliefs, hope, and aspiration. Nurses surely hold responsibility for advancing knowledge of those health-seeking assets. In sum, human beings' health-seeking mechanisms and behaviors, beliefs, and propensities can be classified as biological, psychological (both emotional and cognitive), and sociocultural and as assets of the human spirit; all of them are directly relevant to the natural efforts by humans to seek and attain optimal health. Because so much scientific nursing knowledge remains to be discovered, it is safe to predict that nursing science will likely always represent the largest and most rapidly changing aspect of the discipline. Furthermore, nurses are increasingly recognizing the relevance of scientific knowledge from disciplines not traditionally judged to be relevant for nursing. Included, for example, are concepts, principles, and theories from economics, political science, administration and management, and computer science. The science fundamental to education has long been incorporated as an integral part of the discipline of nursing.

A second important segment of the sphere representing the nursing discipline is historical knowledge (**Figure 2–1b**). Included is knowledge of the heritage of the occupation and the developing profession of nursing, including knowledge of people, circumstances, and events that have shaped that development. Included also is the history of nursing knowledge as it has been transmitted to generations of practitioners.

The third section of the sphere (**Figure 2–1c**) represents philosophic nursing knowledge. Included are the profession's accepted values and codes of professional behavior. Included also should be the several philosophic theories that have been tested, found useful and relevant to nurses' work, and accepted as philosophic guides to practice. Illustrative are selected theories of value, justice and morality, and ethical

theories. Because nurses are encountering increasing numbers of moral and ethical dilemmas and because nurses are increasingly manifesting interest in becoming scholars in the discipline of philosophy, it is predicted that nursing knowledge henceforth will include increasing amounts of tested and relevant philosophic knowledge that will be incorporated into the discipline.

The fourth section of the sphere (**Figure 2–1d**) represents knowledge of nursing strategies, approaches, and technologies along with the scientific and artistic principles essential to their execution. Included also is knowledge of the prevailing health care system. Relationships between the goals and caring functions of nurses and the goals and practice functions of other health professionals in the existing health care systems represent another important segment of the discipline.

Another significant segment of nursing's body of knowledge has always been knowledge of factors that influence the health status, health assets, and health potential of human beings, both favorably and unfavorably (**Figure 2–1e**). Included is knowledge of biological, physical, and cognitive abilities with which people are naturally endowed and knowledge of environmental factors, economic and social circumstances, and changes associated with normal development, including the aging process. In the nursing perspective presented here, pathologies and medical diagnoses and treatments are factors that affect the health of human beings. Nurses must have adequate knowledge of these factors: such knowledge is an integral part of the discipline that must be mastered by nurse practitioners.

There is yet another kind of knowledge that is directly relevant to and essential for nursing practice. It is the knowledge that professionals must gain from relevant data concerning each person being served and that obtained through astute and perceptive observations. Personal knowledge of individuals and groups of persons is needed for nurses to respect the uniqueness of those for whom they provide exemplary services. For that reason, there can be no prescriptive nursing practice theories or professional approaches to nursing care that are universally generalizable.

In summary, conceptualizing the discipline of nursing as an expandable and permeable sphere made up of segments of varying size provides an approach to classifying and organizing the several kinds of knowledge that constitute the nursing discipline. Such an approach demonstrates the vast and growing amounts of knowledge that professionals in the field must master and be able to use selectively, creatively, artistically, humanely, and skillfully to provide exemplary care.

Nursing should be recognized as a learned helping profession and a respected academic discipline. Surely nursing scholars will ensure the attainment of those goals by the beginning of the twenty-first century. Crucial to their attainment is identifying and attaining agreement about the human phenomena that are of particular concern to nurses, enhancing scholarly clinicians' involve-ment in generating promising relevant theories, and testing those theories as the means to discover knowledge through which to continuously improve nursing practices. Such an approach will ensure the availability of valid nursing knowledge in the twenty-first century and its currency during all centuries to come.

References

American Association of Colleges of Nursing. (1986). *Essentials of college and university education for professional nursing.* Washington, DC: Author.

Chinn, P. (1984). From the editor. *Advances in Nursing Science, 6*(2), ix.

Donaldson, S., & Crowley, D. (1978). The discipline of nursing. *Nursing Outlook, 26,* 113–120.

Engel, G. (1977). The need for a new medical model: A challenge for biomedicine. *Science, 196,* 129–136.

Fawcett, J. (1983). Hallmarks of success in nursing theory development. In P. Chinn (Ed.), *Advances in nursing theory development* (pp. 3–17). Rockville, MD: Aspen.

Reverby, S. (1987). A caring dilemma: Womanhood and nursing in historical perspective. *Nursing Research, 36,* 5–11.

Silva, M. (1986). Research testing nursing theory: State of the art. *Advances in Nursing Science, 9*(1), 1–11.

Chapter 3

Fundamental Patterns of Knowing in Nursing

Barbara A. Carper, RN, EdD

It is the general conception of any field of inquiry that ultimately determines the kind of knowledge the field aims to develop as well as the manner in which that knowledge is to be organized, tested, and applied. The body of knowledge that serves as the rationale for nursing practice has patterns, forms, and structure that serve as horizons of expectations and exemplify characteristic ways of thinking about phenomena. Understanding these patterns is essential for the teaching and learning of nursing. Such an understanding does not extend the range of knowledge, but rather involves critical attention to the question of what it means to know and what kinds of knowledge are held to be of most value in the discipline of nursing.

Identifying Patterns of Knowing

Four fundamental patterns of knowing have been identified from an analysis of the conceptual and syntactical structure of nursing knowledge.[1] The four patterns are distinguished according to logical type of meaning and designated as (1) empir-

ics, the science of nursing; (2) esthetics, the art of nursing; (3) the component of a personal knowledge in nursing; and (4) ethics, the component of moral knowledge in nursing.

Empirics: The Science of Nursing

The term *nursing science* was rarely used in the literature until the late 1950s. However, since that time, there has been an increasing emphasis, one might even say a sense of urgency, regarding the development of a body of empirical knowledge specific to nursing. There seems to be general agreement that there is a critical need for knowledge about the empirical world, knowledge that is systematically organized into general laws and theories for the purpose of describing, explaining, and predicting phenomena of special concern to the discipline of nursing. Most theory development and research efforts are primarily engaged in seeking and generating explanations that are systematic and controllable by factual evidence and that can be used in the organization and classification of knowledge.

The pattern of knowing that is generally designated as "nursing science" does not presently exhibit the same degree of highly integrated abstract and systematic explanations characteristic of the more mature sciences, although nursing literature reflects this as an ideal form.

Source: Carper, B. A. (1978). Fundamental patterns of knowing in nursing. *ANS, 1* (1): 13–24. Reprinted with permission from and copyright © 1978 Aspen Publishers, Inc.

Clearly, there are a number of coexisting, and in a few instances competing, conceptual structures—none of which has achieved the status of what Kuhn calls a scientific paradigm. That is, no single conceptual structure is as yet generally accepted as an example of actual scientific practice "which include[s] law, theory, application, and instrumentation together . . . [and] . . . provide[s] models from which spring particular coherent traditions of scientific research."[2(p10)] It could be argued that some of these conceptual structures seem to have greater potential than others for providing explanations that systematically account for observed phenomena and may ultimately permit more accurate prediction and control of them. However, this is a matter to be determined by research designed to test the validity of such explanatory concepts in the context of relevant empirical reality.

NEW PERSPECTIVES

What seems to be of paramount importance, at least at this stage in the development of nursing science, is that these preparadigm conceptual structures and theoretical models present new perspectives for considering the familiar phenomena of health and illness in relation to the human life process; as such, they can and should be legitimately counted as discoveries in the discipline. The representation of health as more than the absence of disease is a crucial change; it permits health to be thought of as a dynamic state or process that changes over a given period of time and varies according to circumstances rather than a static either/or entity. The conceptual change in turn makes it possible to raise questions that previously would have been literally unintelligible.

The discovery that one can usefully conceptualize health as something that normally ranges along a continuum has led to attempts to observe, describe, and classify variations in health, or levels of wellness, as expressions of a human being's relationship to the internal and external environments. Related research has sought to identify behavioral responses, both physiological and psychological, that may serve as cues by which one can infer the range of normal variations of health. It has also attempted to identify and categorize significant etiological factors that serve to promote or inhibit changes in health status.

CURRENT STAGES

The science of nursing at present exhibits aspects of both the "natural history stage of inquiry" and the "stage of deductively formulated theory." The task of the natural history stage is primarily the description and classification of phenomena that are, generally speaking, ascertainable by direct observation and inspection,[3] but current nursing literature clearly reflects a shift from this descriptive and classification form to increasingly theoretical analysis, which is directed toward seeking, or inventing, explanations to account for observed and classified empirical facts. This shift is reflected in the change from a largely observational vocabulary to a new, more theoretical vocabulary whose terms have a distinct meaning and definition only in the context of the corresponding explanatory theory.

Explanations in the several open-system conceptual models tend to take the form commonly labeled functional or teleological.[4] For example, the system models explain a person's level of wellness at any particular point in time as a function of current and accumulated effects of interactions with his or her internal and external environments. The concept of adaptation is central to this type of explanation. Adaptation is seen as crucial in the process of responding to environmental demands (usually classified as stressors) and enables an individual to maintain or reestablish the steady state, which is designated as the goal of the system. The developmental models often exhibit a more genetic type of explanation in that certain events, the developmental tasks, are believed to be causally relevant or necessary conditions for the normal development of an individual.

Thus, the first fundamental pattern of knowing in nursing is empirical, factual, descriptive, and ultimately aimed at developing abstract and theoretical explanations. It is exemplary, discursively formulated, and publicly verifiable.

Esthetics: The Art of Nursing

Few, if indeed any, familiar with the professional literature would deny that primary emphasis is placed on the development of the science of nursing. One is almost led to believe that the only valid and reliable knowledge is that which is empirical, factual, objectively descriptive, and generalizable. There seems to be a self-conscious reluctance to extend the term *knowledge* to include those aspects of knowing in nursing that are not the result of empirical investigation. There is, nonetheless, what might be described as a tacit admission that nursing is, at least in part, an art. Not much effort is made to elaborate or to make explicit this esthetic pattern of knowing in nursing—other than to associate vaguely the "art" with the general category of manual and/or technical skills involved in nursing practice.

Perhaps this reluctance to acknowledge the esthetic component as a fundamental pattern of knowing in nursing originates in the vigorous efforts made in the not-so-distant past to exorcise the image of the apprentice-type educational system. Within the apprentice system, the art of nursing was closely associated with an imitative learning style and the acquisition of knowledge by accumulation of unrationalized experiences. Another likely source of reluctance is that the definition of the term *art* has been excessively and inappropriately restricted.

Weitz suggests that art is too complex and variable to be reduced to a single definition.[5] To conceive the task of esthetic theory as definition, he says, is logically doomed to failure in that what is called art has no common properties—only recognizable similarities. This fluid and open approach to the understanding and application of the concept of art and esthetic meaning makes possible a wider consideration of conditions, situations, and experiences in nursing that may properly be called esthetic, including the creative process of discovery in the empirical pattern of knowing.

ESTHETICS VERSUS SCIENTIFIC MEANING

Despite this open texture of the concept of art, esthetic meanings can be distinguished from those in science in several important aspects. The recognition "that art is expressive rather than merely formal or descriptive," according to Rader, "is about as well established as any fact in the whole field of esthetics."[6(p xvi)] An esthetic experience involves the creation and/or appreciation of a singular, particular, subjective expression of imagined possibilities or equivalent realities that "resists projection into the discursive form of language."[7] Knowledge gained by empirical description is discursively formulated and publicly verifiable. The knowledge gained by subjective acquaintance, the direct feeling of experience, defines discursive formulation. Although an esthetic expression required abstraction, it remains specific and unique rather than exemplary and leads us to acknowledge that "knowledge—genuine knowledge, understanding—is considerably wider than our discourse."[7(p23)]

For Wiedenbach, the art of nursing is made visible through the action taken to provide whatever the patient requires to restore or extend his [sic] ability to cope with the demands of his [sic] situation,[8] but the action taken, to have an esthetic quality, requires the active transformation of the immediate object—the patient's behavior—into a direct, nonmediated perception of what is significant in it—that is, what need is actually being expressed by the behavior. This perception of the need expressed is not only responsible for the action taken by the nurse but reflected in it.

The esthetic process described by Wiedenbach resembles what Dewey refers to as the difference between recognition and perception.[9] According to Dewey, recognition serves the purpose of identification and is satisfied when a name tag or label is attached according to some stereotype or previously formed scheme of classification. Perception, however, goes beyond recognition in that it includes an active gathering together of details and scattered particulars into an experienced whole for the purpose of seeing what is there. It is perception rather than mere recognition that results in a unity of ends and means that gives the action taken an esthetic quality.

Orem speaks of the art of nursing as being "expressed by the individual nurse through her creativity and style in designing and providing nursing that is effective and satisfying."[10(p155)] The art of nursing is creative in that it requires development of the ability to "envision valid modes of helping in relation to 'results' which are appropriate."[10(p69)] This again invokes Dewey's sense of a perceived unity between an action taken and its result—a perception of the means of the end as an organic whole.[9] The experience of helping must be perceived and designed as an integral component of its desired result rather than conceived separately as an independent action imposed on an independent subject. Perhaps this is what is meant by the concept of nursing the whole patient or total patient care. If so, what are the qualities that enable the creation of a design for nursing care that eliminate or would minimize the fragmentation of means and ends?

Esthetic Pattern of Knowing

Empathy—that is, the capacity for participating in or vicariously experiencing another's feelings—is an important mode in the esthetic pattern of knowing. One gains knowledge of another person's singular, particular, felt experience through empathic acquaintance.[11,12] Empathy is controlled or moderated by psychic distance or detachment in order to apprehend and abstract what we are attending to and in this sense is objective. The more skilled the nurse becomes in perceiving and empathizing with the lives of others, the more knowledge or understanding will be gained of alternate modes of perceiving reality. The nurse will thereby have available a larger repertoire of choices in designing and providing nursing care that is effective and satisfying. At the same time, increased awareness of the variety of subjective experiences will heighten the complexity and difficulty of the decision making involved.

The design of nursing care must be accompanied by what Langer refers to as sense of form, the sense of "structure, articulation, a whole resulting from the relation of mutually dependent factors, or more precisely, the way the whole is put together."[7(p16)] The design, if it is to be esthetic, must be controlled by the perception of the balance, rhythm, proportion, and unity of what is done in relation to the dynamic integration and articulation of the whole. "The doing may be energetic, and the undergoing may be acute and intense," Dewey says, but "unless they are related to each other to form a whole," what is done becomes merely a matter of mechanical routine or of caprice.[9]

The esthetic pattern of knowing in nursing involves the perception of abstracted particulars as distinguished from the recognition of abstracted universals. It is the knowing of a unique particular rather than an exemplary class.

The Component of Personal Knowledge

Personal knowledge as a fundamental pattern of knowing in nursing is the most problematic, the most difficult to master and to teach. At the same time, it is perhaps the pattern most essential to understanding the meaning of health in terms of individual well-being. Nursing considered as an interpersonal process involves interactions, relationships, and transactions between the nurse and the patient-client. Mitchell points out that "there is growing evidence that the quality of interpersonal contacts has an influence on a person's becoming ill, coping with illness and becoming well."[13(p4950)] Certainly the phrase "therapeutic use of self," which has become increasingly prominent in the literature, implies that the way in which nurses view their own selves and the client is of primary concern in any therapeutic relationship.

Personal knowledge is concerned with the knowing, encountering, and actualizing of the concrete, individual self. One does not know about the self; one strives simply to know the self. This knowing is a standing in relation to another human being and confronting that human being as a person. This "I–Thou" encounter is unmediated by conceptual categories or particulars abstracted from complex organic wholes.[14] The relation is one of reciprocity, a state of being that cannot be described or even experienced—it can only be actualized. Such personal knowing extends not only to other selves but also to relations with one's own self.

It requires what Buber refers to as the sacrifice of form, that is, categories or classifications, for a knowing of infinite possibilities, as well as the risk of total commitment.

> *Even as a melody is not composed of tones, nor a verse of words, nor a statue of lines-one must pull and tear to turn a unity into a multiplicity—so it is with the human being to whom I say You.... I have to do this again and again; but immediately he is no longer You.*[14(p59)]

Maslow refers to this sacrifice of form as embodying a more efficient perception of reality in that reality is not generalized nor predetermined by a complex of concepts, expectations, beliefs, and stereotypes.[15] This results in a greater willingness to accept ambiguity, vagueness, and discrepancy of oneself and others. The risk of commitment involved in personal knowledge is what Polanyi calls the "passionate participation in the act of knowing."[16(p17)]

The nurse in the therapeutic use of self rejects approaching the patient–client as an object and strives instead to actualize an authentic personal relationship between two persons. The individual is considered as an integrated, open system incorporating movement toward growth and fulfillment of human potential. An authentic personal relation requires the acceptance of others in their freedom to create themselves and the recognition that each person is not a fixed entity, but constantly engaged in the process of becoming. How then should the nurse reconcile this with the social and/or professional responsibility to control and manipulate the environmental variables and even the behavior of the person who is a patient in order to maintain or restore a steady state? If a human being is assumed to be free to choose and chooses behavior outside of accepted norms, how will this affect the action taken in the therapeutic use of self by the nurse? What choices must the nurse make in order to know another self in an authentic relation apart from the category of patient, even when categorizing for the purpose of treatment is essential to the process of nursing?

Assumptions regarding human nature, McKay observes, "Range from the existentialist to the cybernetic, from the idea of an information processing machine to one of a many splendored being."[17(p399)] Many of these assumptions incorporate in one form or another the notion that there is, for all individuals, a characteristic state which they, by virtue of membership in the species, must strive to assume or achieve. Empirical descriptions and classifications reflect the assumption that being human allows for prediction of basic biological, psychological, and social behaviors that will be encountered in any given individual.

Certainly empirical knowledge is essential to the purposes of nursing, but nursing also requires that we be alert to the fact that models of human nature and their abstract and generalized categories refer to and describe behaviors and traits that groups have in common. However, none of these categories can ever encompass or express the uniqueness of the individual encountered as a person, as a "self." These and many other similar considerations are involved in the realm of personal knowledge, which can be broadly characterized as subjective, concrete, and existential. It is concerned with the kind of knowing that promotes wholeness and integrity in the personal encounter, the achievement of engagement rather than detachment, and it denies the manipulative, impersonal orientation.

Ethics: The Moral Component

Teachers and individual practitioners are becoming increasingly sensitive to the difficult personal choices that must be made within the complex context of modern health care. These choices raise fundamental questions about morally right and wrong action in connection with the care and treatment of illness and the promotion of health. Moral dilemmas arise in situations of ambiguity and uncertainty, when the consequences of one's actions are difficult to predict and traditional principles and ethical codes offer no help or seem to result in contradiction. The moral code that guides the ethical conduct of nurses is based on the primary principle of obligation embodied in the concepts of service to people and respect for human life. The discipline of nursing is held to be a valuable and essential social service responsible for conserving life, alleviating suffering, and promoting health, but appeal to the ethical "rule book" fails to provide answers in terms of difficult individual moral choices, which must be made in the teaching and practice of nursing.

The fundamental pattern of knowing identified here as the ethical component of nursing is focused on matters of obligation or what ought to be done. Knowledge of morality goes beyond simply knowing the norms or ethical codes of the discipline. It includes all voluntary actions that are deliberate and subject to the judgment of right and wrong—including judgments of moral value in relation to motives, intentions, and traits of character. Nursing is deliberate action, or a series of actions, planned and implemented to accomplish defined goals. Both goals and actions involve choices made, in part, on the basis of normative judgments, both particular and general. On occasion, the principles and norms by which such choices are made may be in conflict.

According to Berthold, "Goals are, of course, value judgments not amenable to scientific inquiry and validation."[18(p196)] Dickoff, James, and Wiedenbach also call attention to the need to be aware that the specification of goals serves as "a norm or standard by which to evaluate activity . . . [and] . . . entails taking them as values—that is, signifies conceiving these goal contents as situations worthy to be brought about."[19(p422)]

For example, a common goal of nursing care in relation to the maintenance or restoration of health is to assist patients to achieve a state in which they are independent. Much of the current practice reflects an attitude of value attached to the goal of independence and indicates nursing actions to assist patients in assuming full responsibility for themselves at the earliest possible moment or to enable them to retain responsibility to the last possible moment. However, valuing independence and attempting to maintain it may be at the expense of the patient's learning how to live with physical or social dependence when necessary—for example, in instances when prognosis indicates that independence cannot be regained.

Differences in normative judgments may have more to do with disagreements as to what constitutes a "healthy" state of being than lack of empirical evidence or ambiguity in the application of the term. Slote suggests that the persistence of disputes, or lack of uniformity in the application of cluster terms, such as health, is due to "the difficulty of decisively resolving certain sorts of value questions about what is and is not important." This leads him to conclude, "That value judgment is far more involved in the making of what are commonly thought to be factual statements than has been imagined."[20(p220)]

The ethical pattern of knowing in nursing requires an understanding of different philosophical positions regarding what is good, what ought to be desired, what is right; of different ethical frameworks devised for dealing with the complexities of moral judgments; and of various orientations to the notion of obligation. Moral choices to be made must then be considered in terms of specific actions to be taken in specific, concrete situations. The examination of the standards, codes, and values by which we decide what is morally right should result in a greater awareness of what is involved in making moral choices and being responsible for the choices made. The knowledge of ethical codes will not provide answers to the moral questions involved in nursing, nor will it eliminate the necessity for having to make moral choices, but it can be hoped that

> *The more sensitive teachers and practitioners are to the demands of the process of justification, the more explicit they are about the norms that govern their actions, the more personally engaged they are in assessing surrounding circumstances and potential consequences, the more "ethical" they will be; and we cannot ask much more.*[21(p221)]

Using Patterns of Knowing

A philosophical discussion of patterns of knowing may appear to some as a somewhat idle, if not arbitrary and artificial, undertaking having little or no connection with the practical concerns and difficulties encountered in the day-to-day doing and teaching of nursing, but it represents a personal conviction that there is a need to examine the kinds of knowing that provide the discipline with its particular perspectives and significance. Understanding four fundamental patterns of knowing makes possible an increased awareness of the complexity and diversity of nursing knowledge.

Each pattern may be conceived as necessary for achieving mastery in the discipline, but none of them alone should be considered sufficient. Neither are they mutually exclusive. The teaching and learning of one pattern do not require the rejection or neglect of any of the others. Caring for another requires the achievements of nursing science, that is, the knowledge of empirical facts systematically organized into theoretical explanations regarding the phenomena of health and illness, but creative imagination also plays its part in the syntax of discovery in science, as well as in developing the ability to imagine the consequences of alternative moral choices.

Personal knowledge is essential for ethical choices in that moral action presupposes personal maturity and freedom. If the goals of nursing are to be more than conformance to unexamined norms, if the "ought" is not to be determined simply on the basis of what is possible, then the obligation to care for another human being involves becoming a certain kind of person—and not merely doing certain kinds of things. If the design of nursing care is to be more than habitual or mechanical, the capacity to perceive and interpret the subjective experiences of others and to imaginatively project the effects of nursing actions on their lives becomes a necessary skill.

Nursing thus depends on the scientific knowledge of human behavior in health and in illness, the esthetic perception of significant human experiences, a personal understanding of the unique individuality of the self, and the capacity to make choices within concrete situations involving particular moral judgments. Each of these separate but interrelated and interdependent fundamental patterns of knowing should be taught and understood according to its distinctive logic, the restricted circumstances in which it is valid, the kinds of data it subsumes, and the methods by which each particular kind of truth is distinguished and warranted.

The major significances to the discipline of nursing in distinguishing patterns of knowing are summarized as (1) the conclusions of the discipline conceived as subject matter cannot be taught or learned without reference to the structure of the discipline—the representative concepts and methods of inquiry that determine the kind of knowledge gained and limit its meaning, scope, and validity; (2) each of the fundamental patterns of knowing represents a necessary but not complete approach to the problems and questions in the discipline; and (3) all knowledge is subject to change and revision. Every solution of an existing problem raises new and unsolved questions. These new and as yet unsolved problems require, at times, new methods of inquiry and different conceptual structures; they change the shape and patterns of knowing. With each change in the shape of knowledge, teaching and learning require looking for different points of contact and connection among ideas and things. This clarifies the effect of each new thing known on other things known and the discovery of new patterns by which each connection modifies the whole.

References

1. Carper, B. A. "Fundamental Patterns of Knowing in Nursing." PhD dissertation, Teachers College, Columbia University, 1975.

2. Kuhn, T. *The Structure of Scientific Revolutions* (Chicago: University of Chicago Press, 1962).

3. Northrop, F. S. C. *The Logic of the Sciences and the Humanities* (New York: The World Publishing Co., 1959).

4. Nagel, E. *The Structure of Science* (New York: Harcourt, Brace and World, Inc., 1961).

5. Weitz, M. "The Role of Theory in Aesthetics" in Rader, M., ed. *A Modern Book of Esthetics,* 3rd ed. (New York: Holt, Rinehart and Winston, 1960).

6. Rader, M. "Introduction: The Meaning of Art" in Rader, M., ed. *A Modern Book of Esthetics,* 3rd ed. (New York: Holt, Rinehart and Winston, 1960).

7. Langer, S. K. *Problems of Art* (New York: Charles Scribner and Sons, 1957).

8. Wiedenbach, E. *Clinical Nursing: A Helping Art* (New York: Springer Publishing Co., Inc., 1964).

9. Dewey, J. *Art as Experience* (New York: Capricorn Books, 1958).

10. Orem, D. E. *Nursing: Concepts of Practice* (New York: McGraw-Hill Book Co., 1971).

11. Lee, V. "Empathy" in Rader, M., ed. *A Modern Book of Esthetics*, 3rd ed. (New York: Holt, Rinehart and Winston, 1960).

12. Lippo, T. "Empathy, Inner Imitation and Sense-Feeling" in Rader, M., ed. *A Modern Book of Esthetics*, 3rd ed. (New York: Holt, Rinehart and Winston, 1960).

13. Mitchell, P. H. *Concepts Basic to Nursing* (New York: McGraw-Hill Book Co., 1973).

14. Buber, M. *I and Thou.* Translated by Walter Kaufman (New York: Charles Scribner and Sons, 1970).

15. Maslow, A. H. "Self-Actualizing People: A Study of Psychological Health" in Moustakas, C. E., ed. *The Self* (New York: Harper and Row, 1956).

16. Polanyi, M. *Personal Knowledge* (New York: Harper and Row, 1964).

17. McKay, R. "Theories, Models and Systems for Nursing." *Nurs Res* 18:5 (September–October, 1969).

18. Berthold, J. S. "Symposium on Theory Development in Nursing: Prologue." *Nurs Res* 17:3 (May–June, 1968).

19. Dickoff, J., James, P., and Wiedenbach, E. "Theory in a Practice Discipline: Part I." *Nurs Res* 17 (September–October, 1968).

20. Slote, M. A. "The Theory of Important Criteria." *J Philosophy* 63 (April 14, 1966).

21. Greene, M. *Teacher as Stronger* (Belmont, CA: Wadsworth Publishing Co., Inc., 1973).

Chapter 4

Multiple Paradigms of Nursing Science

Elizabeth J. Monti,
MSN, CRNA

Martha S. Tingen,
PhD, RN, ANP, CS

Of the many controversies that have accompanied the growth of nursing as a discipline, few have been debated as long and as vigorously as the question of which paradigm should guide nursing science. Despite more than 20 years of discussion, the question remains unresolved. This article discusses the concept of paradigm, explores the paradigms that influence nursing science, and presents a comparison of the advantages and disadvantages of theoretical unification and multiparadigmism. Additionally, the implications and consequences of multiparadigmism for the present and future development of nursing as a science within a practice discipline are presented.

A discipline is a community of interest that is organized around the accumulated knowledge of an academic or professional group.[1] The discipline of nursing represents the body of knowledge related to the study of caring in human health that encompasses both the science and art of nursing.[1,2] Within the discipline, nursing science is devoted to answering questions of interest to the profession and adding to the body of knowledge. Nursing practice represents the art of the discipline.

The unique perspective of the discipline is exemplified by the metaparadigm, which describes, from a global perspective, the concepts and themes chosen as the focus of the discipline and those that differentiate it from others.[3] The metaparadigm concepts of nursing generally are agreed to be person, environment, nursing, and health; however, these are not exclusive.[2–5] The metaparadigm also reflects the shared values and beliefs of the discipline. For example, nurses subscribe to common values and beliefs, including respect for persons, caring, autonomy of persons, health promotion, illness prevention, professional competence, and ethical conduct.[1,6]

While nursing scientists are in general agreement about the metaparadigm, they often are in disagreement about the paradigms of the discipline. This disagreement stems in part from failure to agree on a single definition of the term; as a result, writers often are describing different concepts. However, the debate also stems from the idea that the discipline must have a predominant paradigm in order to demonstrate progress

Source: Monti, E. J. & Tingen, M. S. (1999). Multiple paradigms of nursing science. *ANS, 21* (4): 64–80. Reprinted with permission from and copyright © 1999 Aspen Publishers, Inc.

as a legitimate science. Because primary paradigms in nursing are considered to represent fundamentally different patterns of knowing and perspectives of reality,[3] these disagreements also focus on the ability of paradigms to answer questions and to explore reality in different ways, the relevance of different types of knowledge for the discipline, and the congruence between paradigm and metaparadigm concepts.

Of the many controversies that have accompanied the growth of nursing as a discipline, few have been debated as long or as vigorously as the question of which paradigm should guide nursing science. Despite more than 20 years of discussion, the question remains unresolved. This article discusses the concept of paradigm, explores the paradigms that influence nursing science, and compares and contrasts the advantages and disadvantages of theoretical unification and multiparadigmism. In addition, the implications and consequences of multiparadigmism for the present and future development of nursing as a science within a practice discipline are presented.

The Nature of Paradigms

Many definitions of the word "paradigm" exist. Webster defines it first as "a pattern, example, or model" and secondarily as "an overall concept accepted by most people in an intellectual community, as a science, because of its effectiveness in explaining a complex process, idea, or set of data."[7(p. 979)] A paradigm also has been described as an abstract view or perspective of a discipline, a set of systematic beliefs, a world view, and a theory.[8] Kuhn,[8] who popularized the term, provided multiple descriptions of a paradigm in the first edition of his book, yet failed to precisely define it. In an effort to resolve the confusion that arose from his varying uses of the term, Kuhn later provided two definitions for a paradigm. In the pri-

mary sense of the word, a paradigm is a "disciplinary matrix," the ordered elements of which are held by the practitioners of a discipline. According to this definition, a paradigm includes symbolic generalizations (laws and definitions), shared beliefs, and shared values. In an alternate use, Kuhn defines paradigms in a more circumscribed manner as exemplars or shared examples. Exemplars are a part of the disciplinary matrix by which students learn to solve problems through the application of concrete solutions.

Nursing authors also have contributed to a lack of coherence about paradigms. Fawcett stated that "...paradigms are represented by diverse conceptual models of nursing that provide distinctive contexts for the metaparadigm concepts and themes."[4(p2)] Newman[9] states that paradigms are pervasive in nature and that a paradigm's values are deeply imbedded in its followers. Kim defines paradigms as "...general scientific perspectives and traditions," because nursing science is developing from various research traditions and the discipline's problems require different perspectives. Lincoln and Guba define a paradigm as "...a systematic set of beliefs, together with their accompanying methods."[11(p15)] Hardy,[12] citing Kuhn, defines the paradigm as a gestalt or world view, a metaparadigm that is broader than theory and precedes it. The definition of paradigm as a world view or philosophy that reflects the values and beliefs embraced by a segment of the discipline does not seem useful for the development of nursing science because values and beliefs seldom are amenable to change and the nature of science is about change. The authors of this article prefer Kim's definition because it infers methods that scientists apply to solve problems regardless of their philosophy and perspective or lens through which phenomena can be viewed. Kim's definition of paradigm is used throughout this article.

Paradigms are important to scientific communities because they not only answer the discipline's most important questions—or puzzles, as Kuhn[8] called them—but also shape the way scientists "do" research. The ontological and epistemological assumptions of a paradigm drive its methodologies. Scientists who share a paradigm "...are committed to the same rules and standards for scientific practice."[8(p11)] A paradigm is useful in that it provides scientists with a general orientation to phenomena, a way of organizing perceptions, criteria for selecting problems, guidelines for investigations and methods, and limitations on possible solutions. Thus, a paradigm provides a guiding framework for resolving problems, conducting research, and deriving theories and laws. For nursing scientists, paradigms direct the perspective from which research questions are asked, problems are investigated, research is designed as well as what methods are used and how data are collected, analyzed, and interpreted.[2]

Paradigms in Nursing

Nursing science is characterized by two predominant paradigms that are broadly classified as the empiricist and the interpretative. These two paradigms represent fundamentally opposing views of knowledge development and reality. Several conceptual frameworks of nursing depict the metaparadigm concepts from the perspective of the different paradigms. The contribution of the primary paradigms to nursing science will be discussed, and examples of conceptual frameworks that are derived from them will be presented. The cardinal features of the two paradigms are presented in **Table 4–1**.

Table 4–1 A COMPARISON OF THE EMPIRICIST AND INTERPRETATIVE PARADIGMS

	Empiricism	Interpretative
Alternative names	Mechanistic Positivism	Organismic
Nursing	Particulate-deterministic	Unitary-transformative
Paradigms	Totality	Simultaneity
Ontology	One reality Reality is independent of context Truth can be determined Certainty is possible	Multiple realities Composite reality Meaning is grounded in experience Truth can never be determined
Epistemology	Reality can be verified by the senses Value-free observations Cognition and perception are separate entities	Knowledge is derived from experience, art, ethics Value-laden observations Cognition, perception and experience affect what is seen or conceptualized Shared meaning
Purpose	Verification and justification Theory testing Identify cause and effect	Discovery and meaning Theory generating Increase understanding and knowledge of lived reality

(Continues)

Table 4–1 A COMPARISON OF THE EMPIRICIST AND INTERPRETATIVE PARADIGMS (CONTINUED)

Human beings are:	Machines The sum of their parts Closed systems	Living organisms Holistic beings Greater than the sum of their parts Open systems
Researcher is	Observer Objective Uninvolved	The instrument Co-creating Involved in the process
Phenomena	Can be reduced to parts	Holistic view Irreducible Context dependent
Behavior	Predictable, linear	Probabilistic Unpredictable
Movement	Organism is passive or at rest Exterior forces cause movement	Active From within organism
Methodologies	Quantitative Observation Control	Qualitative Attention to context and interpretation Interview, observation
Research question	What is the relationship of A and B What is the effect of A on B? Hypothesis testing	What is the meaning of . . . ? What is the structure of the lived experience?
Designs	Experimental Quasi-experimental	Emergent Phenomenology Grounded theory
Sample	Random selection Random assignment Convenience	Purposive Theoretical Volunteer
Data collection techniques	Instrumentation Observation	Interviews Observation Analysis of art, literature, documents
Data analysis	Deductive Statistical analysis	Inductive Interpretation Constant comparative method

Empiricism is based on the assumption that what is known can be verified through the senses.[5] The ontological assumption of empiricism is that there is one reality, which is out there somewhere and can be validated through the senses. In the empiricist paradigm, knowledge is developed through sense observation of the natural world in order to verify and justify theories that describe, predict, and prescribe. Research studies in this tradition focus on the context of justification. Theories depicting reality are reduced into components that can be either validated or disproved empirically in order to justify the relationships set forth. Empiricism also has been described as reductionistic because parts rather than the whole of phenomena are examined and because of the positivistic emphasis on theory reduction.

"The ontological assumption of empiricism is that there is one reality, which is out there somewhere, which can be validated through the senses."

Empiricism has its roots in the logical positivist school of philosophy. Logical positivism, also called logical empiricism and the received view, was espoused by a group of philosophers known as the Vienna school.[11,13,14] Positivists disavowed religious and metaphysical explanations of reality and analyzed theories for logical patterns of reasoning that could be verified in reality.[14] Logical positivism, however, was an extremist variant of empiricism because it espoused the idea that the only reality was that which could be observed in the world.[13,15] Thus, the mind was not an object of study unless the mind could be associated with a physical reality, a position reminiscent of Descartes' theory of mind-body dualism. Positivism also was associated with an antiquated view of the universe that equated it with a machine operated by laws understood only by God.[13] The purpose of science was to discover these laws, or products, in order to be able to explain and predict events in the world. Theories describing reality in formal language either could be verified or disproved by observation of objects in the world. Thus, science resulted in a product, a theory, that could be used to describe, predict, and prescribe.

Positivism fell into disfavor in the 1960s when it was criticized for using defective methods of analysis and having little to do with actual science.[14] Although discredited and recognized as a dead movement since the 1960s,[6,16] many nursing scientists continue to react to contemporary empiricism as though positivism were flourishing. Gortner feels that empiricism has been given short shrift in nursing, because of ". . . continued fallacious identification with logical positivism."[6(p482)] Modern empiricism, also called postpositivism, incorporates a historical approach to science along with empirical methods.[6]

Historicism is concerned with the values and beliefs of scientists as well as the sociological and historical context in which decisions regarding scientific research are made.[16] Historical approaches incorporate the ideas of philosophers such as Laudan, who thought that science should be judged by the number of problems it solved rather than whether or not theories were verified.[16] Thus, postpositivist empirical research retains the empiricist elements of precision, deductive reasoning, objectivity, theory testing, and substantiation of theoretical claims with valid data,[17] while recognizing the impossibility of verification and the value-laden qualities of theory and observation.[6,15] However, postpositivists also recognize that the purpose of scientific investigation in nursing is patient care; that the meaning of relationships can be clarified; that generalizable patterns can be ascertained without full prediction and control; that the conditions or context in which the phenomenon occurs is important; and that the researcher must prevent personal biases from influencing the outcomes of research.[17]

The method associated with empiricism is the scientific method. This method focuses on the experiment, control, objectivity, precise measurement, quantification of data, and description of results in statistical terms. Because empiricists believe that the senses can be used to verify reality, observation is the preferred method of data collection. The scientist uses tools and instruments to measure the phenomenon of concern while remaining a detached observer in order to prevent personal biases from influencing the study results.[18] Numerical values are assigned to data in order to test relationships using statistical methods. The empiricist paradigm is necessary if nursing science is to substantiate claims regarding nursing care and the responses of persons in health and illness situations, provide explanatory models, and test and generate theory.[6,17] The value of the empirical approach to knowledge development lies in its ability to test hypotheses, compare interventions, produce generalizations, and generate confidence intervals that uncover influences.[15] The ability to test hypotheses allows the relationships in theories to be tested and validated.[18] Although no one study ever can verify a relationship, the data collected can offer strong support for the presence of a relationship. Establishment of valid relationships enables theories to be used to explain, predict, and prescribe notions that are essential and relevant for clinical practice.[19] Control limits the problem being researched and attempts to limit extraneous factors so that relationships can be examined more precisely. Random assignment of subjects or treatments also allows factors that may affect the variable of interest to be equally distributed.[15] Generalizability is an important goal of empirical research, as it allows relationships to be extrapolated to a larger population or different situation, a factor that is advantageous in nursing practice.[18] Statistical methods allow for both exploratory and confirmatory analyses of data to describe the data and search for potential relationships.[18] However, discovery of statistical significance does not indicate necessarily clinical significance.[15]

Criticisms of Empiricism

Objectivity and control are aspects of empiricism that have been criticized severely by many nursing researchers. In empirical investigations, researchers control extraneous or confounding variables in order to increase the validity of study results. However, when studying humans, it is impossible to control many factors that might affect the outcome of a study. In addition, excessive control of variables in human studies can remove important contexts that influence a situation and contribute to its meaning. Excessive control produces an artificial situation that bears no resemblance to reality and thus decreases generalizability. Objectivity is also seen as preventing "...full recognition of the other as a person"[20] while experimental conditions can decontextualize the human experience. Thus, the traditional experimental method, in which persons respond to the environment like a machine rather than interacting with the environment, is seen as having a dehumanizing effect.[20]

Some nursing scientists criticize positivism because it does not recognize other forms of knowing besides that that can be verified. Nurses always have recognized the knowledge embedded in practice. Carper[21] identified four fundamental patterns of knowing in nursing: empirics, ethics, esthetics, and personal knowledge. Empirics, or the science of nursing, is concerned with describing, explaining, and predicting phenomena of concern. Esthetics, or the art of nursing, is the expressive and perceptive aspect of nursing that can defy expression. Ethics focuses on moral questions of right and wrong and what ought to be done. Personal knowledge "... is concerned with the knowing, encountering, and actualizing of the concrete, individual self."[21(p251)] The four are not isolated entities but interrelate to form a whole that is greater than the sum of the parts. Thus, knowledge acquisition does not occur as a result of one isolated way of viewing the world but through the simultaneous interaction of the four patterns. Logical positivism ignored aspects of nursing knowledge that were acquired through means other than empirical methods and thus negated a rich source of nursing knowledge.

Prior to the 1950s, nursing research activities were limited.[18] In the 1950s and 1960s, empiricism was the predominant approach to developing nursing knowledge. Strongly influenced by the medical model and education in other disciplines, early nursing scientists favored the empiricist paradigm because they were eager to establish the scientific basis of the profession and demonstrate that nursing was a unique, professional discipline.[22] However, many nursing scientists became frustrated with the positivistic approach and began questioning its use because it often did not reflect the values and beliefs of nursing nor the discipline's focus on holism, person-centered care, and understanding of human experiences in health and disease. Desiring a more humanistic approach that could address the concerns of nurses and their patients, many researchers turned to the methods proposed by phenomenological and existential schools of philosophy that are concerned with the meaning of human experience and understanding the day-to-day experience of individuals.[20]

The Interpretative Paradigm

The interpretative paradigm in nursing science evolved for several reasons. First, many early nurse scientists were educated in disciplines such as philosophy, sociology, and anthropology that exposed them to alternate ways of viewing the world and the methodologies associated with those paradigms. Second, to some nurse scientists, empiricism did not recognize the esthetic, ethical, and personal knowledge inherent in nursing. Interpretative traditions acknowledge that reality has multiple meanings and that knowledge can be derived from sources other than the senses. Thus, other patterns of knowing important to nursing are given credence by interpretative approaches. Third, the interpretative approach was seen as more congruent with the language and beliefs of nursing. Where nursing spoke of holism, individualism, autonomy, and self-determination, the dominating scientific/medical model spoke of reductionism, objectivity, manipulation, prediction, and control.[22] A fourth reason for embracing the interpretative paradigm is that nursing wished to establish a theoretical base for the discipline. The interpretative paradigm provided methods for generating theory that are representative of nursing views rather than borrowed from other professions.[22] Finally, a qualitative approach offers new perspectives and methodologies for answering the questions of the discipline.[23]

The interpretative paradigm is characterized by the ontological assumptions that reality is complex, holistic, and context dependent.[11,24] The focus of investigation is on human experience: thus, subjectivity rather than objectivity is emphasized.[12] Because reality and human experience are variable, multiple ways of knowing are valued to uncover the knowledge that is embedded in human experience. Tacit or intuitive knowledge is recognized in addition to that which is expressed in language or can be observed.[11] Therefore, the method includes techniques that result in extended contact of the researcher with the participant and in mutual interaction. A natural setting is selected because ". . . wholes cannot be understood in isolation from their contexts . . ."[11(p39)] nor can they be separated into parts for study. Inductive reasoning is used to identify patterns of meaning in the data.[11]

Broadly grouped under the term *qualitative research*, interpretative methods include phenomenology, hermeneutics, grounded theory, ethnography, and others. The general goal of interpretative methods is to understand and derive meaning from the human experience; however, instrumentation and conceptualization are other identified purposes.[24] Common features of these research traditions are a holistic approach to questioning, a focus on human experience, purposive sampling, sustained contact with participants, the involvement of the researcher in the process, emergent design, negotiated outcomes, and special criteria for trustworthiness.[11] In-depth interviews with open- ended questions and participant observations are used for data collection. Data analysis proceeds through analysis of written narratives to extract the meaning of the experience.[24]

A strength of the interpretative paradigm is the usefulness of this approach for generating theories. When little is known about a subject, qualitative methods are useful in identifying patterns of experiences and the relationships between them. Relational statements reflecting these relationships can be written and used to develop new theories.[18] For example, grounded theory methods can identify basic social structures or processes (BSP) through the method of constant comparative analysis. These BSPs are then linked into a theory.[24]

Criticisms of the Interpretative Paradigm

Although antipositivist perspectives have been embraced by many nursing researchers, they are not without their limitations for developing knowledge in nursing. While the interpretative paradigm emphasizes humanistic approaches, it ignores the reality of physiological problems that are an integral part of a discipline that deals with health and disease.[6,25] Nursing is not a social science and must acknowledge that physiological and psychosocial phenomena are at the core of the discipline. Nursing science must address the complex clinical problems that prac-

ticing nurses deal with daily. Research traditions that rely solely on interpretation and gaining understanding are not amenable to testing theory.[6] Practitioners need theories that help guide their practice and answer questions posed by clinical situations. Although qualitative methodologies such as grounded theory can present theories describing the knowledge embedded in practice, testing of these nascent theories by empirical methods is required.

Interpretative methodologies have been criticized for a lack of rigor, primarily on the basis of criteria used to judge quantitative studies.[18] However, quantitative criteria are inappropriate for evaluating the rigor of qualitative studies.[11,18] Issues that have been cited as reflecting a lack of rigor include failure to adhere to the philosophy of the method being used, inadequate time spent collecting data, failure to identify values and beliefs that may impinge on the study, and poorly developed methods.[18] Credibility, transferability, dependability, and confirmability are the appropriate criteria for judging qualitative methodologies.[11]

Credibility, transferability, dependability, and confirmability are the appropriate criteria for judging qualitative methodologies.

The results of qualitative studies have been characterized as ". . . a set of interesting stories" that result in isolated findings that do not advance the discipline because they do not form the basis for further work.[25] Although nursing is concerned with the uniqueness of individuals, in daily practice, nurses must identify patterns, look for commonalities, and establish priorities. While the results of qualitative research may serve to uncover some of the aesthetic, ethical, and personal knowledge of nurses, practice demands that this knowledge also be put to use. Knowledge that does not help nurses meet society's needs, understand and explain the concepts and relationships of the metaparadigm and conceptual models, and predict events and effects does not contribute to the discipline.

Various writers have suggested other names for the empiricist and interpretative world views in nursing. Parse characterized the world views of the empiricist and interpretative paradigms as the totality and simultaneity paradigms.[3,26] The simultaneity world view regards the person as more and different than the sum of its parts, an open being, free to choose, in rhythmic interaction with the environment.[3,26] In the totality paradigm, the person is the sum of bio–psycho–social–spiritual parts, and interacts with the environment in a linear manner.[26] Newman[9] proposed the particulate–deterministic, interactive–integrative, and unitary–transformative perspectives. In the first world view, phenomena can be viewed as isolated, reducible entities with measurable properties that have an orderly relationship. The second paradigm is related to the first except that the context of phenomena is considered and reality is understood to be multidimensional. In the third paradigm, human beings are considered to be evolving as unitary self-organizing fields.[9] Fawcett,[26] attempting to integrate these different models, coined the reaction, reciprocal interaction, and simultaneous action world views. Despite the differences in names, the totality, particulate– deterministic, interactive–integrative, and reaction world views are representations of the empiricist or mechanistic paradigm, whereas the others are derived from the interpretative or organismic tradition.

Is Nursing Science a Mature Science?

Does the fact that nursing science lacks a predominant paradigm mean that nursing is not a mature science? Nurses too often attempt to measure the success of the discipline with criteria proposed by others that only serve to highlight the limitations of nursing science and fail to acknowledge its successes.[27] Zbilut states that "perhaps nursing has become a full-fledged professional discipline inasmuch as it succumbs to academic fashion."[28(p188)] Many nursing scientists subscribe to Kuhn's[8] depiction of a mature science. Kuhn characterized science as having three distinct phases: pre-paradigmatic, normal science or postparadigmatic, and transformative periods that he calls "revolutions." The preparadigmatic stage is characterized by ". . . debates over legitimate methods, problems and standards of solution . . ."[8(p. 48)] and the lack of primacy of a particular world view. Change from preparadigm to postparadigm science is characterized by multiple schools of thought giving way to one and science finding a more satisfactory method of "solving puzzles." A period of "normal science" exists when one paradigm emerges as the predominant way of solving problems, members of a scientific community accept the paradigm as foundational, and use the world view espoused by the predominant paradigm to solve problems. Debates about methods, questions for study, and ways of answering questions disappear during periods of normal science. Revolutions occur following a crisis, when scientists begin to see the world differently and debates emerge about the paradigm. Gradually, one paradigm supplants that previously in favor and a new period of normal science begins.

Mature science develops through revolutions that provide a transition from one paradigm to another.[8] According to Kuhn,[8] a mature science is characterized by

1. the scientific community's acceptance of a paradigm
2. approaches to solving the discipline's problems that are driven by the paradigm
3. the presentation of knowledge as research articles in scientific journals rather than books

4. the development of a language that is unintelligible to the uninitiated

A predominant paradigm is the most important criterion.

Using these criteria, nursing science is at a preparadigmatic stage because several paradigms are extant. There is a vigorous, ongoing debate within the nursing scientific community about the appropriateness of philosophies and methodologies for directing and conducting research as well as about the questions of relevance to the discipline. However, nursing does meet Kuhn's requirements for shared values, a unique language, scientific journals, and reporting of research findings in articles. A review of the numerous scientific nursing journals indicates that nursing has developed a language of its own and that a significant body of scholarly activity has been accumulated. However, Kuhn,[8] a physicist by training, has been criticized as providing an inaccurate account of the history of science and evaluating science from a positivist perspective due to his emphasis on facts, empiricism, experimentation, and natural science. This positivist perspective is inappropriate and too narrow for a human science such as nursing that confronts a variety of problems.[27,29] Other ways of evaluating scientific progress may be more useful to nursing science.

Meleis[27] proposed a theory of integration for evaluation of progress in nursing science that is more congruent with the tortuous path by which the discipline has developed. Diversity, theory development, competition, creativity, innovation, openness, flexibility, and change are characteristics of a mature discipline according to Meleis. She states that nursing has achieved disciplinary status when evaluated by these criteria.[27]

Fawcett[4] identified three areas of success in nursing research and suggested yard sticks for measuring future progress in nursing science. She recognized "hallmarks of success" that nursing has achieved as identification of the boundaries of research, the types of research required by the discipline, and the types of research activities appropriate for nurses with different educational preparation. Goals for the 21st century are elimination of obstacles to nursing research, acceptance of multiple methods of inquiry, and utilization of research findings in practice. Whether or not nursing science achieves these goals or nursing scientists are in agreement about these criteria, they are important because they provide a nursing perspective of what is important to the discipline rather than applying qualifications developed by those unfamiliar with the history and advances of nursing science.

Single or Multiple Paradigms?

Kuhn's[8] conceptualization of an overarching paradigm that directs the scientific endeavors of a discipline is the basis for the idea of theoretical unification in nursing. This idea is reminiscent of the positivist philosophy of theoretical reduction and reflects his philosophical underpinnings. Paradigmatic supremacy represents the outmoded positivist viewpoint that considers theory reduction an important goal of science.[16] This philosophy assumes that there is one inclusive theory that can reveal the characteristics of reality.[16] However, the concept of unification suggests the mingling of paradigms rather than the dominance of one over the other. Given that the empiricist and interpretative paradigms represent opposing ontological and epistemological views, it is impossible to reconcile the differences underlying the two paradigms to form a unified paradigm.

Several authors suggest that theoretical unification is beneficial to the profession. The advantage of one paradigm lies in its simplicity and parsimony, as there are fewer concepts and relationships to be examined.[16] Hardy suggests that one possible reason for adopting a predominant paradigm is to define the boundaries of the profession or "turf."[12(p92)] Others believe that a unified focus ". . . has the potential for claiming the shared vision of nursing."[2(p5)] Reed believes that accepting multiple paradigms is contrary to the idea of holism and ". . . nursing may be sacrificing coherence for diversity."[30(p78)] Reed[30] advocates a "meta-narrative" or overarching ideal of nursing to direct knowledge development in the profession. While a metanarrative offers potential for discourse and reflection, it does not offer resolution for the differences between the interpretative and empiricist paradigms.

A disadvantage of theoretical unification or the ascendancy of one world view is the narrowness of vision afforded by such a perspective. Kuhn describes the paradigm as an "inflexible box,"[8(p24)] which directs periods of normal science. In this respect, the purpose of normal science is not to examine new phenomena; rather, the aim of normal science is to articulate ". . . the phenomena and theories that the paradigm already supplies."[8(p24)] Because a paradigm directs the work of a community of scientists, selection of one perspective narrows the focus of vision to examining in detail only those phenomena it recognizes. However, when the paradigm becomes too restrictive, scientists "behave differently" and change the nature of their research problems. Thus, theoretical unification can be likened to the idea of the young child who enthusiastically scribbles in a coloring book, only to be told to stay within the lines. Initial enthusiasm for the task quickly becomes discouragement. The challenges confronting practitioners of nursing art and science are too numerous and pressing to permit disenchantment for change or challenge to occur by the unqualified acceptance of a single paradigm.

The existence of multiple paradigms in nursing science indicates a strong and flourishing science. Multiple paradigms are indicative of a "healthy" scientific community because they encourage creativity, stimulate debate and the exchange of ideas, provide diversity of views,[10,31] promote productivity,[1] and keep open avenues of inquiry.[31]

Creativity is a vital and necessary source of ideas in science. Multiple paradigms stimulate creativity by providing different points of view from which to examine a problem or question.[13] Because nursing deals with human behavior, one viewpoint is not sufficient to explain the variety of phenomena and relationships nurses encounter.[27] Theoretical unification focuses vision in one plane, like a microscope, but multiple paradigms expand vision, like a wide-angle lens. Because the goal of nursing science is not simply to add to the discipline's knowledge base, but to develop theories that explain, predict, and prescribe numerous ways of conceptualizing ideas and examining phenomena are beneficial. Multiple paradigms encourage "thinking outside the box" rather than in the box like theoretical unification.

Debate is stimulated by the existence of multiple paradigms. According to the theory of integration, it is debate and competition of theories and ideas that make a discipline scholarly.[27] Compendiums of articles such as *Perspectives on Nursing Theory*[32] offer a window through which to view debate within the discipline. A review of these articles reveals the intensity with which authors have supported and defended their particular world view, resulting in clarification, codification, and modification of views. The active exchange of opinions and ideas through discourse stimulates growth and development.[31] Just as a growing organism achieves maturity through rapidly dividing and multiplying, so can a discipline grow through a multiplicity of paradigms. Selection of one world view can be considered analogous to the loss of variability that accompanies aging and death in complex physiological systems.[33]

Diversity of view points has been likened to a cable that is strengthened by multiple strands.[34] Nursing is a complex profession with many providers with differing educational preparation and areas of specialization caring for many types of clients in varying situations. How can one paradigm for nursing science possibly reflect this diversity? Just as people have been urged to celebrate their differences, so should nursing science rejoice in the fact that within nursing is a rich and varied assortment of threads that, when woven together, draw a strong, resilient, whole tapestry. The problems of nursing are so diverse that multiple answers and solutions to a question can be appropriate. Multiple perspectives encourage appreciation of the uniqueness of individual nurses and patients by finding multiple answers to common problems. Problems may be erroneously considered solved and questions answered if one perspective for developing knowledge is selected.

Different paradigmatic views may increase productivity. Reliance on one perspective may limit a scientist to repeatedly investigating the same problem from the same approach in different populations. However, applying different viewpoints provides new insights to formulate new ideas to old questions. For example, the continual use of a phenomenological approach will result in many studies about the meaning of an experience. However, for both the discipline and the investigator to advance in knowledge, those studies must be used as a foundation on which to build others that generate and test theory. Other perspectives are needed to channel these initial findings into further studies. In addition to maximizing the strengths and minimizing the weakness of each method, combining or triangulating methods can involve more than one investigator in a research project, resulting in more discussion, more ideas, and more projects.[35]

> *"Different paradigmatic views may increase productivity."*

Premature closure also may result from the selection of one paradigm. Cognitive dissonance may not be noted if only those phenomena that are congruent with a single perspective are examined.[3] In other words, a single perspective is similar to wearing blinders: phenomena that might attract attention are not seen, as they are outside the field of vision. Thus, opportunities to go somewhere more interesting or follow a different path are thwarted.

Multiple paradigms also have disadvantages for nursing science in that practitioners may become confused and divided over the conflicting claims of different view points.[30] Many in the profession find continuing debate over such matters inconclusive, frustrating, and not germane to the business of nursing. Students can become confused if exposed to new, untested ideas, and even experienced practitioners may find the seemingly never-ending debate mystifying.[28] For example, it is difficult to reconcile the pragmatic aspects of everyday nursing with ideas espoused by interpretative paradigms. If each individual is unique, why are standard care plans devised? What does it mean for a person to be an open system and how can this be evaluated? Why do nurses assess patients systematically if they are holistic beings? How can the accomplishments of empiricism be accepted while its methods are condemned as controlling and dehumanizing? If empiricism is abandoned, what will replace it?

Implications of Multiparadigmism for Nursing Science

A change of perspective is required for nursing science to reconcile the philosophical differences between the two extant paradigms. A perspective that emphasizes inquiry rather than paradigmatic supremacy or unification is more advantageous to nursing as a discipline. Dzurec and Abraham[36] noted that there were few real differences between quantitative and qualitative methods of research. Although specific techniques may vary between methods. ". . . the findings generated by both . . . are based on description, probability, and inference."[36(p74)] The results of both empirical and interpretative studies are due to interpretation of raw data by the investigator.[36] The authors argue that neither method is more scientific than the other and that the process of inquiry is the same despite the methods used to acquire knowledge. Therefore, nursing scientists can take heart in the thought that careful adherence to the principles and philosophy of the method they chose will result in valid and reliable findings that will add to the body of knowledge of the discipline.

Integration of qualitative and quantitative methods has been suggested as advancing nursing science.[20,35,36] Research traditions from the empirical and interpretative paradigms are complementary as each presents a different approach.[15] Qualitative methods can describe phenomenon of interest in nursing and generate theories that propose relationships between identified concepts. Quantitative methods can test the relationships of qualitatively developed theories and suggest whether the theory should be accepted or revised. The different perspectives presented by the empiricist and interpretative paradigms can examine different dimensions of a phenomenon.

Collaboration toward solving problems is more beneficial for the discipline than acrimony and competition over which tradition is most useful.[16] Collaboration will result in increased opportunities for all nursing scientists. For example, critical multiplism, a strategy similar to triangulation, has been recommended as an approach for nursing research.[34] This strategy is "...based on the premise that...thoughtful choices are the approach most likely to yield an objective body of knowledge."[34] Multiple multiples are involved: of researchers, institutions, frameworks, research questions, issues, methods, and data collection and analysis modes. The approach increases efficiency by spreading the workload and increases utility by studying more than

one question at a time.[34] Methods such as this offer greater opportunities for collaboration and discourse than traditional, single-investigator approaches.

When paradigms are associated with values and beliefs, polarization occurs between different views, with little hope of bridging the gulf between the sides. Acceptance of multiple paradigms as perspectives and research traditions rather than as values has the potential to lessen the division between the academic and scientific communities. Practicing nurses often are blind to the relevance of theoretical arguments for the everyday practice of nursing. However, clinicians readily understand that there are many ways to accomplish the same goal and that a nurse uses whatever method he or she is most comfortable with or whatever works best in a particular situation.

Presenting research as a system of inquiry that can be accomplished in several ways may also improve the palatability of research in educational programs. Both baccalaureate and masters students often are overwhelmed by research courses and rate their usefulness to practice as low. However, student interest in research may be spurred by courses that emphasize principles of sound inquiry rather than the vagaries and quirks of different paradigmatic approaches. Just as students learn sound principles of nursing care on which to build their nursing practice, so must they learn basic principles of inquiry that recognize the equality of all methods. Presenting a system of inquiry rather than a philosophy also will require that instructors provide a more balanced view of different research traditions.

A variety of paradigms allows the development of more theories for nursing. Different perspectives of nursing practice enhance the ability to understand and interpret the meaning in different practice situations, identify relationships, and develop theories. Laudan[37] recommends a process of integration of different research traditions with the goal of expanding the number of theories in order to solve the problems of the discipline.

The feasibility and importance of a multiparadigmatic approach ultimately will be established through its usefulness in practice. If differing perspectives can generate and test theories that provide faithful representations of practice and are useful in practice settings, they will flourish. As a pragmatic profession, nurses choose the method that works best to provide the critical services clients require. Practice will indicate those aspects of a perspective that are not useful and discard or revamp them into a new variant. Applying different paradigms together in practice situations can help to determine whether the perspective offered by opposing perspectives results in different nursing actions. According to history, often that which is not useful does not survive. If the multiparadigmatic approach is not congruent with practice, it too, may become obsolete or extinct.

Summary

The discussion about theoretical unification or multiparadigmism is reminiscent of the debate over single or multiple conceptual frameworks for nursing. Interestingly, that debate has been abandoned as the discussion shifts to paradigms. The war of words over single or multiple paradigms cannot be won easily. However, multiparadigmism is an approach to the development of nursing knowledge that offers greater promise for the discipline than theoretical unification. Multiparadigmism recognizes the differences inherent in opposing world views while celebrating the possibilities that each offers and the way that each complements the other. Downplaying paradigmatic differences while enhancing the value of scholarly inquiry through multiple approaches is paramount for the advancement of nursing science.

References

1. Donaldson SK, Crowley DM. The discipline of nursing. In: Nicoll LH, ed. *Perspectives on Nursing Theory*, 3rd ed. Philadelphia, PA: Lippincott; 1997.

2. Newman MA, Sime AM, Corcoran-Perry SA. The focus of the discipline of nursing. *ANS*. 1991;14:1–6.

3. Fawcett J. *Analysis and Evaluation of Conceptual Models of Nursing*, 2nd ed. Philadelphia, PA: F.A. Davis Company; 1989.

4. Fawcett J. Hallmarks of success in nursing research. *ANS*. 1984;8:1–11.

5. Chinn PL, Kramer MK. *Theory and Nursing: A Systematic Approach*, 4th ed. St. Louis, MO: Mosby; 1995.

6. Gortner SR. Nursing's syntax revisited: a critique of philosophies said to influence nursing theories. *Int J Nurs Studies*. 1990;30:477–488.

7. *Webster's New World Dictionary*, 3rd college ed. New York: Webster's New World; 1988.

8. Kuhn TS. *The Structure of Scientific Revolutions*, 2nd ed. Chicago: The University of Chicago Press; 1970.

9. Newman MA. Prevailing paradigms in nursing. *Nurs Outlook*. 1992;40:10–13.

10. Kim HS. Theoretical thinking in nursing: Problems and prospects. In: Nicoll LH, ed. *Perspectives on Nursing Theory*, 3rd ed. Philadelphia, PA: Lippincott; 1997.

11. Lincoln YS, Guba EG. *Naturalistic Inquiry*. Newbury Park, CA: Sage; 1985.

12. Hardy ME. Perspectives on nursing theory. In: Nicoll LH, ed. *Perspectives on Nursing Theory*, 3rd ed. Philadelphia, PA: Lippincott; 1997.

13. Jacox AK, Webster G. Competing theories of science. In: Nicoll LH, ed. *Perspectives on Nursing Theory*, 3rd ed. Philadelphia. PA: Lippincott; 1997.

14. Suppe F, Jacox AK. Philosophy of science and the development of nursing theory. In: Werley H, Fitzpatrick J, eds. *Annual Review of Nursing Research*. New York: Springer; 1985.

15. Poole K, Jones A. A re-examination of the experimental design for nursing research. *J Adv Nurs*. 1996;24:108–114.

16. Silva MC, Rothbart D. An analysis of changing trends in philosophies of science on nursing theory development and testing. In: Nicoll LH, ed. *Perspectives on Nursing Theory*, 3rd ed. Philadelphia, PA: Lippincott; 1997.

17. Weiss SJ. Contemporary empiricism. In: Omery A, Kasper CE, Page GG, eds. *In Search of Nursing Science*. Thousand Oaks, CA: Sage; 1995.

18. Burns N, Grove SK. *The Practice of Nursing Research: Conduct, Critique, & Utilization*, 3rd ed. Philadelphia, PA: W. B. Saunders; 1997.

19. Schumacher KL, Gortner SR. (Mis)conceptions and reconceptions about traditional science. *ANS.* 1992;14:1–11.

20. Holmes CA. Alternatives to natural science foundations for nursing. *Int J Nurs Studies.* 1990;27:187–198.

21. Carper BA. Fundamental patterns of knowing in nursing. In: Nicoll LH, ed. *Perspectives on Nursing Theory*, 3rd ed. Philadelphia, PA: Lippincott; 1997.

22. Munhall PL. Language and nursing research. In: Munhall PL, Boyd CO, eds. *Nursing Research: A Qualitative Perspective*, 2nd ed. New York: National League for Nursing; 1993.

23. Bramlett MH, Gueldner SH, Boettcher JH. Reflections on the science of unitary human beings in terms of Kuhn's requirement for explanatory power. *Visions.* 1993;1:22–35.

24. Boyd CO. Philosophical foundations of qualitative research. In: Munhall PL, Boyd CO, eds. *Nursing Research: A Qualitative Perspective*, 2nd ed. New York: National League for Nursing; 1993.

25. Downs FS. New questions and new answers. *Nurs Res.* 1989;38:323.

26. Fawcett J. From a plethora of paradigms to parsimony in world views. *Nurs Sci Q.* 1993;6(2):56–58.

27. Meleis AI. *Theoretical Nursing: Development & Progress*, 3rd ed. Philadelphia, PA: Lippincott; 1997.

28. Zbilut JP. Contradictions of nursing in a postmodern world. *Image.* 1997;38:188–189.

29. Fry ST. Science as problem solving. In: Omery A, Kasper CE, Page GG, eds. *In Search of Nursing Science.* Thousand Oaks, CA: Sage; 1995.

30. Reed PG. A treatise on nursing knowledge development for the 21st century: beyond postmodernism. *ANS.* 1995;17:70–84.

31. Ramos MC. Adopting an evolutionary lens: an optimistic approach to discovering strength in nursing. In: Nicoll LH, ed. *Perspectives on Nursing Theory*, 3rd ed. Philadelphia, PA: Lippincott; 1997.

32. Nicoll LH. *Perspectives on Nursing Theory*, 3rd ed. Philadelphia, PA: Lippincott; 1997.

33. Lipsitz LA, Goldberger AL. Loss of "complexity" and aging: potential application of fractals and chaos theory to senescence. *JAMA.* 1992;267:1806–1809.

34. Knaft KA, Pettengill MM, Bevis ME, Kirchhoff KT. Blending qualitative and quantitative approaches to instrument development and data collection. *J Prof Nurs.* 1988;4:30–37.

35. Dzurec LC, Abraham IL. The nature of inquiry: linking quantitative and qualitative research. *ANS.* 1993;16:73–79.

36. Laudan L. *Progress and Its Problems: Towards a Theory of Scientific Growth.* Berkeley: University of California Press; 1977.

37. Kim HS, Holter IM. Critical theory for science of nursing practice. In: Omery A, Kasper CE, Page GG, eds. *In Search of Nursing Science.* Thousand Oaks, CA: Sage; 1995.

Chapter 5

What Constitutes Nursing Science?

John R. Phillips,
RN, PhD

Science is an organized body of knowledge concerning human beings and their worlds; it encompasses "the attitudes and methods through which this body of knowledge is formed" (Chernow & Vallasi, 1993, p. 2452). Chernow and Vallasi (1993) also state that since scientific methods do not always guarantee scientific discovery, other factors such as intuition, experience, and good judgment "contribute to new developments in science" (p. 2452). In addition, a survey of the evolution of knowledge shows that abstract thinking is integral to the advancement of science. This broad view of science is essential in understanding the development of any particular science and its phenomena of concern.

This is especially true for nursing science with its unique body of knowledge. Controversy arises, however, when attempts are made to identify this body of knowledge, where some nurses make little distinction between nursing knowledge and the knowledge of other sciences, such as medicine. Too, some nursing models and theories still include knowledge from other sciences that has not been transposed into a nurs-

ing perspective. Furthermore, it must be determined how or if these nursing models and theories can be used to generate nursing knowledge that constitutes nursing science.

Some nurses may say this is a moot point and probably not worthy of further pursuit. However, one needs to realize that it is nursing science that gives direction to the further generation of nursing knowledge, and it is nursing science that provides the knowledge for all aspects of nursing. Moreover, it is through the art of nursing, "the imaginative and creative use of knowledge" (Rogers, 1988, p. 100), that nurses can know and understand the health care needs of people. How adequately can this be achieved if nursing science is not constituted with nursing knowledge?

Fawcett (1993, 1995) in her metaparadigm of nursing has helped to provide an understanding of what constitutes nursing science. Her analysis and evaluation of nursing models and theories make it clear that there is a particular perspective of the metaparadigm concepts for each of the nursing models and theories. For example, the definitions of person, environment, health, and nursing are different for each model and theory. Since each nursing model and theory has a different philosophical and theoretical foundation,

Source: Phillips, J. R. (1996). What constitutes nursing science? *Nursing Science Quarterly, 9*(2): 48–49. Reprinted by permission of and copyright © 2002 Sage Publications, Inc.

nurses who use them have different realities of nursing. How are these differences related to what constitutes nursing science?

Parse (1987) and Newman (1992) in their paradigms of nursing and Fawcett (1993) in her worldviews of nursing address these differences and provide for further understanding of what constitutes nursing science. The use of these paradigms and worldviews reveals that some nursing models and theories are composed of conflicting philosophical and theoretical foundations. Too, some nursing models and theories overlap more than one paradigm or worldview. If a nursing model or theory lacks coherence within its philosophical and theoretical foundation and overlaps more than one paradigm or worldview, then a close examination of it is needed to determine whether it constitutes nursing science. Will a time come when particular nursing models or theories will no longer be appropriate to constitute nursing science?

Nursing models and theories provide multiple diverse and divergent nursing realities. These realities foster creative ideas and insights that are essential to the methods that are used to discover knowledge. It is time, however, to evaluate how the various scientific methods contribute to the development of nursing science. Realizing, for example, that statistics is only one language of science, nurses can no longer be satisfied with only the traditional scientific methods that often give a cloudy vision of what nursing science is. Nurses must emerge from the womb of other sciences so as to give birth to scientific methods that give a clear vision of what nursing is and can be, knowing that today there is only an inkling of the future of nursing science.

Nurses can design these new methods through a creative synthesis of the various aspects of science and the human processes such as intuition and lived experiences. Some of our current nursing scientific methods already provide for imaginative, abstract, and logical reasoning processes that are required to discover knowledge to develop nursing science. Such scientific methods will give unity to nursing science through the diversity of nursing models and theories. This assumption is acceptable when Moody (1990) quote of Bronowski is considered: "Science is nothing else than the search to discover unity in the wild variety of nature or . . . in the variety of our experiences" (p. 18).

A cumulative body of knowledge that is flexible and open to change flows from the unitary nature of nursing science. The wholeness of this knowledge provides further understanding of the ambiguity and uncertainty found in the multiple realities of nursing models and theories. This understanding will reveal the rigid and static nature of knowledge from other sciences, which in many instances is outdated and not from a nursing perspective. However, as nurses develop knowledge through the use of nursing models and theories, they must remain in doubt and be open to changes in it (Wilson, 1985). This is essential if nurses are to advance a nursing science that provides the knowledge for the changing art of nursing, where there is concern for the wholeness of people.

Questions of what constitutes nursing science have revealed an evolving phenomenon in nursing. The revelation is that facts alone do not constitute nursing science, however important they may be; it is the pattern of knowledge that gives unity to nursing science. As the pattern is revealed, nurses are being challenged to relook at what constitutes nursing science. Needless to say, the focus on the pattern of knowledge brings a profound provocation to create a new vision of nursing science, a vision that will eventually sever the umbilical cord of subjugation to the knowledge of other sciences. This new vision may save some of the nursing models and theories from becoming obsolete, even extinct.

The recognition and use of the pattern of knowledge is moving nursing science to the forefront of science in general. This new, prominent position enables nurses to respond to the public's desire for quality health care, where the concern is the healing of the whole person. In such an arena of health care, nurses will not compete with other health care providers since they will be using nursing knowledge for the practice of nursing, rather than knowledge from other sciences, particularly medicine. Can we say that the "gap" between theory and practice will disappear as nurses continue to use nursing models and theories that constitute the nursing science for their practice?

Yes, nursing models and theories do constitute nursing science. Nurses must not accept the perennial denigration of nursing models and theories and the call to abandon them for the knowledge from other sciences. If nurses do, nursing will become a wasteland filled with "illiterate nurses" where all of humanity will suffer in immeasurable ways.

Nursing models and theories are the savior of nursing science, and nurses' ravenous use of them will bring redemption from a wasteland composed of knowledge from other sciences. This is the power that nursing models and theories give nurses in determining what constitutes nursing science, its knowledge, and its scientific methods. As nurses continue to use nursing models and theories, nursing science will no longer be invisible in the world of science.

References

Chernow, B. A., & Vallasi, G. A. (1993). *The Columbia encyclopedia* (5th ed.). New York: Columbia University Press.

Fawcett, J. (1993). *Analysis and evaluation of nursing theories*. Philadelphia: Davis.

Fawcett, J. (1995). *Analysis and evaluation of conceptual models of nursing* (3rd ed.). Philadelphia: Davis.

Moody, L. E. (1990). *Advancing nursing science through research*, Vol. 1. Newbury Park, CA: Sage.

Newman, M. A. (1992). Prevailing paradigms in nursing. *Nursing Outlook, 40*, 10–13, 32.

Parse, R. R. (1987). *Nursing science: Major paradigms, theories, and critiques*. Philadelphia: Saunders.

Rogers, M. E. (1988). Nursing science and art: A prospective. *Nursing Science Quarterly, 1*, 99–102.

Wilson, H. S. (1985). *Research in nursing*. Menlo Park, CA: Addison-Wesley.

Part Two

NURSING SCIENCE IN THE NEW MILLENNIUM

The turn of the millennium offered all humankind an opportunity to reflect on the past and anticipate the future. Nurses greeted the new century as a full-fledged profession for the first time, as the largest acknowledged health profession in contemporary society, and quite possibly as the profession that carries within it the greatest potential for the transformation of healthcare practice for the new millennium. In Part Two of this text, a number of authors offer their assessments of nursing science at the turn of the millennium.

In Chapter 6, Fawcett offers one view of nursing science, rooted in the value for nursing theory-guided practice and research. Fawcett finds the contemporary literature lacking in this regard and actually expresses fear for the survival of the discipline. Even a casual observer of nursing can easily discern that Fawcett's assertions are accurate regarding the dearth of nursing science in the greater portion of "nursing" research and "nursing" practice in contemporary society. What, then, does the dearth of nursing science in the activities of professional nurses mean for the future of nursing? For Fawcett, it represents an opportunity to issue a rallying cry for all nurses to become nurse scholars and for commensurate changes in our educational structures and processes. Certainly it is clear that mastery of the complexities and subtleties inherent in values-based practice and evidence-based care requires education and scholarship that is both broad and deep. Readers are invited to picture a world in which all nurses are prepared as scholars to achieve that mastery.

In Chapter 7, Silva has a turn at reconceptualizing nursing science for the 21st century, starting not from what nursing science itself *is*, but from what demands the 21st century places on all scholarship. For example, linear logic may not serve nursing science well any longer, as many phenomena of interest may not be susceptible to

it. Silva is concerned above all with the pace of change in the contemporary world, leading her to assert the importance of "letting go, moving on, and making a difference in nursing science."

In Chapter 8, Parse explores the transformation of nursing practice when it is guided by the human becoming school of thought. Nursing practice from this frame of reference is explicitly based on values and beliefs. Parse writes, "The *form* of nursing in the transformational practice guided by the human becoming principles is true presence: a non-routinized way of being with others that honours the others' views and choices on changing health patterns and quality of life." Parse asserts that nurses as professionals have an ethical responsibility to practice from an explicitly nursing frame of reference. She cites literature that documents changes in quality of life when care is delivered from the human becoming framework. Readers are invited to reflect on how their adoption of a nursing framework impacts (or would impact) the values on which their practice is based and their use of evidence as the basis for care.

In Chapter 9, Bunkers delineates the portrait of the 21st century nurse scholar as committed to human freedom and choice, openness, meaning, and social justice; pursuing an understanding of health as process, community as process, and the nature of suffering; believing in the power of personal presence; and focused on ethics and quality of life while acknowledging the centrality of mystery and uncertainty in human experience. Bunkers's nurse scholar, a kind of renaissance person for the new millennium, would surely be well prepared to explore the depths of values-based practice and the intricacies of evidence-based care and is, therefore, an excellent role model for the reader of this book who is likely a graduate student or doctoral student in nursing.

In Chapter 10, Wuest provides a historical and feminist perspective on the notion of professionalism in nursing. In lieu of the received view of professionalism, which is the more familiar view, Wuest argues for value laden feminist epistemologies and methodologies that generate and apply knowledge in a manner that values people and freedom. In Chapters 11 and 12, three scholars offer international perspectives on nursing science and the dominance of Western (North American) perspectives therein. These chapters suggest that a value for people and their quality of life mandates a focus within the discipline that is different from that which currently obtains.

Taken together, the chapters in this section offer readers the opportunity to appreciate current developments in nursing science in a forward-looking way, to picture the professional practice of nursing befitting the onset of a new millennium, and to consider the philosophical and theoretical basis necessary for underpinning that practice.

Chapter 6

The State of Nursing Science: Hallmarks of the 20th and 21st Centuries

Jacqueline Fawcett,
RN, PhD, FAAN

Science generally is regarded as the systematic, controlled, empirical, and critical activities undertaken to generate and test theories. Nursing science, therefore, comprises those systematic, controlled, empirical, and critical activities undertaken to generate and test nursing theories. This column focuses on my view of the state of nursing science circa 1999. My comments reflect countless hours of solitary thought, as well as 35 years of dialogue with colleagues and students in classrooms and at local, regional, national, and international workshops and conferences. I have become increasingly troubled by the state of our science but have retained sufficient optimism to accept the invitation to write this column and share my vision of what we can do if we want to save our discipline and advance our science.

Hallmarks of 20th-Century Nursing

During the 1980s, I published a trilogy of articles that reflected my excitement with the state

Source: Fawcett, J. (1999). The state of nursing science: Hallmarks of the 20th and 21st Centuries. *Nursing Science Quarterly*, 12(4): 311–315. Reprinted by permission of and copyright © 1999 Sage Publications, Inc.

of nursing science and my optimism for the future of the discipline of nursing. In the first article, I identified four hallmarks of success in nursing theory development (Fawcett, 1983). In the second article, I identified three hallmarks of success in nursing research (Fawcett, 1984). In the third article, a colleague and I identified four hallmarks of success in nursing practice (Fawcett & Carino, 1989).

The four hallmarks of success in nursing theory development that I identified were specification of a metaparadigm for nursing, explication of conceptual models of nursing, explication of unique nursing theories, and theories shared with other disciplines. The meaning and content of the nursing metaparadigm, conceptual models, and unique nursing theories most likely are well known to readers. Shared theories may require some explanation. Simply put, a shared theory is one that has been borrowed from another discipline and then tested to determine its empirical adequacy in nursing situations. If the theory is found to be empirically adequate in legitimate nursing situations, it may be considered to be a shared theory.

The three hallmarks of success in nursing research that I identified were specification of the boundaries of nursing research, explication of the types of research needed by the professional discipline of nursing, and delineation of research activities appropriate for nurses according to educational preparation. The boundaries of nursing research were, I maintained, set by the metaparadigm of nursing and by the rules of research that are inherent in each conceptual model of nursing. The metaparadigm sets the global boundary for research as examination of nursing's efforts to facilitate person–environment interactions having to do with health. Each conceptual model of nursing provides an interpretation of that boundary and presents more circumscribed boundaries in the form of a set of conceptual and methodologic rules for research.

Drawing from the notion that nursing is a professional rather than an academic discipline, I maintained that basic, applied, and clinical types of research are required. An academic discipline has as its mission only the development and dissemination of knowledge. A professional discipline, in contrast, has as its mission the development, dissemination, and utilization of knowledge. Basic research focuses only on development of knowledge, without regard to its later use; this type of research is conducted by the members of both academic and professional disciplines. Applied research focuses on determination of the practical limits of knowledge, that is, determination of the range of practical situations in which each theory is empirically adequate. Applied research also is conducted by members of both academic and professional disciplines. Clinical research focuses on the effects of actual implementation of theories in clinical practice situations; this type of research is conducted only by members of professional disciplines.

For the third hallmark of success in nursing research, delineation of research activities appropriate for nurses according to educational preparation, I drew from the American Nurses' Association Commission on Nursing Research 1981 statement of guidelines for the investigative functions of nurses. The commission issued guidelines for participation in a wide range of research-related activities that took into account distinct differences in research capabilities between the graduates of associate degree nursing programs, baccalaureate nursing programs, master's degree nursing programs, practice-oriented doctoral programs (DNSc), and research-oriented programs (PhD).

The four hallmarks of success in nursing practice that Carino and I identified were the use of conceptual models of nursing to guide nursing practice, development of classification systems, establishment of formal linkages between nursing education and nursing service, and recognition of clinical scholars and clinical scholarship. The first three hallmarks are self-explanatory. The fourth hallmark characterizes clinical scholarship as a professional imperative and the consequent emergence of nurse clinicians as clinical scholars. Clinical scholarship takes many forms, including the development and testing of assessment formats and intervention protocols and the application of clinical nursing research findings in daily clinical practice. Clinical scholars are nurse clinicians who practice nursing in an increasingly thoughtful manner. "They continually contemplate situations and stretch their minds toward insights into nursing practice and helping people to improve their health. Nurses who are true clinical scholars are noted for their ability to make novel connections between things or ideas—mental leaps and intuitive lunges that improve nursing practice and, therefore, enhance the well-being of their patients" (Fawcett & Carino, 1989, p. 6).

Current Trends in Nursing Science

Throughout the 1990s, my excitement about the advances in nursing science that led to the trilogy of hallmark articles has been progressively dampened. I have been particularly discouraged because I have seen little that might indicate a need for updates in those hallmark works. That is, although I do not see any evidence of a loss of ground for the existing hallmarks, I do not see any progress either. Even more to the point, I have seen nothing that might qualify as a new hallmark of success in nursing theory development, nursing research, or nursing practice. Moreover, my early optimism has turned to pessimism, reflecting a very real concern for the continued existence of the discipline of nursing.

Research conducted by nurses has increased in quantity and, some might argue, in quality in recent years, but I can no longer support the maxim that research conducted by nurses is, by definition, nursing research. That is because the current trend in research by nurses signals a major threat to the very survival of our discipline. More specifically, much of the research conducted by contemporary nurse researchers (i.e., those nurses who are academically qualified to advance science through research) has not been nursing research and has done nothing to advance nursing science. Instead, much of the research has employed nonnursing methodologies to generate new theories guided by nonnursing conceptual frameworks and to test theories developed by members of other disciplines. Note, for example, that just 6 of the 73 studies (8%) reported in Nursing Research and Research in Nursing and Health in 1998 involved the generation or testing of nursing theories using nursing methodologies. However, 2 of the 6 studies were designed to test ad hoc theories that combined concepts from nursing and some other discipline, and another 2 of the 6 tested ad hoc nursing theories developed from an interdisciplinary literature exclusive of nursing. Thus, just 2 of the 73 studies (3%) were guided by widely recognized nursing theories, namely, Leininger's theory of culture care diversity and universality and Pender's theory of health promotion. Clearly, much science was produced in 1998, but very little nursing science.

The argument could be advanced that the studies that were guided by nonnursing conceptual frameworks and theories were focused on the development of shared nursing theories, which I previously identified as a hallmark of success in nursing theory development (Fawcett, 1983). However, the investigators who reported those studies did not identify the development of shared theory as a goal, nor did they explicitly discuss any modifications in the original theories that might be required for their use in legitimate nursing situations.

Turning to practice, services offered by nurses have become seemingly more comprehensive and sophisticated, but I can no longer support the maxim that practice by nurses is, by definition, nursing practice. That is because the current trend in practice by nurses, especially by so-called advanced practice nurses, signals another major threat to the survival of our discipline. More specifically, many of the services offered by contemporary nurse practitioners (i.e., those nurses academically and professionally qualified to utilize science through practice) have not been based on nursing science and have done nothing to inform nursing science. Instead, nurse practitioners increasingly base their practice on medical science and perform tasks "traditionally within the domain of medical practice" (Orem, 1995, p. 41). Note, for example, that nurse practitioners are said to resemble physicians' assistants (Martha Rogers, cited in Huch, 1995), junior doctors (Meleis, 1993), or pseudo-doctors (Kendrick, 1997) engaged in nursing qua medicine (Watson, 1996).

The reasons for the current trends in research and practice most likely are many and complex. With regard to research, perhaps editors and peer reviewers think that the use and testing of nonnursing conceptual frameworks and theories will increase the visibility of research conducted by nurses among members of other disciplines and the public. Perhaps researchers who base their studies on conceptual models of nursing and nursing theories do not submit their reports to the two journals cited here because they think that such studies are not published in those journals. I would be remiss, then, if I did not mention that almost every report of research based on an explicit conceptual model of nursing that I have submitted to either journal has been published. Thus, it is unlikely that systematic bias against nursing science is operating. However, in contrast to *Nursing Science Quarterly and Visions: The Journal of Rogerian Nursing Science*, neither of the other two journals cited requires research to reflect advances in nursing science through the testing of a conceptual model of nursing or a nursing theory.

With regard to practice, perhaps practitioners think that if they emulate medical practice, their services will be more highly valued by the public and other health professionals, or perhaps many nurses feel so oppressed by physicians that they, like virtually all oppressed persons, have a disdain for the science of their own discipline and identify with the science of the perceived oppressor, medicine.

The Hallmark of 21st-Century Nursing: A Prediction

While in the depths of pessimism, I began to think of a way to save our discipline. It has become increasingly clear to me that the discipline of nursing can survive if, and only if, we end our romance with medical science and the conceptual frameworks, theories, and methodologies of nonnursing disciplines. We see evidence of that romance every day in the reports of studies conducted by nurses but guided by nonnursing conceptual frameworks, theories, and methodologies. We also see evidence of that romance in advertisements for either a nurse practitioner or a physician's assistant—as if they were interchangeable professions. And, perhaps most disturbing, we see evidence of that romance every time that nurse practitioners are featured in the news media, including the nursing media, and talk about how they provide the same services as primary care physicians and receive—or hope to soon receive—the same reimbursement as physicians for those services from third-party payers. No wonder, then, that physicians claim that nurses are infringing on medical turf. No wonder, then, that we tolerate and even support Nurse Practice Acts that require supervision of nurse practitioners by a licensed physician.

If we do not end the romance with nonnursing disciplines. I predict that we will not survive as a distinct discipline. If, however, we do end the romance, we have a chance at survival but only under certain conditions. Those conditions, I believe, involve embracing nursing science through the integration of research and practice, which will require a change in the educational preparation of all nurses and will mandate a change in the employment conditions of nurses. More specifically, I believe that our discipline will not only survive but flourish through rapid advances in nursing science if all nurses become nurse scholars. I envision nurse scholars as nurses who integrate nursing science versions of the roles of nurse researcher and nurse practitioner. Today's separate roles of nurse researcher and nurse practitioner will no longer exist. Rather, all nurses will perform a single role—that of nurse scholar. The immediate and obvious advantage of a single role is the elimination of the so-called research-practice gap. If actualized, I predict that the single role of nurse scholar will become the one hallmark of the success of 21st-century nursing.

I envision nurse scholars as academically and professionally qualified to develop and utilize nursing science. More specifically, I envision nurse scholars as qualified to conduct nursing discipline-specific research and to practice from a nursing discipline-specific perspective. Nurses will focus on discipline-specific research and practice and employ nursing methodologies to generate, test, and apply nursing theories within the context of conceptual models of nursing. Only when that occurs can the research and practice activities of nurses be said to advance nursing science, and only then can research and practice be said to contribute to the discipline of nursing.

All nurse scholars will actively engage in integrated research-practice activities, using nursing methodologies to test and apply conceptual models of nursing and nursing theories in the provision of nursing services to people. Clearly, nurse scholars are not the nurse researchers or nurse practitioners of today but, rather, are nursing practitioners (Orem, 1995) or senior nurses (Meleis, 1993) who are engaged in nursing qua nursing (Watson, 1997). Inasmuch as nurse scholars constantly conduct nursing discipline-specific research and engage in nursing discipline-specific practice, they advance nursing science continuously.

Nurse scholars are initially prepared for their integrated role responsibilities in postbaccalaureate doctorate of nursing (ND) programs. I believe that today's diversity in entry levels cannot continue to exist if our discipline is to survive. Thus, I envision the ND as the entry level for all nursing. Moreover, given the holistic, comprehensive nature of nursing discipline-specific practice, I envision no need for unlicensed assistive nursing personnel. ND-prepared nurse scholars want to be at the patient's side, which is the only place where they can perform integrated research and practice role activities.

ND-prepared nurse scholars use nursing methodologies, which are derived from explicit conceptual models of nursing and nursing theories, to guide their integrated research and practice activities. The integration of research and practice is evident as ND-prepared nurse scholars use the data obtained from every encounter with a patient for nursing research purposes. Every nurse-patient encounter, then, becomes a case study, with an individual patient serving as his or her own control (Wood, 1978). Thus, each case study is an experiment that tests the efficacy of the conceptual model and theories used to guide the nurse-patient encounter. In other words, ND-prepared nurse scholars use the clinical data available to them in every patient situation to determine the credibility of existing conceptual models of nursing and the empirical adequacy of existing nursing theories, thereby contributing constantly to nursing science.

Rather, their area of expertise or specialization is in a particular conceptual model of nursing or nursing theory. These scholars carry out their role responsibilities with the individuals, families, and/or communities regarded as legitimate patients within the context of that particular conceptual model of nursing or nursing theory. In addition, they apply the relevant nursing methodology to the full range of conditions and situations encompassed by the conceptual model or theory.

ND-prepared nurse scholars receive advanced preparation in doctor of philosophy (PhD) programs. The focus of PhD programs in nursing science is on the use of nursing methodologies, derived from conceptual models of nursing and nursing theories, with groups of patients rather than with individual patients. More specifically, PhD-prepared nurse scholars use aggregate data obtained from multiple encounters with patients to determine the credibility of various existing conceptual models of nursing and the empirical adequacy of various existing nursing theories. They also use those data to develop new conceptual models of nursing, nursing theories, and nursing methodologies. In other words, they combine single case studies to advance nursing science.

Rather than specialize in a particular conceptual model of nursing or nursing theory, PhD-prepared nurse scholars are generalists who examine the differential efficacy of two or more conceptual models of nursing or nursing theories with diverse patients with diverse conditions in diverse situations. The results of such examinations ultimately will lead to a better understanding of the "fit" of a particular intellectual perspective with a particular patient and, therefore, a substantial advance in nursing science.

ND- and PhD-prepared nurse scholars function as "attending nurses," that is, nurses who are with patients continuously wherever they are "in and outside of institutions, schools, homes, clinics, and community settings" (Watson, 1996, p. 163). Thus, each patient always has his or her own nurse scholar, who collaborates with other health professionals when the patient requires services from others. Attending nurses, of course, carry out integrated research and practice role responsibilities. As attending nurses, ND- and PhD-prepared nurse scholars may work in nurse corporations, which are made up of nurse scholars in equal partnership with one another, or they may elect to be self-employed. Nurse corporations contract with individuals, families, communities, medical centers, community and specialty hospitals, home care agencies, hospices, and other agencies and organizations for the provision of distinctively nursing services guided by conceptual models of nursing, nursing theories, and nursing methods. The idea of nurse corporations was proposed by Sills (1983), who explained this:

> The conceptual key to the corporation proposal is that it changes the fundamental nature of the social contract. The professional nurse would no longer be an employee of the hospital or agency, but rather a member of a professional corporation that provides nursing services to patients and clients on a fee-for-service basis. . . . Such a change in the nature of the social contract is, it seems to me, fundamentally necessary for the survival of nursing as a profession rather than

> an occupational group of workers employed by other organizations. (p. 573)

Sills viewed nurse corporations as a solution to the problem of collective bargaining by nurses and an organizational way to address the economics of nursing practice.

I envision nurse corporations as extending beyond the provision of nursing services to the provision of programs of nursing education. In this case, nurse corporations contract with universities to design and implement ND and PhD programs. Universities, of course, have the right and responsibility to appoint only those partners in the nurse corporation who meet the university's criteria for faculty. Furthermore, universities, as well as clinical agencies, might elect to contract with more than one nurse corporation. Self-employed nurse scholars are entrepreneurs who contract directly with universities for appointment to the faculty and with clinical agencies for practice and research privileges. Alternatively, they engage in private practice, contracting directly with patients for certain nursing services, with students for such educational services as tutoring and mentoring, and with nurse corporations for the continuing education of the partners.

Conclusion

Achievement of the proposed hallmark of 21st-century nursing depends on our individual and collective willingness to take potentially enormous risks and "have the courage to take a position about why people need nursing and about what nursing can and should be" (Orem, 1995, p. 414). Clearly, if we want to ensure the survival of our discipline, all of us must fall in love with nursing science now and develop a passion for the destiny of the discipline of nursing.

References

Fawcett, J. (1983). Hallmarks of success in nursing theory development. In P. L. Chinn (Ed.), *Advances in nursing theory development* (pp. 3–17). Rockville, MD: Aspen.

Fawcett, J. (1984). Hallmarks of success in nursing research. *Advances in Nursing Science, 7*(1), 1–11.

Fawcett, J., & Carino, C. (1989). Hallmarks of success in nursing practice. *Advances in Nursing Science, 11*(4), 1–8.

Huch, M. H. (1995). Nursing and the next millennium. *Nursing Science Quarterly, 8*, 38–44.

Kendrick, K. (1997). What is advanced nursing? *Professional Nurse, 12*(10), 689.

Meleis, A. I. (1993, April). Nursing research and the Neuman model: Directions for the future. Panel discussion at the Fourth Biennial International Neuman Systems Model Symposium, Rochester, NY.

Orem, D. E. (1995). *Nursing: Concepts of practice* (5th ed.). St. Louis: C. V. Mosby.

Sills, G. M. (1983). The role and function of the clinical nurse specialist. In N. L. Chaska (Ed.), *The nursing profession: A time to speak* (pp. 563–579). New York: McGraw-Hill.

Watson, J. (1997). The theory of human caring: Retrospective and prospective. *Nursing Science Quarterly, 10*, 49–52.

Watson, M. J. (1996). Watson's theory of transpersonal caring. In P. H. Walker & B. Neuman (Eds.), *Blueprint for use of nursing models: Education, research, practice, and administration* (pp. 141–184). New York: NLN Press.

Wood, K. W. (1978). Casework effectiveness: A new look at the research evidence. *Social Work, 23*, 437–458.

Chapter 7

The State of Nursing Science: Reconceptualizing for the 21st Century

Mary Cipriano Silva, RN, PhD, FAAN

As nurses begin their exodus from the familiar landscapes of the 20th century and enter into the unknown landscapes of the 21st century, I challenge you to pause and consider the following two questions: Within the realm of known nursing knowledge, what do you see as the present state of nursing science? What do you envision as the future state of nursing science? These questions are explored through a brief discussion of the following five themes: respecting nursing science as past and as prologue; questioning the "what is" of nursing and nursing science; questioning the necessity of logic in nursing science; reconciling "opposites" in nursing science; and letting go, moving on, and making a difference in nursing science.

Respecting Nursing Science as Past and as Prologue

Nurses should appreciate the visionary nurse scholars of the past and their seminal scholarship

Source: Silva, M. C. (1999). The state of nursing science: Reconceptualizing for the 21st Century. *Nursing Science Quarterly*, 12(3): 221–226. Reprinted by permission and copyright © July 1999 of Sage Publications, Inc.

that, within the context of a given time, advanced nursing science. Too often, however, the scholarship of an earlier time has been decontextualized, resulting in disparaging comments about nursing science past. One area in which this trend has been particularly prevalent is that of the so-called grand nursing theories that began to emerge as a movement in the 1950s. Today's critics often find them meaningless, irrelevant, or even worse, impeding the progress of nursing science. The grand nursing theories were not without their flaws (no theory is), but what contemporary critics fail to understand is that, as a whole, these theories were largely responsible for moving nursing away from the then well-entrenched medical model into other ways of visioning nursing that were more in keeping with nursing values and phenomena.

However, of even greater concern today are those nurses and other persons who would eliminate all nursing theory because it does not speak to them. I agree with three scholars who believe that practice or research without a philosophy or theory (including nursing theory) is shortsighted (Nolan, Lundh, & Tishelman, 1998). I would go one step further and predict that theory in general and nursing theory in particular will be more essential for nursing's prominence in the 21st century than in the 20th century. As more and more knowledge is generated and disseminated at a faster pace, nurses must be able to understand and articulate clearly the theoretical bases of their discipline, past and present, and the rapid changes within it in order to work with transdisciplinary scholars and practitioners in the 21st century.

Nursing theory and science past and present is prologue to nursing theory and science future. Therefore, nurses must commit themselves to nursing theory and science in a positive and productive way. What does this mean? First, all nurses (whether nurse scientists, educators, administrators, clinicians, and/or students) must understand that a major goal of science is to generate theory; therefore, nurses cannot afford to disparage what is a generally accepted scientific maxim without looking foolish. Second, to communicate better with ourselves and with the transdisciplinary teams that we expect to work with in the 21st century, we must simplify and/or eliminate contrived or convoluted language in existing nursing theories that only speaks to a few (Rutty, 1998).

Questioning the "What Is" of Nursing and of Nursing Science

What is nursing? What is nursing science? These questions have been raised hundreds of times in nursing, and many scholars still claim that nursing or nursing science cannot advance until these questions are answered. In response, at least two other questions must be raised: (1) Can one give good nursing care or contribute to the body of good nursing science without defining nursing or nursing science, and (2) is the "what is" question the right one to ask?

Regarding question 1, I believe the answer to be no. Virtually every semester, doctoral students

raise issue with the importance of answering the "what is nursing" and the "what is nursing science" questions before nursing can advance. With rare exception, all of these students at one time or another have practiced nursing at the bedside or in the community with clients and consider the care they gave to be good. How could these nurses (or any nurses) give good nursing care and at the same time be clueless about what nursing and nursing science are? The point is that nurses are not clueless. They have been socialized into and have internalized the essences of nursing and nursing science, and they are able to define them if and when asked. Is there universal agreement among their definitions? No, but there is a constancy of response that speaks to the "what is" of nursing and of nursing science and not to the "what is" of another discipline. It is unrealistic (not to mention deadly dull and creatively stifling) to expect unanimous agreement on all aspects of a definition of nursing or of nursing science, a definition that is not the critical matter. Nursing will be best remembered not for what nurses defined but for what nurses did or failed to do.

Regarding question 2, "Is the 'what is' [nursing or nursing science] question the right one to ask?" I believe the answer to be no. In a Scholarly Dialogue column of *Nursing Science Quarterly* ("What is Nursing Science?" 1997), the "what is nursing science?" question was posed to nine well-educated registered nurses representing eight countries worldwide. The question was raised in the present tense, and all nurses responded likewise. Yet, I do not believe the "what is" question (if we must continue to ask this question!) gives nurse scientists the most useful information because it is focused on the present. The present constitutes only a moment in time and then rapidly becomes the past. Therefore, I believe the more compelling and right question is this: "How should nursing science be defined?" This question is an ongoing search for the best of nursing science and is futuristic; such an orientation will better prepare nurse scientists to make the transition into the 21st century.

Questioning the Necessity of Logic in Nursing Science

In most of the literature focusing on the worth of nursing science, logic is a necessary condition (e.g., Bishop, 1998, p. 35; Copnell, 1998; Ray, 1998). Logic suggests the use of the mind to reason in a systematic way that makes sense to self and others. Although logic plays an important role in furthering much of nursing science, at times it can become an impediment. It will become an even greater impediment in the 21st century when the acceleration of information produced surpasses the human mind's ability to understand it.

Traditionally, one goal of science is to understand, and most scientists use considerable logic to do so, but now, and even more so in the future, humans will be confronted with events that defy logic and linear reasoning. Now, and even more so in the future, humans will be confronted with events that defy making sense. Now, and even more so in the future, humans will be confronted with events that occur outside of the scientific mainstream. Examples of such events involve the paranormal (Phillips, 1996) and the power of prayer to heal (Silva & DeLashmutt, 1998).

The question, then, is what to make of events of these types within nursing science. Is nursing inquiry leading to nursing knowledge possible with such events? To the nurse scientist who ascribes primarily to logical empiricism, the answer is probably no. To the nurse scientist who is challenged by the inexplicable and the unpredictable, the answer is probably yes. Whereas the former nurse scientist can reject or dismiss any outlier events such as the paranormal, the latter nurse scientist is fascinated with them. But, fascination does not a nursing science make.

What is needed is not only the passion to explore largely uncharted and controversial nursing phenomena but also the methods to do so. Such methods cannot rely primarily on traditional logic or linearity, as these types of phenomena but also the methods to do so. Such methods cannot rely primarily on traditional logic or linearity, as these types of phenomena defy both. Therefore, what is in order are creative, nonlinear research methods that explore in-between spaces and places. Beginning departures from traditional logic include the use of retroductive reasoning when serendipity occurs and the use of fuzzy logic theory when reasoning cannot be exact (Bishop, 1998, pp. 38–42). In addition, the nurse scientist should not feel compelled to use an up-front plan; instead, the nurse scientist should follow the phenomena wherever they lead no matter how illogical. The result may be untidy, but it may also be breakthrough nursing science in which the logical takes a well-deserved back seat to the illogical and the fuzzy in the 21st century.

Reconciling Opposites in Nursing Science

The thesis put forth here is that so-called opposites in nursing science frequently attract. Theory exists in practice, and practice exists in theory. Qualitative research exists in quantitative research, and quantitative research exists in qualitative research. Related-discipline sciences exist in nursing science, and nursing science exists in related-discipline sciences. It is this last controversial thesis that I reflect on in answering three questions.

First, should reconciling opposites in nursing science and related-discipline sciences occur? No easy response exists. One's response rests on many factors. Philosophical beliefs and degrees of commitment to them, advances in theory and science, social-cultural-political climate, what one believes to be in the best interest of nursing (both as discipline and as practice), and what one believes to be in the best interest of clients (that is, what makes a positive difference to human health) are major considerations. One's response also rests on which of the preceding (or other) factors are used in combination to answer the question and what the potential strengths and pitfalls of one's combination of factors are. My own response is that so-called opposites should be reconciled if such reconciliation advances nursing science and practice in a meaningful way.

Second, what form(s) could the reconciling nursing science and related-discipline sciences take in the 21st century? Five conceptual possibilities are suggested here:

1. Synchronizing. *Synchronizing* means that nursing science and the related-discipline sciences coexist; that is, they occur at the same time and place but retain their separate identities (metaphor: think duet).

2. Overlapping. *Overlapping* means that nursing science extends over and covers a part of the related-discipline sciences and vice versa. In overlapping, both nursing science and the related-discipline sciences maintain a part of themselves that is unique (metaphor: think hand-drawn star).

3. Overlaying. *Overlaying* means that the nursing science is attached to and placed over and/or under the related-discipline sciences (metaphor: think lacquered wood).

4. Synthesizing. *Synthesizing* means combining the parts of nursing science and of the related-discipline sciences into a whole. In synthesizing, parts of nursing sciences are attached to and intertwined with the related-discipline sciences to make a whole (metaphor: think woven basket).

5. Blending. *Blending* means to combine nursing science smoothly with related-discipline sciences so that they are inseparable and indistinguishable one from the other (metaphor: think non-primary colors).

Third, what degree of importance could be attached to reconciling nursing (NS) and related-discipline sciences (RDS)? The following nine possibilities are suggested based on a 3 × 3 matrix using levels of high, medium, and low: high degree of importance to both NS and RDS, high degree of importance to NS and medium degree of importance to RDS, high degree of importance to NS and low degree of importance to RDS, medium degree of importance to NS and high degree of importance to RDS, medium degree of importance to both NS and RDS, medium degree of importance to NS and low degree of importance to RDS, low degree of importance to NS and high degree of importance to RDS, low degree of importance to NS and medium degree of importance to RDS, and low degree of importance to both NS and RDS. If you believe in the reconciling of so-called opposites, which of the preceding forms and degrees of importance would you support, if any, between nursing science and the related discipline sciences? My response would be that both the form and the degree of importance would vary depending on the phenomena being reconciled.

In the 21st century, with the explosion of science (especially genetic science) and technology (especially computer technology), more antithetical phenomena will occur. Whether dealing with nursing science or related-discipline science, it seems prudent to seize the day and reflect on our beliefs about reconciling so-called opposites and about the forms, degrees of importance, and short- and long-term impact of our decisions.

Letting Go, Moving On, and Making a Difference in Nursing Science

Letting go in nursing science refers to the giving up of some aspect of nursing science and moving on with another aspect of it when the timing seems right. Letting go and moving on are influenced by, among other factors, one's temperament, the degree of investment in and commitment to a nursing science goal, the ability to see what is timely and cutting edge not only in one's own discipline but also in other human and hard science disciplines, in the arts and humanities, and in the social-cultural-political environments. Nurses cannot be isolationists in the 21st century, for certainly we will hurt no one but our profession and ourselves. To astutely let go and move on requires courage, impeccable timing, hard work, and a clear vision that what one is moving on to will make a positive difference for nursing science and for nursing.

What are some impediments to letting go and moving on? Perhaps the most crippling one is oneself. The more highly invested one is with a nursing theory or a nursing science thesis, the more difficult it may be to let go and move on. However, advances in science move on as do advances in nursing science; thus, the nurse theorist and/or scientist who cares about the state of nursing science must move on too.

Apart from impediments inflicted on oneself, other impediments may be generally accepted maxims about nursing science that one has bought into without question, and therefore, one does not know when to let go and move on. Two of many such impediments are described.

Build a systematic research program. The flaw with this maxim is that it is outdated for the 21st century. Building a systematic research program takes time, with several studies each building on the other. A long-term commitment that expands several decades may be necessary to accomplish such a goal. With the rapid explosion of new human and health science knowledge that is expected to occur in the 21st century, the nurse scientist must be able to plan, conduct, and disseminate (not to mention apply to practice) research at a pace in keeping with the advances in science and in nursing science. If the nurse scientist is unable to keep pace, her or his work will become obsolete and incapable of making a difference. (Moral of the story: The tortoise may never get to the finish line.)

Develop a passion for nursing knowledge. Passion suggests strong feeling. Although feeling passionate about nursing knowledge has its strengths, it is not without its flaws. One flaw with this maxim is that a person becomes emotionally attached to (and sometimes even addicted to) that about which she or he feels strongly. Considerable human knowledge and nursing knowledge are ephemeral and will become even more so in the 21st century. If a nurse scientist becomes addicted via passion to use of certain types of nursing knowledge, will that nurse scientist be able to let go and move on when she or he should? At the turn of this century, it seems prudent to ask for less passion about nursing knowledge and more questioning and nonembeddedness about it. (Moral of the story: You cannot teach an embedded dog new tricks.)

Conclusion

Is the present state of nursing science in need of reconceptualization? After reflecting about the past, present, and possible future states of nursing science as presented in the five identified themes related to nursing (i.e., respecting nursing science as past and as prologue; questioning the "what is" of nursing and nursing science; questioning the logic in nursing science; reconciling opposites in nursing science; and letting go, moving on, and making a difference in nursing science), the conclusion is an unequivocal "yes." Based on this reflection and conclusion, the following reconceptualization comes to mind: If the past and present can be characterized as a continuing search for the knowledge within the meaning of nursing science, than a productive future state of nursing science can be conceptualized as a creative but challenging transformation of nursing science through social, political, technological, scientific, artistic, and spiritual forces that will shape the 21st century.

References

Bishop, S. M. (1998). Logical reasoning. In A. M. Tomey & M. R. Alligood (Eds.), *Nursing theorists and their work* (4th ed., pp. 35–42). St. Louis: Mosby.

Copnell, B. (1998). Synthesis in nursing knowledge: An analysis of two approaches. *Journal of Advanced Nursing, 27,* 870–874.

Nolan, M., Lundh, U., & Tishelman, C. (1998). Nursing's knowledge base: Does it have to be unique? *British Journal of Nursing, 7,* 270, 272–276.

Phillips, J. R. (1996). Inquiry into the paranormal. *Nursing Science Quarterly, 9,* 89–91.

Ray, M. A. (1998). Complexity and nursing science. *Nursing Science Quarterly, 11,* 91–93.

Rutty, J. E. (1998). The nature of philosophy of science, theory and knowledge relating to nursing and professionalism. *Journal of Advanced Nursing, 28,* 243–250.

Silva, M. C., & DeLashmutt, M. (1998). Spirituality and prayer: A new age paradigm for ethics. *Nursing Connections, 11*(2), 13–17.

What is nursing science? An international dialogue. (1997). *Nursing Science Quarterly, 10,* 10–13.

Chapter 8

Nursing Science: The Transformation of Practice

Rosemarie Rizzo Parse, RN, PhD, FAAN

World-wide transformations in nursing practice are evolving as more nurses are embracing extant nursing theories and frameworks in order to fortify their unique contributions to the healthcare system. This article specifies the importance of and the ethical considerations arising when using nursing knowledge from within the school of thought of the discipline to guide practice.

The ideas set forth are in stark contrast to the general nursing process with its medical model-driven diagnostic systems now proliferating in nursing practice in the global healthcare community. Both challenges and opportunities are present in the transformation of practice to a nursing knowledge base.

Introduction

Transformations are evolutionary; they are gradual and incremental. The word transformation comes from the Latin *transformation* (Oxford English Dictionary, 1986), which means to change or metamorphose in the structure and form of something familiar. Form refers to the distinguishing characteristics that shape something, and structure refers to the whole configuration of relationships in a system. Nursing has begun to transform from traditional medical science-based practice, where nursing is considered an applied science, to nursing as a basic sci-

Source: Parse R.R. (1999). Nursing science: The transformation of practice. *Journal of Advanced Nursing, 30*(6), 1383–1387. Reprinted with permission of Blackwell Science Ltd.

ence practice. Thus, it is changing in structure and form.

The structure of nursing world-wide has been and for the most part still is connected closely to and is in fact under the purview of medicine (Parse, 1981, 1993, 1994). Although nursing is growing in stature as a unique basic-science discipline, the medical-model applied-science nursing still predominates in practice. This takes the form of a mechanistic approach to humans as biopsycho–social–spiritual beings who can be fixed through diagnostic and intervention methods that objectify the human being. The *structure* of this practice focuses on the nurse as an expert in guiding people on what is best for their healthcare. The *form* of the practice is through the general nursing process (assess, diagnose, plan, implement, and evaluate).

This diagnostic process is reductionistic; it places on human beings labels that arise from objective judgments by nurses. Health-promoting actions are often taken by nurses based on the labels rather than on individual descriptions given by the persons themselves. The configuration of relationships revolves around clearly defined tasks embedded in a view that posits nursing as an applied science, one that combines physiology, psychology, sociology, and other sciences but has no specific knowledge base of its own (Parse, 1987; Cody, 1994b). In other words, nursing knowledge is a collection of ideas from other sciences (Huch, 1988, 1995). How can this be so, when nursing knowledge is, in fact, specified in the extant theories and frameworks?

Some nurse authors (Rogers, 1970; Parse, 1981, 1998; Phillips, 1996) take issue with this traditional stance of nursing as an applied science and posit nursing as a basic science embracing a unified body of knowledge with the human–universe–health process as the phenomenon of concern to the discipline. The notion of basic-science nursing as a guide to practice is a relatively new one, and the impetus to embrace it is now unfolding in light of the global health-care reformation (Parse, 1987, 1992; Paplau, 1987). The unsettledness in health care delivery systems provides nurses with opportunities to fortify their unique contributions to the health-care of society by deliberately and explicitly continuing to transform nursing practice. This transformation or metamorphosis happens through the use of nursing knowledge based on a unitary perspective of the human being (Parse, 1995, 1998; Rogers, 1994).

Basic-science nursing in the simultaneity paradigm has two schools of thought: the human becoming school (Parse, 1987, 1997b, 1998) and the science of unitary human beings (Rogers, 1970). This paradigm espouses the belief that the human is unitary in mutual process with the universe and that health is a process and a set of values (Parse, 1981, 1998; Rogers, 1994). The notions of unitary, mutual process, and health as a process are unique and different from traditional applied-science nursing beliefs (Parse, 1995, 1997a). Unitary refers to the human as whole, recognized through patterns, whereas the notion of biopsycho–social–spiritual refers to an applied-science view based on a separation of the biological, psychological, sociological, and spiritual parts of the human being (Parse, 1987, 1992).

The focus of this article, the human becoming school of thought (Cody, 1994a; Parse, 1997a, 1997b, 1998) within the simultaneity paradigm, has an ontology and methodologies. The ontology contains philosophical assumptions and the principles. The principles (described in detail in Parse, 1981, 1998), often referred to as the theory (Parse, 1998, p. 34), follow:

1. Structuring meaning multidimensionally is co-creating reality through the languaging of valuing and imaging.
2. Co-creating rhythmical patterns of relating is living the paradoxical unity of revealing–concealing and enabling–limiting while connecting–separating.
3. Cotranscending with the possibles is powering unique ways of originating in the process of transforming.

The methodologies are the research and practice processes congruent with the ontology. The phenomena for research with this method are universal lived experiences of health surfacing in the human–universe process reflecting being–becoming, value priorities, and quality of life, such as joy–sorrow, grieving, persisting while wanting to change, and hope. The findings are structures of the remembered, the now-moment, and the not-yet, all-at-once. The structures are the lived experiences as described by participants, and these structures enhance understanding of human becoming (Parse, 1987, 1997a, 1999). The understandings gained from research expand the knowledge that nurses use in practice.

With the human becoming principles (Parse, 1981, 1992, 1995) as a guide to practice, nurses are with persons as they enhance their own quality of life. Nurses do not focus only on persons who are ill, as is often the case with the practice of traditional nursing (Cody, 1994b; Parse, 1997a). The *structure* of human becoming nursing occurs within nurse-person and nurse-group configurations. Nurse–group situations may be with families or communities (Parse, 1987, 1996). Family refers to those persons with whom one is closely connected, not just nuclear family members, as is usually the case in traditional nursing (Parse, 1981).

Community refers to the universe, the galaxy of human connectedness present through face-to-face engagement, reading of printed material, use of telecommunication networks, and through imaginings with people, ideas, objects, and situations (Parse, 1996). Again, community here is defined differently than in applied-science nursing. The nurse may participate with person, family, and community for a variety of reasons arising from the specific desires of the persons in the situation. The participation of the nurse is not guided by traditional societal norms. The setting may be a home, hospital, hospice, day care center or health center, in the context of telephone conversation or computer e-mail, and wherever else persons and nurses meet.

If documentation is required as part of the structure in the specific setting where nurses and persons meet, the reporting includes the person's descriptions of their experiences, the situations from their views, and the hopes, dreams, and intents related to what is most important to them at the moment. This type of documentation is quite different from standard assessment forms that usually focus on the illness process rather than the meaning of the situation from the person's own view. The person's meanings of situations are shown in the descriptions. For example, the person's own words are used to provide a health description. Emerging paradoxical patterns of preference in living health are apparent in the descriptions and may be documented by the person and nurse. Activities and plans may also be documented but always from the persons', families', or communities' perspectives.

The *form* of nursing in the transformational practice guided by the human becoming principles is true presence: a nonroutinized way of being with others that honors the others' views and choices on changing health patterns and quality of life (Parse, 1995, 1996, 1997a). Honoring the person's views means abiding by their wishes and not forcing a standardized plan of care on them (Parse, 1981, 1987, 1992). True presence is lived by nurses whose beliefs are consistent with the principles of human becoming—that is, persons know the way and choose their health situation and their quality of life (Parse, 1990). True presence arises in the living of the principles as the nurse is with person, family, or community. To be in true presence, the nurse centers and prepares to attend to the other through the process of coming-to-be-present, gentling down, and lifting up to focus on others as they illuminate meaning, synchronize rhythms, and mobilize transcendence (Parse, 1990). The nurse readies himself or herself to be available to the other without judging or intending to label the other. The nurse is available to be with the person as the person changes his or her health patterns. This is very different from the traditional practice of nursing where the nurse as an expert on health informs persons what to do to achieve certain health norms. The dimensions and processes of the practice methodology in the human becoming school of thought (Parse, 1998, pp. 69–70) are as follows:

- Illuminating meaning is explicating what was, is, and will be. *Explicating* is making clear what is appearing now through languaging.

- Synchronizing rhythms is dwelling with the pitch, yaw, and roll of the human–universe process. *Dwelling* with is immersing with the flow of connecting–separating.
- Mobilizing transcendence is moving beyond the meaning moment with what is not-yet. *Moving beyond* is propelling with envisioned possibles of transforming.

This means that the nurse in true presence goes along with persons as they make choices about changing health priorities (illuminating meaning, synchronizing rhythms, and mobilizing transcendence). In illuminating meaning, synchronizing rhythms and mobilizing transcendence, persons share only what they wish with the nurse, and the nurse respects what is said as the persons' structured reality. No effort is made by the nurse to tell persons what to do—but the nurse does listen carefully and answers questions and refers persons to other healthcare providers when appropriate. Health teaching is not a predetermined process where all persons receive the same information, as it often is in traditional nursing practice. Rather, the teaching arises as persons indicate readiness to learn by asking questions or indicating curiosity about something of importance to them. In human becoming practice, there are no standardized teaching plans such as those in traditional practice (for example the plans for persons with diabetes or heart disease).

Clearly, nursing practice takes on a unique identity when guided by the human becoming theory, which specifies for those within and without the discipline how nurses contribute to healthcare delivery in a way different from professionals in other disciplines (Parse, 1993). There is not effort to emulate medicine; nursing is a unique discipline when lived from a human becoming perspective. For example, the nurse does not place a diagnostic label on the person as physicians do. The uniqueness lies in what nurses know; what nurses know about human beings and health always guides what they do. The activities of nurses reflect their belief systems, and if these are in concert with human becoming theory, then nursing as a basic science and performing art is recognized, as other disciplines are, by its unique knowledge base. In this case, the unique knowledge is the belief system that encompasses views of humans as unitary and health as a continuously changing process chosen by the person.

It is logical to conclude, then, that if unique nursing knowledge really guides research and practice, the practice modalities must flow from the ontology of the schools of thought and cannot be the general nursing diagnostic system which is commonly known as the nursing process (assessing, diagnosing, planning, implementing, and evaluating). The nursing diagnostic system was a useful way to organize practice in the 1950s and 1960s when nurses had not yet specified the knowledge base of nursing, but it is not acceptable in the 21st century to utilize an outmoded system that is based on medical rather than nursing science. There are a number of nursing diagnostic systems that are offspring of the North American Nursing Diagnostic Association system vying for attention in the global nursing community. In fact, there are not only computerized nursing diagnoses but also intervention strategies and expected outcomes now prescribed and tested that further categorize people as objects. These systems did not arise from the schools of thought within the discipline but have been modeled after medicine's diagnostic system and do not support the advancement of nursing science-based practice (Barrett, 1993; Hall, 1996; Parse, 1987). The nursing diagnostic systems tend to be reductionistic and dehumanizing (Parse, 1992, 1995; Taylor, 1988).

Yet, some nurses say they wish to be eclectic and use the diagnostic system and whatever general or nursing theory seems most appropriate for the situation. This belies the whole notion of nursing knowledge-based practice. To say that nursing frameworks or theories can be used whenever the appropriate occasion arises relegates nursing knowledge to someplace outside the nurse as person. For example, following the person's perspective only when it is convenient and making demands toward a goal emanating from the nurse on other occasions mixes paradigms and confuses the person receiving nursing care.

Nurses as unitary beings live their beliefs about the human–universe–health process, and therein lies the knowledge upon which they practice. Nursing knowledge-based practice is not something "I put on." It shows itself in "what I am" to the other. The performing art of nursing is based on its science and is the explicit and tacit articulation of beliefs about the human–universe–health process. What one believes about human beings and health permeates one's actions consistently; thus, the human becoming nurse lives a different practice from nurses who believe in other views of humans and health. Eclecticism in nursing practice is scientifically unsound, serves to foster confusion, and undermines the notion of nursing as a discipline with its own knowledge base, as well as raising some issues for ethical consideration.

Ethical Considerations

What responsibility do nurses have to practice within a school of thought of the discipline? If nursing is indeed a discipline focusing on the human–universe–health process with its own unique body of knowledge concerning health services for people, then do not nurses have an ethical responsibility to offer the services guided by that knowledge? Should not nursing practice be governed by the principles of the extant theories and frameworks in the discipline instead of

by procedures or diagnoses emanating from medical science? Conversely, if nursing does not have a unique knowledge base, is it a discipline, and should doctor of philosophy degrees in nursing continue to be granted? Or should the substantive content of nursing remain primarily with medical science and nurses practice from a medical-model base as assistants to physicians?

If the body of knowledge guiding the nurse is the human becoming school of thought, then the ethical responsibility flows from the values that constitute the ethic of that belief system. These values flow from the ontology; thus, the performing art of nursing brings to life the ethic of this school of thought. For example, a fundamental belief in the human becoming theory is that humans choose health in mutual process with the universe, consistent with their own value priorities, and only they can change their patterns of health as their values change (Parse, 1990, 1997a). The inherent ethic here requires that the person's value priorities be respected. The human becoming nurse, then, would not label, diagnose, plan care for, make judgments about, or exert pressure to change a person's way of living, as is often true with other guides to nursing practice. Thus, the ethic embedded in the ontology of the human becoming school of thought is lived out in the nurse's practice. This way of nursing practice is an alternative to the traditional one.

Challenges and Opportunities

Living basic-science nursing from a human becoming perspective is a weighty challenge with opportunities. The *challenge* arises in two main areas: (a) the human becoming school of thought requires a shift in belief systems from traditional applied science-based nursing to basic science-based nursing and gaining this knowledge requires the nurse's desire, time, and effort; and (b) the healthcare settings are often not prepared for this unique nursing practice but continue to foster the notion of nursing as part of medical science rather than nursing as a unique discipline guided by extant nursing theories and frameworks. Nurses with the desire are willing to take the time and effort to learn a different way to enhance human quality of life, and some of these nurses have conducted research studies with the human becoming perspective as a guide to practice (Jonas, 1995; Mitchell, 1995; Santopinto & Smith, 1995). These evaluation studies have shown that human becoming is a viable mode of practice.

Nurses, persons, families, and other healthcare providers state that they are more satisfied with human becoming nursing care, and these findings are substantiated in the published works of several nurses whose practice is guided by the human becoming theory (Mitchell & Pilkington, 1990; Quiquero et al., 1991; Rasmusson et al., 1991). For example, in the research studies on human becoming practice (Jonas, 1995; Mitchell, 1995; Santopinto & Smith, 1995) persons and their families remarked that they felt listened to and respected (which they had not felt before); human becoming nurses did not tell people what they had to do but, rather, discussed with them what their own desires and goals were regarding health. They were not labeled with diagnoses or forced to follow a preplanned regime, but rather, their own desires were honored (Quiquero et al., 1991; Rasmusson et al., 1991). The persons in the research studies recognized the differences between human becoming nursing practice and traditional practice (Jonas, 1995; Mitchell, 1995; Santopinto & Smith, 1995). Thus, evidence from research shows that the nontraditional practice of human becoming is successful. Although this is remarkable, further research must be done to illustrate more clearly the value of human becoming nursing practice.

Nurses must also assume responsibility to educate healthcare systems about the meaning of a practice based on human becoming views The opportunities involved in guiding nursing practice from a human becoming perspective are afforded to nursing, nurses, and humankind. Through practice guided by the human becoming school of thought, nursing is enhanced and can be recognized as a discipline with a unique knowledge base. This fortifies nursing's position in university and healthcare settings. Nurses have opportunities to contribute uniquely to the health of humankind by focusing on quality of life from the person's, family's, and community's perspectives. People are afforded the opportunity to be treated with dignity by having their values respected without judgment by others.

Recommendations

The transformation of nursing requires a true metamorphosis underpinned with the commitment of nurses throughout the world to practice differently and conduct research to ensure that the practice of nursing serves people in a unique way. The possibilities are unlimited when basic-science nursing guides the practice, as the form and structure will change for the betterment of humankind. The metamorphosis of nursing resides with nurses who accept the responsibility to learn and live basic-science nursing practice so that it blossoms and grows in the 21st century and beyond.

References

Barrett, E. A. M. (1993). Nursing centers without nursing frameworks: What's wrong with this picture? *Nursing Science Quarterly, 6*, 115–117.

Cody, W. K. (1994a). The language of nursing science: If now when? *Nursing Science Quarterly, 7*, 98–100.

Cody, W. K. (1994b). Nursing theory-guided practice: What it is and what it is not. *Nursing Science Quarterly, 7*, 144–146.

Hall, B. A. (1996). The psychiatric model: A critical analysis of its undermining effects on nursing in chronic mental illness. *Advances in Nursing Science, 8*, 16–26.

Huch, M. H. (1988). Theory-based practice: Structuring nursing care. *Nursing Science Quarterly, 1*, 6–7.

Huch, M. H. (1995). Nursing science as a basis for advanced practice. *Nursing Science Quarterly, 8*, 607.

Jonas, C. M. (1995). Evaluation of the human becoming theory in family practice. In *Illuminations: The Human Becoming Theory in Practice and Research* (Parse, R. R., ed.). New York: National League for Nursing Press, pp. 347–366.

Mitchell, G. J. (1995). Evaluation of the human becoming theory in practice in acute care setting. In *Illuminations: The Human Becoming Theory in Practice and Research* (Parse, R. R., ed.). New York: National League for Nursing Press, pp. 367–399.

Mitchell, G. J., & Pilkington, B. (1990). Theoretical approaches in nursing: A comparison of Roy and Parse. *Nursing Science Quarterly, 3*, 81–87.

Oxford English Dictionary. (1986). Oxford: Oxford University Press.

Paplau, H. E. (1987). Nursing science: A historical perspective. In *Nursing Science: Major Paradigms, Theories, and Critiques* (Parse, R. R., ed.). New York: Saunders, pp. 13–29.

Parse, R. R. (1981). *Man-Living Health: A Theory of Nursing.* New York: Wiley.

Parse, R. R. (1987). *Nursing Science: Major Paradigms, Theories and Critiques.* Philadelphia: Saunders.

Parse, R. R. (1990). Health: A personal commitment. *Nursing Science Quarterly, 3*, 136–140.

Parse, R. R. (1992). Human becoming: Parse's theory of nursing. *Nursing Science Quarterly, 5*, 35–42.

Parse, R. R. (1993). Nursing and medicine: Two different disciplines. *Nursing Science Quarterly, 6*, 109.

Parse, R. R. (1994). Charley Potatoes or mashed potatoes? *Nursing Science Quarterly, 7*, 97.

Parse, R. R. (1995). *Illuminations: The Human Becoming Theory in Practice and Research.* New York: National League for Nursing Press.

Parse, R. R. (1996). Community: A human becoming perspective. *Illuminations: The Newsletter of the International Consortium of Parse Scholars 5*, 1–4.

Parse, R. R. (1997a). The human becoming theory: The was, is, and will be. *Nursing Science Quarterly, 10*, 32–38.

Parse, R. R. (1997b). The language of nursing knowledge: Saying what we mean. In *The Language of Theory and Metatheory* (Fawcett, J., & King, I. M., eds.). Indianapolis, Indiana: Sigma Theta Tau Monograph, pp. 73–77.

Parse, R. R. (1998). *The Human Becoming School of Thought: A Perspective for Nurses and Other Health Professionals.* Thousand Oaks, CA: Sage.

Parse, R. R. (1999). *Hope: An International Human Becoming Perspective.* Sudbury, MA: Jones and Bartlett.

Phillips, J. R. (1996). What constitutes nursing science? *Nursing Science Quarterly, 9*, 48–49.

Quiquero, A., Knights, D., & Meo, O. (1991). Theory as a guide to practice: Staff nurses choose Parse's theory. *Canadian Journal of Nursing Administration, 4*(1), 14–16.

Rasmusson, D., Jonas, C. M., & Mitchell, G. J. (1991). The eye of the beholder: Parse's theory with homeless individuals. *Clinical Nurse Specialist, 5*(3), 139–143.

Rogers, M. E. (1970). *An Introduction to the Theoretical Basis of Nursing.* Philadelphia: Davis.

Rogers, M. E. (1994). The science of unitary human beings: Current perspectives. *Nursing Science Quarterly, 7*, 33–35.

Santopinto, M. D. A., & Smith, M. C. (1995). Evaluation of the human becoming theory in practice with adults and children. In *Illuminations: The Human Becoming Theory in Practice and Research* (Parse, R. R., ed.). New York: National League for Nursing Press, pp. 309–346.

Taylor, S. C. (1988). Nursing theory and nursing process: Orem's theory in practice. *Nursing Science Quarterly, 1*, 111–119.

Chapter 9

The Nurse Scholar of the 21st Century

Sandra Schimdt Bunkers,
RN, PhD, FAAN

The professional nurse of the 21st century is called to be a nurse scholar. *Webster's Ninth New Collegiate Dictionary* (1990) defines scholar as '1. One who attends school or studies under a teacher; 2. a: one who has done advanced study in a special field; b: a learned person' (p. 1051). The professional nurse of the 21st century must be learned, must be mentored by wise and knowledgeable teachers, and must have the academic foundation for advancing the scholarship of service to humankind.

Nursing: A Call to Scholarship

Professional nursing today is a call to scholarship. Suggesting that the 21st century nurse be a nurse scholar implies that the discipline has a unique knowledge base from which one can draw on in the service of humankind. Nursing's history denotes a productive evolutionary journey of such knowledge development. Nursing began as a human service called into being by society. The knowledge base of our discipline

was built as nurses, beginning with Florence Nightingale, carefully collected data on how to solve human health problems. Nurse scholar Marilyn Rawnsley (1999) points this out in writing the following:

It is the profession of nursing legitimized as a responsive human service that engendered the science of nursing. Nursing research, perhaps beginning with Nightingale's systematic data collection, was launched to solve problems encountered in practice. Nursing science as a legitimate academic endeavor, with theories aimed at understanding and explaining phenomena central to the discipline, evolved almost a century later. (p. 316)

It is true that nursing science has evolved. We are now at the point as a scientific discipline of having developed nursing theories encompassing more that one paradigm (or world-view to guide nurses in understanding the human health process). Nurse theorist Rosemarie Rizzo Parse identifies two competing worldviews in nursing, which she names the totality paradigm and the simultaneity paradigm. Parse (1996b) writes

The discipline of nursing encompasses the knowledge in the extant frameworks and theories that are embedded in the totality and simul-

Source: Bunkers, S. S. (2000). The nurse scholar of the 21st century. *Nursing Science Quarterly, 13*(2): 116–123. Reprinted with permission and copyright © 2000 by Sage Publications, Inc.

taneity paradigms. These theories and frameworks explicate the nature of nursing's major phenomenon of concern, the human–universe–health process. (p. 275)

Nurse scholars of the 21st century must be accountable for understanding these nursing theories and conceptual frameworks and utilizing them in guiding practice, research, education, and regulation. It is our challenge as nurse leaders today to merge the professional practice science (the problem solving for human health issues) and the academic science (the creation of theories and conceptual frameworks) of our discipline. This merging of professional science and academic science is brought about in the formation of nursing theory–based education, practice, and regulation models. Examples of such models include The Health Action Model for Partnership in Community (Bunkers, Nelson, Leuning, Crane, & Josephson, 1999), an education-practice model originating in the Department of Nursing at Augustana College in Sioux Falls, South Dakota; a human becoming nursing theory-based parish nursing model created at First Presbyterian Church in Sioux Falls (Bunkers & Putnam, 1995); the nursing theory-based South Dakota Board of Nursing Regulatory Decisioning Model (Damgaard & Bunkers, 1998); and a model for teaching-learning based on the theory of human becoming (Bunkers, 1999b). These models are prototypes for nursing, providing a blueprint for creating nursing theory-guided practice, education, research, and regulation.

The demand to educate responsive, ethical, and intelligent knowledge-guided nurses has been echoed through time. Constance Schuyler (1992) writes in a commentary on Florence Nightingale the following:

Nightingale believed that nursing education should develop both the intellect and the character of the nurse. Accordingly, she gave her stu-

dents a solid background in the sciences to enable them to understand the theory behind their care. To develop character, she assigned readings in the humanities to increase their understanding of human ethics and morals. She believed that nurses should never stop learning. She wrote to her student, 'To nurse is a field of which one may safely say: there is no end in what we may be learning every day.' (p. 11)

Nightingale was known to be brilliant. However, intellectual pursuits were not enough. She had a drive for action and this coupled with her brilliance spurred her on 'to be one of the greatest reformers of the 19th century' (Schuyler, 1992, p. 16). In addressing human suffering, Nightingale writes in 1859:

No mockery in the world is so hollow as the advice showered upon the sick. It is of no use for the sick to say anything, for what the adviser wants is, not to know the truth about the state of the patient, but to turn whatever the sick may say to the support of his own argument, set forth, it must be repeated, without any inquiry whatever into the patient's real condition. . . . How little the real sufferings of illness are known or understood. (p. 57)

The scene is now around 1992. Nurse theorist Martha Rogers (1992) writes concerning the development of nursing knowledge:

Over-emphasis on technology tends to overshadow therapeutic modalities that can have real significance. Nurses must recognize that they do not create change in people, rather they participate in the process of change to the extent that they bring knowledge to the situation and recognize that the healing process has the potential for healing beyond that which we tend to recognize today. The answer to health will not be found in more drugs, more technology, or more hospitals. (p. 61)

In 1992, nurse theorist Callista Roy (1992) writes addressing her focus for nursing:

I can amass in a week more evidence of human pain and suffering than Nightingale perceived in her lifetime. . . . Nightingale would be sure to respond in her characteristic way, noting that she need not wait until she fully understood the phenomena, nor definitively prove that a given approach could relieve such suffering, but rather she would use everything at her disposal, and all that she could garner from others, to relieve such suffering and find ways to prevent it. She would organize and teach nurses to work with people around the world to create life-giving environments, to free human bodies and spirits from all that hinders full life potential. (p. 69)

The date is 1997. Discussing the evolution of nursing science and in particular the human becoming theory's focus on quality of life from the person's perspective, nurse theorist Rosemarie Rizzo Parse (1997a) writes

The journey of the evolution of the human becoming theory has not been simply an easy movement from one port to another, but, like all journeys, it has been an ebb and flow of intense and quiet moments, pleasures and challenges all-at once. The journey is one of forging new paths for the discipline of nursing and other health-related disciplines and living with opportunities that arise when daring to question the prevailing paradigm. The author is open to the new, the mysteries of the yet-to-be discovered possibles in the quest for preserving the uniqueness of nursing in its contributions to the quality of life for humankind. (p. 36)

These nurse theorists are among many that are actively engaged in the continual scientific endeavor of knowledge development for the discipline of nursing. However, nursing needs to frame this nursing knowledge within an umbrella of values and beliefs.

Framing Nursing Knowledge

The knowledge base of nursing science, with an emphasis on the betterment of humankind, is composed of ideas concerning the person, health, the environment, the universe, and the focus of nursing. 'The core substance of nursing, like all other disciplines, resides in its theories and frameworks, historically created and developed by nurses' (Parse, 1995, p. 51). Along with this unique nursing knowledge, the discipline draws on the natural sciences, human sciences, arts, and humanities to understand phenomena. Although specific knowledge in these areas needs to be known so as to be a competent practitioner of nursing knowledge content changes. Knowledge is in a variety of settings, as time and society evolves, constantly being created and is an interchange between the knower and the known (Palmer, 1993).

Parker Palmer in *To Know as We Are Known* (1993) suggests three sources of knowledge:

History suggests two primary sources for our knowledge. . . . One is curiosity; the other is control. The one corresponds to pure, speculative knowledge, to knowledge as an end in itself. The other corresponds to applied science, to knowledge as a means to practical ends. (p. 7)

Palmer (1993) goes on to identify one other source of knowledge: 'This is a knowledge that originates not in curiosity or control but in compassion, or love—a source celebrated not in our intellectual tradition but in our spiritual heritage' (p. 8). He suggests that the goal of knowledge arising from love 'is the reunification and reconstruction of broken selves and worlds' (p. 8).

All three sources of knowledge identified by Palmer are relevant to nurse scholars. All three sources of knowledge are sources of truth. Palmer (1993) suggests that truth is personal and truth is communal: it exists in relationship. He writes

Truth is neither 'out there' nor 'in here,' but both. Truth is between us, in relationship, to be found in the dialogue of knowers and knowns who are understood as independent but accountable selves. (p. 56)

As independent and accountable selves, nurses must identify foundational values or tenets to guide the teaching–learning processes that will engage nursing's quest for truth in the 21st century. And, teaching-learning in the discipline is the responsibility of all nurse leaders.

Foundational Tenets in Guiding the Framing of Nursing Knowledge

In educating nurse scholars, this author suggests 16 foundational tenets that can frame nursing curriculum and guide nursing education, practice, and research in the 21st century.

These 16 tenets need to be grounded in the theories and conceptual frameworks of nursing (see **Table 9–1**).

Honoring Human Freedom and Choice

The nurse scholar of the 21st century must seek to understand the interconnection between health and human freedom. This tenet implies that the nurse be a student of philosophy as well as a student of science. Jean-Paul Sartre (1956) writes in *Being and Nothingness*, 'Human freedom precedes essence in man and makes it possible; the essence of the human being is suspended in her/his freedom. What we call freedom is impossible to distinguish from the *being* of human reality' (p. 60). Sartre's existential position is that humans are free to choose in situations. Parse's (1998) theory of human becoming posits that humans are open beings, freely choosing meaning in situations and bearing responsibility for these choices. 'The human is responsible for all outcomes of reflective–prereflective choices, even though many are

---

TABLE 9–1 TENETS FOR FRAMING NURSING KNOWLEDGE

1. Honoring human freedom and choice.
2. Cultivating an attitude of openness to uncertainty and difference.
3. Appreciating the meaning of lived experiences of health.
4. Understanding the nature of suffering.
5. Committing to social justice.
6. Believing in the imagination as a source of knowledge.
7. Recognizing the significance of language in structuring mean and reality.
8. Understanding health as process.
9. Understanding community as a process.
10. Believing in the power of personal presence.
11. Participating in scientific inquiry.
12. Asserting the ethics of individual and communal responsibility.
13. Emphasizing living in the present moment.
14. Respecting life and nature.
15. Acknowledging mystery.
16. Focusing on quality of life.

unknown when making decisions' (Parse, 1998, p. 21). Nurse scholars must acknowledge and understand the role human freedom and choice play in persons cocreating patterns of health.

Cultivating an Attitude of Openness to Uncertainty and Difference

Nurse scholars need to cultivate an attitude of openness, openness to new ideas, changes in worldviews and to the unexpected. Jacob Bronowski in his book *The Origins of Knowledge and Imagination* (1978) writes

> *Science is essentially a self-correcting activity. But more important, scientists are people who correct the picture of the moment with another one, as a natural evolution towards a 'true' picture of the world. We have spoken enough about truth to know that we are not going to get a final picture of the world. Nobody is going to find the truth one fine day, as I say, like a hat or an umbrella. . . . The creative personality is always one that looks on the world as fit for change and on herself/himself as an instrument for change. Otherwise, what are you creating for? If the world is perfectly all right the way it is, you have no place in it. The creative personality thinks of the world as a canvas for change and of herself/himself as a divine agent of change. (pp. 122–123)*

Parse (1998) suggests that 'the human aspires and reaches beyond to that which is not-yet' (p. 46). The nurse scholar of the 21st century must look at differing views and differing lifestyles as an invitation to discover opportunities for new knowledge and creative growth for the self and the larger community. With such an attitude of openness to uncertainty and difference, unique possibilities will emerge in healthcare for the betterment of humankind.

Appreciating the Meaning of Lived Experiences of Health

Victor Frankl in his classic work *Man's Search for Meaning* (1984) suggests that the essence of human existence is to find meaning in life. This meaning of life 'always changes but never ceases to be' (Frankl, 1984, p. 115). According to Frankl, we can discover meaning in life 'in three different ways: (1) by creating a work or doing a deed; (2) by experiencing something or encountering someone; and (3) by the attitude we take toward unavoidable suffering' (p. 117). Nurse theorist Rosemarie Parse's human becoming theory and practice and research methodologies focus on understanding the meaning of lived experiences of health. 'Each human's reality is the meaning of the situation' (Parse, 1996b, p. 56).

For the nurse scholar of the 21st century, understanding the meaning the individual or community gives to their health experiences will make it possible for the nurse to work with others' reality. 'Understanding the meaning of the lived experience of another is the essence of coming to know another and valuing the other as a unique human being' (Bunkers, 1998, p. 62). Understanding is the basis for reflective, knowledgeable action.

Understanding the Nature of Suffering

Suffering, in most health literature, is connected with loss, pain, disfigurement, defeat, or harmful events (Daly, 1995). Philosopher Thich Nhat Hanh (1998) identifies suffering in such 'problems of the world like hunger, war, oppression, and social injustice' (p. 31). Hanh also connects suffering with lack of communication or using words that are untruthful or words of hatred or division. Perhaps the most important understanding of suffering is that suffering is unique to each person. Mitchell (1991) views suffering 'as a lived experience which is multidimensional and which can be understood only from the perspective of the individual living it' (p. 101). Newman (1994a) suggests that 'suffering offers us the opportunity to transcend a particular situation' (p. 142). She suggests, 'The need is to let go, embrace our experience, and allow the expansion of consciousness to unfold' (Newman, 1994a, p. 142). Parse (1996a) suggests concerning suffering that 'joy–sorrow is a paradoxical rhythm lived by all human beings' (p. 80). In a study on joy–sorrow, Parse (1997b) found that participants talked about adversities, but also there were 'always pleasures, either remembered or in the immediate moment' (p. 85).

The nurse scholar of the 21st century must attend carefully to others' suffering and be aware of the meaning of the joy–sorrow rhythm in people's lives. By bearing witness to suffering and being with others in moments of joy and moments of pain and sorrow, the nurse will discover new ways of providing comfort and quality of life.

Committing to Social Justice

The commitment to social justice runs throughout the history of knowledge development in nursing. Starting with Florence Nightingale, considered one of the leading reformers of the 19th century, this history includes Margaret Sanger, Lillian Wald, and Livina Dock (Chinn, 1991). Margaret Sanger developed knowledge of birth control and fought against great resistance to distribute birth control to women desperate for it. Her attempts to develop support for family planning remains with us today in the development of theoretical constructs informing women's health. Lillian Wald was concerned for the extremely poor immigrants crowded in housing in New York City. She developed the House on Henry Street from which emerged concepts of community health nursing. Livina

Dock, who was an active organizer in the House on Henry Street, worked for over 20 years to give women the right to vote (Chinn, 1991). Newman (1994b) suggests, 'It is necessary to connect all parts of the system, to integrate the similar and the dissimilar, unleashing the power of creativity' (p. 45). Such creative activity involves the human becoming concept of originating (Parse, 1998), which 'is inventing new ways of conforming—not conforming in the certainty–uncertainty of living' (p. 49).

The nurse scholar of the 21st century must be aware of the social and political forces of uncertainty influencing healthcare and quality of life. The nurse scholar must develop the ability to work with individuals, families, governmental systems and countries, not conforming to what has been but, instead, creating new ways for addressing human health challenges.

Believing in the Imagination as a Source of Knowledge

To imagine is to think of what can be. It is the process of imagining that generates new ideas and new ways of being in the world. Goleman, Kaufman, and Ray in *The Creative Spirit* (1992) suggest creativity is akin to leadership: 'A successful leader is someone who can persuade people to change their ideas or behavior. A successful creator is someone who gives other people a different way of looking at a world' (p. 26). These authors go on to suggest the art of creativity involves the capability to sift important information, selectively combine relevant information, and draw comparisons and analogies. 'The ability to see things in a fresh way is vital to the creative process, and that ability rests on the willingness to question any and all assumptions' (Goleman et al., 1992, p. 36). Parse (1998) suggests that through the process of imaging, reality is constructed: 'The human is a questioning being, however, and all that is imaged explicitly–tacitly is an answer to a question, and the questioning is a searching for certainty in knowing' (p. 36).

The nurse scholar of the 21st century must be prepared to question everything and use imaging as a means of addressing the known and the unknown, of creating what is yet to be. Daring to be different and inventing new ways of viewing the familiar holds the potential for transforming nursing knowledge.

Recognizing the Significance of Language in Structuring Meaning and Reality

Edward Murray in *Imaginative Thinking and Human Existence* (1986) writes, 'Without words, no thing may be; with words, much may be…. It will be remembered that language operates within the horizon sketched out or drawn by the human imagination' (p. 83). Human language exists both in speaking–being silent and moving–being still (Parse, 1995). Gemma Fiumara (1990) in *The Other Side of Language: A Philosophy of Listening* calls for a society that 'pays heed' to each other through active listening. Such listening Fiumara (1990) refers to as 'life-enhancing' (p. 17). Newman (1999) cites the importance of listening and silence in relating with the pattern of others: 'If we want to get in touch with this pattern, we need to listen to the silence, to listen with our hearts, as we attune ourselves to the rhythm of the other person' (p. 227). Parse (1998) suggests

Languaging is not just the content of what a person says with words, but how the whole message is uncovered in the context of the situation. It is the rhythmical moments of silence, the choice of words of syntax, the intonation, the facial expressions, the gestures, the posture, and that which is not said and movements that are not made that con-

stitute the symbolic expression characteristic of languaging as a concept of structuring meaning multidimensionally. (p. 40)

The nurse scholar of the 21st century must learn to use the languaging of speaking—being silent and moving—being still carefully and constructively. This scholar needs to develop the skill of listening multidemensionality to what is said and what is left unsaid in the human interconnectedness with others and the universe. The careful and deliberate use of language is vital in expanding understanding of human health experiences.

Understanding Health as a Process

Nursing and other disciplines have come to explore health as much more than the absence of disease. Ferguson (1980) describes health as an attitude that reflects accepting responsibility for self in developing purpose in life. Dossey (1982) describes health as a shared phenomenon created by the person with the environment. Newman (1994a) describes health as a process of expanding consciousness, which is the ability of the individual to interact with the environment. Parse defines health as a process of personal becoming; it is a living of value choices (Parse, 1990). These encompassing definitions of health as process reflect the complexity of human life and the opportunity nurses have to work with people in a variety of settings to address changing patterns of health.

The nurse scholar of the 21st century must understand health as the way one chooses to live and be attuned to the choices involved in living one's patterns of health. The nurse scholar will need to continue to seek ways of working with individuals and groups as they choose ways of living with complex health issues.

Understanding Community as a Process

Community is much more than a place. Community is a process of 'living in relationship' (Bunkers et al., 1999, p. 92). Such community interconnectedness involves the interrelationship of ideas, people, places, events, and personal histories (Parse, 1999a). Newman (1994a) suggests 'that the focus of our discipline is the unitary field that combines person–family–community all at once' (p. xix). Parse (1996a) posits that community, in its most abstract sense, is viewed as 'the universe, the galaxy of human connectedness' (p. 4). Parse (1999a) suggests that 'no engagement with another is without community. The individual is community, the family is community, the group is community, the world is community' (p. 120).

The nurse scholar of the 21st century must understand the connections–disconnections occurring in human relationships in community. For example, nursing practice must respond to 'the relational connection–disconnection issues of those underserved by health and human resources' (Bunkers et al., 1999, p. 93). The nurse scholar needs to be prepared to work with the complexity of community, knowing that it is not a place one goes to, but is a unitary process of relationship that one engages in.

Believing in the Power of Personal Presence

The power of the personal presence of the nurse is cornerstone for nursing practice in the 21st century. Philosopher Kabir Helminski (1992) writes

Presence signifies the quality of consciously being here. It is the activation of a higher level of awareness that allows all our other human functions—such as thought, feeling, and action—to be known, developed, and harmonized. Presence is the way in which we occupy

space, as well as how we flow and move. (p. viii)

Scholars of nursing have long written about and developed theoretical constructs concerning the importance of presence in nursing. Peplau (1952/1991) in her landmark book *The Nurse–Patient Relationship* detailed clearly for the first time the healing quality of the nurse's presence with those struggling with emotional issues. Watson (1997) writes about the 'transpersonal caring relationship' as core to nursing. Newman (1994a) identifies authentic presence as key in working with others and states,

The new paradigm of health, essential to nursing, embraces a unitary pattern of changing relationships. . . . The task is not to try to change another person's pattern but to recognize it as information that depicts the whole and relate to it as it unfolds. (p. 13)

Parse posits that the nurse–person process is the core of nursing and is lived in true presence. True presence is an intentional, reflective way of being with others in bearing witness to their changing health patterns. Parse (1997a) writes,

The nurse in true presence joins the reality of the person at all realms of the universe and is open to him or her without judging or labeling. The person at all realms of his or her universe experiences the intent of the nurse, which is to bear witness to changing health patterns. The intent of the nurse is languaged in his or her whole being, in all realms of the universe, so words are not necessary to live true presence in the nurse–person process. (p. 35)

These examples of the importance of the nurse's presence indicate that it is the quality of the relationship between the nurse and other, not the quantity nor the task conducted, that is of central importance. Quality of presence implies competence in the tasks/skills needed in the setting in which a nurse has selected to practice. However, even more than this, it implies competence in the nurse–person process. It is critical that the nurse scholar of the 21st century be exposed to beliefs and values that elevate the power of the nurse's personal presence.

Participating in Scientific Inquiry

Scientific inquiry in nursing is critical to the ongoing development of the discipline. Nurse scholar Judy Norris (1999) states, '*Inquiry* can be thought of as a transformative act accomplished by intentionally expending cognitive effort in activities such as discourse, reflection, reading, writing, or analysis' (p. 197). And, the goal of the discipline of nursing is 'to expand knowledge about human experiences through creative conceptualization and research' (Parse, 1999b, p. 275). It must also be remembered that the practice of science is both an individual and a social activity, for even great minds cannot work in isolation (Bronowski, 1978).

The nurse scholar of the 21st century must be mentored within a community of scholars. This community of scholars needs to focus on developing scientific inquiry that will continue to advance nursing science. The nurse scholar will need skills in creatively conceptualizing, dialoguing, utilizing research findings, and conducting either basic or applied research. The challenge of generating new knowledge for the discipline will be an ongoing one.

Asserting the Ethics of Individual and Communal Responsibility

The development of nursing knowledge and the role of the nurse scholar must be grounded in integrity and honesty. Bronowski (1978) points out,

> Knowledge cannot be gained unless you behave in certain ways. . . . Once you regard truth (truth in detail) as the cement of the scientific

community, then it follows at once that people have got to behave so that the truth shall be apparent. (pp. 129–130)

Bronowski (1978) goes on to identify personal values necessary for science to be carried out: individual values of sensitivity, tolerance, and respect, and the community values of honesty, integrity, dignity, and authenticity— 'which bind the scientific community together' (Bronowski, 1978, p. 132).

The nurse scholar of the 21st century must provide leadership in advancing the knowledge base of the discipline. Values reflecting individual and communal responsibility for knowledge development must be reflected in the education and practice of nurses. Fawcett (1999) suggests that it is the discipline of nursing's responsibility to see that 'nurse scholars will actively engage in integrated research-practice activities, using nursing methodologies to test and apply conceptual models of nursing and nursing theories in the provision of nursing services to people' (p. 313).

Emphasizing Living in the Present Moment

Philosopher Thich Nhat Hanh (1998) writes concerning life being available only in the present moment. He posits that living fully in the moment requires mindfulness:

> The Chinese character for mindfulness has two components: heart, or mind, and present moment. To be mindful means to be fully present in the moment—not one part of you washing the dishes while another part is wondering when the work will be finished. . . . Conscious breathing is the vehicle that brings us back to the present moment and keeps us here. . . . Mindfulness leads to concentration and wisdom. . . . Mindfulness makes life real, deep, and worth living. It helps us be in the here and now where true life

can be encountered. It helps us get in touch with refreshing and healing elements within and around us. (pp. 37–38)

The nurse scholar of the 21st century will need to understand the power of attending to what is happening here and now. Focusing on the now bids us to not hold on to what was or try to force what will be. Newman (1994a, p. 68) suggests, 'There is not basis for rejecting any experience as irrelevant. The important factor is to be fully present in the moment.' Parse (1998) writes about focusing on the moment in true presence as 'a special way of 'being with' in which the nurse is attentive to moment-to-moment changes in meaning as she or he bears witness to the person's or group's own living of value priorities' (p. 71). The nurse scholar must be prepared to practice a mindfulness that cultivates sensitive encounters with others in the present moment and cultivates the development of wisdom.

Respecting Life and Nature

The unitary interconnectedness of all that is summons nursing to be concerned with and attend to the health of the universe. Sylvia Earle in the book *Sea Change: A Message of the Oceans* (1995) conveys an urgent call to action to do something about the damage being done to our global environment and the universe. Earle writes passionately about her concern for oceanic life:

> There's plenty of water in the universe without life, but nowhere is there life without water. . . . The living ocean provides the cornerstone of the life-support system for all creatures on our planet, from deep-sea starfish to desert sagebrush. That's why the ocean matters. If the sea is sick, we'll feel it. If it dies, we die. Our future and the state of the oceans are one. (p. xii)

The nurse scholar of the 21st century must be concerned with the treatment and care of nature.

This scholar must study the interrelationship of life on this planet with the universe. Parse (1998) posits that the human–universe–health process is a mutual process and that 'quality of life is the meaning one gives to one's life at the moment in cocreation with the universe' (Parse, 1994b, p. 18). Respect for life and nature must coexist with respect for the advances of modern science and civilization.

Acknowledging Mystery

It is important for nurse scholars of the 21st century to know that there is much we do not know or understand. 'Acknowledging mystery involves recognizing that there is a power greater than ourselves present in the universe' (Bunkers, 1999a, p. 29). Nursing in the 21st century must work with the mystery of not knowing and acknowledge 'that not knowing is simply the first step toward truth' (Palmer, 1993, p. 72). Parse (1998) suggests that fundamental to understanding humans is 'the notion of the human as mystery—an appreciation of the unexplainable in human becoming' (p. 43). Acknowledging mystery and the unexplainable provides the nurse scholar of the 21st century with the foundation for developing questions for advancing nursing science.

Focusing on Quality of Life

The meaning individuals give experiences constitutes their quality of life (Parse, 1994a). Frankl (1984) suggests that meaning 'boils down to becoming aware of a possibility against the background of reality or . . . to becoming aware of *what can be done* about a given situation' (p. 145). Gioiella (1994) writes about quality of life from an international perspective. She suggests quality of life is seen as a universal human goal: 'Nursing has a commitment internationally to work to achieve this goal' (p. 1). Theory development in nursing demonstrates various definitions of quality of life. Peplau (1994) suggests, 'Human relationships are a major determinant of quality of life' (p. 10). Leininger (1994) suggests that quality of life 'is culturally constituted and patterned' (p. 22). Parse (1994a) posits that quality of life 'is what the person *there* living the lie says that it is' (p. 17); 'the unitary perspective is essential to capture the meaning of quality of life now and in the next millennium' (p. 20).

The nurse scholar of the 21st century must be prepared to understand the meanings persons give to life experience, thus being in concert with their quality of life issues. As Florence Nightingale addressed the challenges to quality of life posed to her by the meanings she gave experiences in the Crimean War, so too will the nurse scholar of the 21st century be challenged to respond to quality of life issues for the betterment of humankind.

Conclusion

The development of the nurse as scholar is a journey, a journey that began over a century ago. Parse (1994b) identifies three crucial processes involved in scholarship: 'perpetual curiosity, a focused commitment, and a willingness to risk challenge' (p. 143). On this journey of scholarship, perpetual curiosity must be fostered in those who will question and who wish to discover the new. A focused commitment must be modeled by mentors of the discipline and lived in their day-to-day practice of both the art and science of nursing. A willingness to risk challenge calls for courage to push forward with nursing theory and model development in expanding nursing science. Are we, the nursing community of today ready for this challenge of scholarship? Florence Nightingale (1859) wrote in Notes on Nursing, 'For it may safely be said, not that the habit of ready and correct observation will by itself make us useful nurses, but that without it we shall be useless with all our

devotion' (p. 63). A habit of ready and correct observation, a habit of continual scholarship, is the call for nursing in the 21st century.

References

Bronowski, J. (1978). *The origins of knowledge and imagination*. London: Yale University Press.

Bunkers, S. S. (1998). Considering tomorrow: Parse's theory-guided research. *Nursing Science Quarterly, 11*, 56–63.

Bunkers, S. S. (1999a). Emerging discoveries and possibilities in nursing. *Nursing Science Quarterly, 12*, 26–29.

Bunkers, S. S. (1999b). The teaching-learning process and the theory of human becoming. *Nursing Science Quarterly, 12*, 227–232.

Bunkers, S. S., Nelson, M., Leuning, C., Crane, J., & Josephson, D. (1999). In E. Cohen & V. De Back (Eds.), *The outcomes mandate: Case management in health care today* (pp. 92–100). St. Louis: Mosby.

Bunkers, S. S., & Putnam, V. (1995). A nursing based model of health ministry: Living Parse's theory of human becoming in parish nursing. In *Ninth Annual Westberg Parish Nurse Symposium: Parish nursing: Ministering through the arts* (pp. 197–212). Northbrook, IL: Advocate Health Care.

Chinn, P. (1991). *Theory and nursing: A systemic approach*. St. Louis: Mosby.

Daly, J. (1995). The view of suffering within the human becoming theory. In R. R. Parse (Ed.), *Illuminations: The human becoming theory in practice and research* (pp. 45–59). New York: National League for Nursing Press.

Damgaard, G., & Bunkers, S. S. (1998). Nursing science-guided practice and education: A state board of nursing perspective. *Nursing Science Quarterly, 11*, 142–144.

Dossey, L. (1982). *Space, time and medicine*. Boulder, CO: Shambhala.

Earle, S. (1995). *Sea change: A message of the oceans*. New York: Fawcett Columbine.

Fawcett, J. (1999). The state of nursing science: Hallmarks of the 20th and 21st centuries. *Nursing Science Quarterly, 12*, 311–315.

Ferguson, M. (1980). *The Aquarian conspiracy: Personal and social transformation in the 1980s*. Los Angeles: J. P. Tarcher.

Fiumara, G. C. (1990). *The other side of language: A philosophy of listening*. New York: Routledge.

Frankl, V. (1984). *Man's search for meaning*. New York: Simon & Schuster.

Gioiella, E. C. (1994). Quality of life: An international commitment. *Nursing Science Quarterly, 7*, 1.

Goleman, D., Kaufman, P., & Ray, M. (1992). *The creative spirit*. New York: Dutton.

Hanh, T. N. (1998). *Interbeing*. Berkeley, CA: Parallax Press.

Helminski, K. E. (1992). *Living presence*. New York: Putnam.

Leininger, M. (1994). Quality of life from a transcultural nursing perspective. *Nursing Science Quarterly, 7*, 22–28.

Mitchell, G. (1991). Nursing diagnosis: An ethical analysis. *Image: Journal of Nursing Scholarship, 23*, 99–103.

Murray, E. (1986). *Imaginative thinking and human existence*. Pittsburgh: Duquesne University Press.

Newman, M. (1994a). *Health as expanding consciousness* (2nd ed.). New York: National League for Nursing Press.

Newman, M. (1994b). Into the 21st century. *Nursing Science Quarterly, 7*, 44–46.

Newman, M. (1999). The rhythm of relating in a paradigm of wholeness. *Image: Journal of Nursing Scholarship, 31*(3), 227–229.

Nightingale, F. (1859). *Notes on nursing*. London: Harrison.

Norris, J. R. (1999). The Internet: Extending our capacity for scholarly inquiry in nursing. *Nursing Science Quarterly, 12*, 197–201.

Palmer, P. (1993). *To know as we are known*. San Francisco: Harper-Collins.

Parse, R. R. (1990). Health: A personal commitment. *Nursing Science Quarterly, 3*, 136–140.

Parse, R. R. (1994a). Quality of life: Sciencing and living the art of human becoming. *Nursing Science Quarterly, 10*, 16–21.

Parse, R. R. (1994b). Scholarship: Three essential processes. *Nursing Science Quarterly, 7*, 143.

Parse, R. R. (1995). Building the realm of nursing knowledge. *Nursing Science Quarterly, 8*, 51.

Parse, R. R. (1996a). Community: A human becoming perspective. *Illuminations: The Newsletter of the International Consortium of Parse Scholars, 5*(1), 1–4.

Parse, R. R. (1996b). The human becoming theory: Challenges in practice and research. *Nursing Science Quarterly, 9*, 55–60.

Parse, R. R. (1997a). The human becoming theory: The was, is, and will be. *Nursing Science Quarterly, 10*, 32–38.

Parse, R. R. (1997b). Joy-sorrow: A study using the Parse research method. *Nursing Science Quarterly, 10*, 80–87.

Parse, R. R. (1998). *The human becoming school of thought*. Thousand Oaks, CA: Sage.

Parse, R. R. (1999a). Community: An alternative view. *Nursing Science Quarterly, 12*, 119–121.

Parse, R. R. (1999b). Nursing: The discipline and the profession. *Nursing Science Quarterly, 12*, 275–276.

Peplau, H. E. (1991). *Interpersonal relations in nursing*. New York: Springer Publishing Company. (Original work published 1952).

Peplau, H. E. (1994). Quality of life: An interpersonal perspective. *Nursing Science Quarterly, 7*, 10–15.

Rawnsley, M. (1999). Response to Fawcett's 'The state of nursing science.' *Nursing Science Quarterly, 12*, 315–318.

Rogers, M. (1992). Nightingale's notes on nursing: Prelude to the 21st century. In D. Carroll (Ed.), *Notes on Nursing by Florence Nightingale* (Commemorative edition) (pp. 58–62). Philadelphia: J. B. Lippincott Company.

Roy, C. (1992). Vigor, variables, and vision: Commentary of Florence Nightingale. In D. Carroll (Ed.), *Notes on Nursing by Florence Nightingale* (Commemorative edition) (pp. 63–71). Philadelphia: J. B. Lippincott Company.

Sartre, J. P. (1956). *Being and nothingness*. New York: Philosophical Library, Inc.

Schuyler, C. (1992). Florence Nightingale. In D. Carroll (Ed.), *Notes on Nursing by Florence Nightingale* (Commemorative edition) (pp. 3–17). Philadelphia: J. B. Lippincott Company.

Watson, J. (1997) The theory of human caring: Retrospective and prospective. *Nursing Science Quarterly, 10*, 49–52.

Webster's ninth new collegiate dictionary. (1990). Springfield, MA: Merriam-Webster.

Chapter 10

Professionalism and the Evolution of Nursing as a Discipline: A Feminist Perspective

Judith Wuest,
RN, MN

The evolution of nursing knowledge and nursing as a practice discipline has been stunted by the quest for professionalism. Liberal and socialist feminist theory clarifies the hazards inherent in the masculine institution of professionalism for a predominately female discipline. Socialist feminist theoretical perspectives facilitate a vision of nursing that includes altering social structure such that caring is valued.

The development of nursing as a discipline has been dominated by the hegemony of the patriarchal institutions of professionalism. Feminism can broadly be defined as seeking to end the domination of women (Jaggar, 1983). Nursing, historically a women's occupation, has been a vehicle of both liberation and oppression. The lens of liberal and socialist feminist theory provides a perspective for examining the evolution of nursing as a discipline. Professionalism has played a key role in marginalizing nursing and in constraining knowledge development. Feminism with its emphasis on praxis illuminates possible future directions in knowledge development for nursing as a practice discipline.

Source: Wuest, J. (1994). Professionalism and the evolution of nursing as a discipline: A feminist perspective. *Journal of Professional Nursing, 10*(6): 357–367. Reprinted with permission from W.B. Saunders. Copyright © 1994.

Feminist Theoretical Perspectives

Feminist theories have defined the causes of women's oppression and offer a means for eliminating it (MacPherson, 1991). Alison Jaggar (1983) clearly distinguished between liberal and socialist feminism.

Liberal Feminist Theory

"Liberal feminism rests on a conception of human nature that is radically individualistic" (Jaggar, 1983, p. 355). Impartiality is a key tenet of liberal feminism. Thus, all individuals should be treated equally, and women should receive no special privileges. The focus of liberal feminism is on eliminating oppression by seeking equal opportunity for women, not on determining the factors that lead to women's oppression (MacPherson, 1991). The major approach to knowledge development is logical positivism, a legacy of Cartesian dualism. Adequacy of scientific theory is based on objectivity, scientific method, and value-free criterion. Within the liberal tradition, judgments must be impartial to the perspective of a particular group or individual.

Socialist Feminist Theory

Socialist feminism adopts the Marxist view that individual existence requires interaction with other humans and the nonhuman world. Knowledge development occurs in the process of human activity that is influenced by society. Knowledge is not value free and is always shaped by the perspective of the class from which the knowledge emerges. In contrast to the Marxist view that the perspective of the working class is most adequate, socialist feminism asserts that the standpoint of women is most valid because women's social position gives them access to a reality not accessible to men and because women have no vested interest in maintaining the status quo of a patriarchal society. Although this is a similar position to that of radical feminists, the difference lies in how the knowledge is acquired. Socialist feminists do not accept that the standpoint of women is expressed in "women's naive and unreflective worldview" (Jaggar, 1983, p. 371) because this is distorted by male-dominated structure and ideology. Instead, women's standpoint is continually evolving through scientific and political struggle. Jaggar acknowledged that individual women's standpoints may differ especially by race and class but suggested that this diversity contributes to a representation of reality that is continuously unfolding. Women's standpoint evolves in a matrix operation in which women's distinctive social experience guides the pattern of research in a particular discipline and the outcomes of the research are then

tested within the social reality of women. Knowledge is deemed useful if it helps to reconstruct a world in which women's interests are not subordinate to those of men.

Feminism, Professionalism, and Nursing

Until recently, nursing links with feminism have been tenuous. A brief historical look at both the women's movement and the growth of professionalism in North America will shed light on the development of the discipline of nursing. From a socialist feminist perspective, examining historical context is essential; however, this examination reveals that any links between nursing and feminism have largely been in the liberal feminist tradition of seeking equality.

Early Women's Movement

Cott (1987) identified three foci in the women's movement of the 19th century: service and social action performed by charitable, altruistic women who felt their gender gave them a special mandate and who found new strength in their collectivity and self-assertion; women's rights action performed by individually motivated women who wanted "rights equivalent to those men enjoyed on legal, political, economic, and civic grounds" (p. 16); and action for self-determination through "emancipation from structures, conventions and attitudes enforced by law and custom" (p. 16). Regardless of specific beliefs, "the spectrum of ideology in the women's movement had a see-saw quality" (Cott, 1987, p. 19). At one end were elimination of limitations and the attainment of equal rights, a liberalist perspective. At the other was the desire to value the unique qualities and abilities that women had to offer society. This valuing resulted either in acceptance of the unique but subservient status of women's existing social order or in adoption of a socialist feminist approach to change the existing social order to one that valued women in different ways. "No collective resolution of these tensions occurred and seldom even did individuals resolve them in their own minds" (Cott, 1987, p. 20).

Nursing's Early Development in North America

The three positions of maintaining the status quo, seeking equality, and seeking to change the social order can be seen in nursing's development. "Nursing's identity has been inextricably bound to the very word and notion of nurturance as well as to the myth that women exist to be mothers" (Church, 1990, p. 7). Initially, nursing was simply one of the many domestic roles that women were expected to fulfill on the basis of love and obligation (Reverby, 1987). "To practice it [nursing] at home was to fulfill the true calling of womanhood" (O'Brien, 1986, p. 14). By the mid 1800s in North America, despite the desire of middle class women to be ladies, many found themselves economically in need of work. The affluent could afford to hire others to take on many of their domestic responsibilities. Hence, the emergence of the professed nurse.

They brought to the bedside only the authority their personalities and community stature could command. Neither credentials nor a professional identity gave weight to their efforts. Their womanhood and the experience it gave them, defined their authority and taught them to nurse (Reverby, 1987, p. 6).

In contrast to factory work, "the nature of nursing with its roots deep in the domestic world of the family, muted the dramatic shift in self-perception that women in factory work experienced" (O'Brien, 1986, p. 13).

Reverby (1987) noted that within the hospital setting, working class women attempted to exert control on working conditions and relationships with physicians, despite their lack of formal training and subservient class position.

The sense of rights of working class womanhood gave them authority to press their demands. The necessity to care and their perception of its importance to patient outcome also structured their belief that demanding the right to be relatively autonomous was possible (Reverby, 1987, pp. 6–7).

Nevertheless, these women were unsuccessful largely because of class differences between nurses and hospital administrators, paternalism, and very demanding work.

Few nurses at this time were engaged in trying to change the social order. Lavinia Dock was a pioneer in nursing history who was labeled a suffragist, a pacifist, and a Marxist. Her overriding concern was self-determination for women, nurses, and nursing (Church, 1990). Throughout her life, she challenged nurses to fight against male dominance but was considered by the majority of nurses as deviant. Dock urged nursing leaders to involve public and political activism (Ashley, 1976). A more widely known nurse feminist was Margaret Sanger, birth control agitator, who championed women's rights to control their sexuality regardless of church or state (Cott, 1987). These nurses made a significant contribution to the development of nursing but were representative of a minority view within nursing.

During this time period, Nightingale's philosophy of nursing education, legitimated by her successes in the Crimea, was developing a following in North America. Her intentions were to establish autonomous schools of nursing, under the control of nurses who would ultimately share power with physicians in the health care setting. Although this approach was admirable from the liberalist feminist perspective, her intended hierarchy within the nursing school eliminated the possibility of equality among nurses (Reverby, 1987). Nightingale's vision was distorted in its implementation by the physicians and hospital superintendents in North America who viewed schools of nursing as vehicles for obtaining cheap labor. They supported the establishment of apprenticeship schools and in doing so gained control over nurse's labor (Melosh, 1982). Nightingale indicated that nurses were prepared by developing womanly virtue. Thus, she legitimized paid work by embodying in it 19th century social values and needs (O'Brien, 1986). From a socialist feminist perspective, nursing is an example of household work shifted to the outside world of production. Because this work was not valued when it took place within the home, it similarly received little economic or status reward when practiced publicly (Miller, 1991). Coburn (1987) noted that despite the desire of upper-class Nightingale nurses to attract refined women to nursing, the difficult working conditions and unpleasant work deterred many. The majority of recruits were working-class women whose only other option was factory work.

> *The school's emphasis on high moral character constituted an imposition of upper-class values on working-class women. The socialization process during training rested largely in the hands of middle- and upper-class nursing educators— women whose financial and social position allowed them to receive the necessary qualifications to teach (Coburn, 1987, p. 447).*

This was the beginning of a class system within nursing: the elite educators and administrators versus the bedside practicing nurses. From a socialist feminist perspective, many of the decisions made from this point forward ensured the continuation of this division.

Ashley (1976) suggested that the apprenticeship system of nursing educations entrenched the dominations of nurses by physicians and hospital administrators.

> *Convinced of their inferiority and of the need for their subordination to the medical profession, many nurses identified with the system that oppressed them and worked to support its continuing existence. Nurses learned to believe in the virtues of hospital training. Early conditioning within these institutions intensified the capacity of women to aid the cause of their oppressors (Ashley, 1976, p. 32).*

Nursing training was rigid, orderly, and disciplined and students were overworked. Nevertheless, standards of care were established, nurses developed pride in their skills, had their idealism nurtured, and felt empowered to care (Reverby, 1987).

> *. . . nurses have emphasized perceived womanly qualities and differences from men by stressing a role complementary to that performed by men. This position, often labelled anti-feminist, has led present-day feminists to disregard nursing because it tends to epitomize a set of characteristics and problems from which women are attempting to distance themselves. (Kirkwood, 1991, p. 53)*

In this sense, nursing embodies the dilemma of early (and present day) feminists who, by seeking equality, deny the very uniqueness of their contribution to society, but nursing was being controlled by forces beyond simply their desire to care.

> *. . . caring was shaped not simply by women's psychological identity but by the social and political context in which nursing developed. It was a duty to care directed by a male medical hierarchy, not an ethic of care in which nurses would be able to make more autonomous judgments about the kind of care patients should receive. (Baines, 1991, p. 63)*

Nurses and Physicians

At the turn of the century, the medical profession was not well established in North America and was open to competition from nurses, pharmacists, and other allied occupations (Torrance, 1987). Medical students had no internship and nursing students in training schools had greater opportunity to observe and to care for the sick. Although the training system had established physicians as dominant, their position was not secure. In 1904 through 1905, Abraham Flexner, a sociologist, visited and assessed Canadian and American medical schools. His report, published in 1910, was highly critical of schools that lacked the facilities to teach laboratory-based scientific medicine and resulted in the closure or reorganization of 92 medical schools. "The Flexner Report . . . helped to consolidate the dominance of the allophatic practitioners and to establish laboratory-based scientific medical education and practice. This mechanistic-individualistic conception is currently pervasive in medical practice and research" (Bolaria, 1988, p. 3). The alliance of medicine with science and the subsequent entrenchment of medical education in the university resulted in the definition and domination of the health care field by the physicians. Flexner's study led also to a definition of "profession" and that had significant implications for the future of nursing.

Professionalism

In 1915, Flexner presented a paper that identified the criteria for characterizing professions from an analysis of the universally acknowledged professions of law, medicine, and clergy (Parsons, 1986).

> *Professions involve essentially intellectual operations; they derive their raw materials from science and learning; this material they work up into a practical and definite end; they possess an educationally communicable technique; they tend to self-organization; they are becoming increasingly altruistic in motivation (Flexner, 1915, p. 904).*

This definition stressed rationalism, scientific standards, and objectivity, all characteristics that embodied the masculine ethos. His masculine, sociological view was never questioned and the criteria became the sociological standard for distinguishing professions (Parsons, 1986). Professions were dominated by men and "a culture developed that affirmed male-centered values of order, efficiency, and hierarchical division of labour" (Baines, 1991). Flexner's paper also suggested that occupations could alter their status and become professions by developing the traits that were lacking.

Professions, reinforced by their scientific credibility, became sources of power and prestige. Professionalization offered white, middle-class men a means of carving out new roles and obtaining monopoly on their services (Baines, 1991). Women who entered women-dominated professions were more motivated by an ethic of service or care than by a desire for power (Baines, 1991). "The bases for women's special expertise and place within the professions continued to rest on an ideology of service that lionized caring as a virtue particular to women" (Baines, p. 55). The norm of professionalism is historically and socially unacceptable to women because of their exclusion from its conception (Parsons, 1986). Cott (1987) noted that although women professionals were seen as leaders before obtaining the vote, once the vote was attained, the bond that held them together was gone. A barrier developed between women professionals and nonprofessionals. To progress within the professions, and hold the tenets of nonbias, objectivity, and impersonality, women were required to abandon allegiance to feminism and create a community of interest with professional men rather than nonprofessional women (Cott, 1987). Glazer and Slater (1987) noted that professionals scorned nurturant, expressive, and familial interaction, valuing expertise and monopoly over an ethic of service.

Nursing and Professionalism

"Prior to Flexner, American nurses . . . were secure in their identity as professionals" (Parsons, 1986, p. 273). However, nursing did not measure up to Flexner's criteria. By 1936, there were articles in nursing journals that indicated nursing was a developing profession (Parsons, 1986). Nursing had a limited body of scientific knowledge defined as nursing and exclusive of other disciplines. Because the phenomena unique to nursing had not been articulated and studied, nursing lacked control over practice and was subordinate to the medical profession (Lyon, 1990). Varying levels of educational preparation resulted in the absence of pervasive ideology and monopoly over work. Roberts (1984) asserted that nurses, once autonomous, became oppressed through societal forces and now exhibit the characteristics of an oppressed group. "Nurses have also accepted the fact that if they could only attain the characteristics of the powerful, or professional status, they too would be powerful" (Roberts, 1984, p. 26).

In the early 20th century, women who wanted recognition for nurses as significant health care providers readily accepted Flexner's assertion that an occupation could become a profession. Acceptance of professional ideology can be viewed as a strength from a liberal feminist perspective. It pushed nurses to sever the link with domestic labor and establish standards of paid work, to refuse the limitations of gender in their own lives and in goals for nursing profession, and to challenge the traditional constraints on women in the workforce (Melosh, 1982). Because nursing was a women's profession, women had the potential monopoly and power to effect change. What nurses and other women striving for more traditional professions failed to recognize was that the criteria that they were trying to meet were established by men. The rightness of these criteria was not questioned. In fact, by accepting these criteria, and striving to meet them, nursing was supporting the existing patriarchal order. This decision resulted in securing privileges for few nurses at the expense of many (Melosh, 1982).

Knowledge Development

Professionalism and Knowledge Development

When nursing leaders decided to respond to the Flexner report by seeking to meet his criteria of profession, they recognized that nursing had to establish a scientific knowledge base. Because professionals had to be scientific, and the only academic preparation for nurses at that time was at the Columbia Teacher's College, most study and research related to education and administration and not to clinical practice (Baer, 1987). Thus, academically prepared nurses were further divided from those practicing at the bedside, and there was much debate about whose work was the most meaningful. This divisiveness is characteristic of the horizontal violence of oppressed groups. Roberts (1984) noted that whether nurses were in the hospital or the academic setting they were (and are) rewarded for being marginal and taking on the characteristics of the dominant groups. As nursing programs opened up in universities in Canada and the United States, nurses struggled to have their knowledge and experience validated as scholarship. "A knowledge base for nursing stemming from women's private, domestic sphere was suspect within the male-dominated culture of the university, which took pride in intellectual scientific achievements" (Kirkwood, 1991, p. 54).

World War II opened opportunities for nurses to expand their practice roles and to have advanced university study in post-war years; however, Baer (1987) noted that all nurses were not enthusiastic about these openings. Nurses seeking professionalization were anxious to upgrade their educational preparation, but this was very threatening to nurses who had trained under the hospital system. Hospital educators, anxious to support apprenticeship, failed to grasp post-war opportunities for upgrading. This further developed the class system in nursing.

Research became an issue for nurses as they attempted to establish a scientific knowledge base. Nurses ignored gender issues and moved away from its domestic heritage. "Nurses believed that, if they met university demands to demonstrate nursing was a scholarly discipline with a unique scientific base, nurses would be accorded the same professional respect as others in the university" (Kirkwood, 1991, p. 61). Hughes (1990, p. 31) noted that the development of nursing as a discipline is often equated with its evolution as a profession, but history "suggests that professional status is not likely to evolve passively from nursing's recognition as a scholarly discipline." However, it is significant that "by successfully developing and maintaining university nursing education, nurses have to some extent undermined the patriarchal structure of the university by locating work, traditionally assigned to women in the public sphere of higher education dominated by men" (Kirkwood, 1991, p. 62).

In November 1951, the *American Journal of Nursing* announced the publication of *Nursing Research*, noting that research was essential for knowledge development in nursing (Baer, 1987). It was 1976 before over half the articles published focused on clinical practice rather than education because most of the researchers were nursing faculty whose higher education had been in education. Whereas their institutions required that they participate in scholarly activity to meet criteria for tenure and promotion, service agencies and hospitals did not encourage such activity from practicing nurses (Baer, 1987). Hence, the gap widened with

practitioners viewing educators as more and more removed from the real world of nursing.

Nursing's major goal in fostering research was to achieve recognition of its professional status. Some individual nurses certainly saw research as a means, a method through which they could answer questions and expand their ideas, but for most nurses, it was an end, a criterion of professionalism they yearned to attain (Baer, 1987, p. 24).

Research and Theory Development

Early approaches to research followed the reductionistic methods of the biomedical model as the surest way to be credible as scientists (Nagle & Mitchell, 1991). Nursing adopted the empirical ethic of science through a research tradition "that concentrates on objectivity, facts, measurement of smaller and smaller parts, and issues of instrumentality, reliability, validity, and operationalization to the point that nursing is in danger of exhausting the meaning, relevance, and understanding of the values, goals, and actions that it espouses in its heritage and ideals" (Watson, 1988, p. 17). Researchers have only recently begun to recognize that the scientific method is insufficient for addressing many of nursing's concerns and are beginning to embrace more diverse, qualitative approaches to research.

Concern for nursing's lack of theory base developed in the 1960s when nurses began to study at a doctoral level in other disciplines. The embryonic nursing science was attached to other sciences and fed on their theories, methods, and instruments (Stainton, 1982). Much debate developed surrounding such issues as whether nursing theory should be borrowed from other disciplines, single versus multiple theories, and whether theories should influence or be influenced by practice.

At early nursing theory conferences, the views of theory development expressed by such leaders as Dickoff and James and Abdellah supported the logical empiricist tradition for the development of nursing science (Silva & Rothbart, 1983). "Early nurse theorists such as Roy and Orem maintained the status quo of objective reductionism by focusing on problems and defining health according to medical and/or societal norms" (Nagle & Mitchell, 1991, p. 18). Although nurses were strongly supporting this approach, the philosophers of science from where this tradition stemmed were seriously questioning the limitations of this approach (Silva & Rothbart, 1983; Webster & Jacox, 1985). Nurse researchers and theorists recognized the limitations of the received view in theorizing about people's experiences with health and illness; however, the drive for professionalism and scientific legitimacy resulted in nursing, as an emerging discipline, holding on to this respectable approach.

In the 1960s, the unity and political and academic power of the received view theorists were sufficiently great that lip service had to be paid to their basic beliefs. Now we are free to choose among the insights of the received view and select only those that we find useful and sound for our purposes in constructing nursing theory (Webster & Jacox, 1985, p. 27).

These authors suggest that nursing is free to develop its own philosophy of science. Evidence of changing views about the philosophy of science is in the works of such theorists as Watson (1988) and Parse (1981).

Theory and Nursing Practice

Theory is argued to be important in the establishment of the unique body of knowledge essential for nursing to be recognized as a profession and as a means of fostering communication and improving patient care. Theory development

through creative conceptualization expanded nursing knowledge. However, the language of theory is frequently abstract and there is much discussion among theorists and those attempting to understand and apply nursing theories to practice. "There are serious credibility gaps between the ideal prescriptive theory that is taught and the practical knowledge used by practitioners" (Aydelotte, 1990, p. 10).

Resultant debates have tended to develop into a vicious circle, with theorists berating practitioners for their lack of concern with the conceptual basis for their actions, whilst practitioners bemoan theoretical approaches which are seen as having little or no relevance to their daily work (Nolan & Grant, 1992).

Fawcett (1992) asserted the existence of a reciprocal relationship between conceptual models and nursing practice, but she was adamant that the models come first and are tested for their credibility and refined in the field of clinical practice. This position fails to consider the fact that many practitioners find the conceptual model too obscure to enter into that reciprocity.

Nagle and Mitchell (1991) noted that nursing is being driven by professional licensing bodies and accreditation bodies to adopt a single theory as a base for practice within their agency. They suggested that this is a paternalistic action that denies nurses the autonomy of choosing their own theoretic base for practice consistent with their unique worldview. This suggestion assumes that most practicing nurses have articulated a worldview and is further evidence of the rift between practitioners and those nurses with advanced education. This imposition may give practicing nurses a means for voicing what they do and do not like about practicing within a specific, theoretical framework. This may be the key to Fawcett's reciprocity.

Feminism: Looking to the Future for Nursing

The acceptance of patriarchal professionalism has resulted in nursing adopting liberalist traditions for the development of research and practice. "Feminism, in its liberal form, appears to give nursing a political language that argues for equality and rights within the given order of things" (Reverby, 1987, p. 10). Nurses have often been criticized for rejecting liberal feminism.

> *From a feminist perspective, the individualism and autonomy promised by this rights framework often fails to acknowledge collective social need, to provide a way for adjudicating conflict over rights, or to address the reasons for the devaluing of female activity (MacPherson, 1991, p. 30).*

Reverby (1987) suggested that nursing will have to create the social climate that values caring. This implies the need for a socialist feminist approach in which nursing takes a more active role in altering social structure.

Professionalization has objectified those for whom nurses care. "A feminist ethos of professionalism needs to be based on an ideology that integrates an ethic of care and forms a more equal partnership with the cared for" (Baines, 1991, p. 67). Feminism offers some revolutionary ideas for nursing (Chinn, 1987). "Feminism values and endorses women, critiques male thinking, challenges patriarchal systems, and focuses on creating self-love and respect for all others and all forms of life" (Chinn, 1987, p. 23).

Knowledge Development

Dorothy Smith (1990) addressed the impact that hegemony has on knowledge development by influencing the issues that are valued and by dictating an approach to those issues based on the conceptual view of those institutions rather than the lived experienced of the people involved. As people are educated to take up roles within institutions, they are exposed to a "conceptual imperialism" (Smith, 1990, p. 15) that ensures a perpetuation of the worldview of the institution under the guise of objectivity. People have two ways of knowing, experiencing and doing: one on a local, immediate, bodily level, and one that is at an objective, conceptual level. The objective account, giving the appearance of neutrality and impartiality, in fact conceals class, gender, and race and puts forward the ideology of the governing groups. The objectified text has power because of the way it organizes social relations. People read the objectified text as fact and repress their own lived experience. Thus, people begin to see things the same way. "Objectified knowledge, as we engage with it, subdues, discounts, and disqualifies our various interests, perspectives, angles, and experience, and what we might have to say speaking from them" (Smith, 1990, p. 80).

Smith's account sheds some light on the current division that exists between nursing theory and practice. Nursing theory has been developed by the elite and educated, the nurses who have wielded power in the development of nursing as a profession. The separation of these nurses from those at the bedside has been well documented. These nurses identified a professional route for the development of nursing knowledge and endorsed the patriarchal structure. Hence, the approaches to nursing theory reflect the dominant culture rather than the lived experience of nurses at the bedside.

Smith (1990) argued that women must create a reflexive critique through investigation that is grounded in the lives of women and people. This requires an exploration of women's everyday experience with socially organized practices and an examination of how women's practices contribute to and are articulated with the relations that rule our lives. This emphasis on praxis is most consistent for the development of nursing knowledge that reflects the human experience of nursing. However, a major barrier exists. Many nurses who wield educational and administrative power within nursing have a vested interest in maintaining their current positions of power and this is readily accomplished through Smith's "conceptual imperialism." For a significant change to occur nurse leaders and educators must be conscious of this oppression.

There is evidence that nursing is beginning to consider some more revolutionary approaches to knowledge development. Critical scholarship, a pattern of thought and action that challenges institutionalized power relations in the social reality of nursing has been suggested by Thompson (1987) as one means of addressing the issues that nursing faces. She urged nurses to question the assumption that underlie our liberal undergraduate education such as the logical positivist approach to science, the functionalist framework of the social world, and professional ideology because these assumptions foster acceptance of the status quo. "Critical scholarship in nursing can speak about the process of reweaving, regaining confidence in new reality, regaining a commitment to new definitions of nursing practice, and feeling grounded in new value orientations" (Thompson, 1987, p. 37). Anderson (1991, p. 2) noted that feminism and poststructuralist perspectives

> challenge us to extend our analysis of phenomena relating to the lives of clients or patients beyond the micro level of analysis to an examination of the broader social processes that influence health and illness behaviour. This has the potential for the development of nursing science that will be inclusive of the complex socioeconomic, historical, and political nexus in which human experience is embedded.

Silva and Rothbart (1983), drawing on the work of Laudan, suggested that nursing theory development is currently in a state of transition, that it will never result in a static set of truths but will always be evolving.

> Data for nursing theory development and testing will include the common practices of nurse clinicians, the social and psychological factors affecting the profession of nursing, the widely held beliefs of the community of nurses, and the reasoning patterns of individual nurse theorists. A result of integrating these data will be a nursing theory that more explicitly addresses the human dimension of nursing (Silva & Rothbart, 1983, p. 11).

The test for adequacy of theory will be more focused on solution of nursing care problems than on truth and error. This is very consistent with socialist feminist theory for which the criteria of adequacy is usefulness. These approaches hold promise for future development of nursing research and theory development.

Feminist Epistemology and Research Methodology

Jaggar and Bordo (1989, p. 4) indicated that feminist epistemology shares the critique of many philosophers that "the Cartesian framework is fundamentally inadequate, an obsolete and self-deluded world view badly in need of reconstruction and revisioning" borrowing from other traditions such as Marxist historicism, psychoanalytic theory, literary theory, and sociology of knowledge to support its claim. Contemporary feminism's arguments differ from others in the assertion that the Cartesian framework is not gender neutral. Feminist epistemology is not about women being able to conduct science in its current form as well as men can. "Rather its position is that women who have come to recognize and accept feminist assumptions about the world will practice science differently in a world that legitimates these assumptions. . ." (Farganis, 1989, p. 208). Belenky, Clinchy, Goldberger, and Tarule (1986) have identified that the epistemological perspectives that influence how women see and know the world are different from those of men.

Farganis (1989) suggested that feminism acknowledges that each person has a different position from which they view the world but does not accept that each view is equally good. Feminism has a moral dimension that opposes normative relativism. Because of their experiences as marginal persons and their experiences of care and concern, "women can offer an epistemically sounder and politically and morally better position" (p. 217). Rose (1988) supported this view urging that knowledge gained through the practice of caring be a base for a science that values people. Harding (1986) went one step further and suggested that the hierarchy of positivism should be reversed with studies directed by such moral emancipatory interests as the elimination of sexist, racist, and classist understandings of social life being most valued.

In the health care field, patriarchal standards have reigned and the personal experience of professional caregiving has been devalued. "Feminist ideology holds that marginal persons in society are those whose roles threaten those in power" (Miller, 1991, p. 49). Nursing can be considered marginal and this results in "the development of care modalities that are unspoken, unrecognized, and unappreciated by the dominant groups and, therefore, by society at large" (Miller, 1991, p. 49). Feminist approaches to science support the development of a nursing science based on the knowledge that nurses have gained through practice.

A further contribution that feminism makes to nursing knowledge development is direction for research. Fonow and Cook (1991) distilled four common, interdisciplinary themes of feminist epistemology and methodology that are helpful for nursing research.

REFLEXIVITY

This is the practice of reflecting on, examining critically, and exploring analytically the research process and using it to understand the underlying assumptions about gender relations. Consciousness raising is one method of reflexivity

that is reflected in the increased consciousness of the researcher of the effects of the research process on the researcher's identity, the impact of the research on the subjects, and finally as a feminist research method. Collaboration between women researchers is another focus of reflexivity:

> . . . there is also the expectation among some scholars that feminist collaboration will bring about a deeper intellectual analysis, an original approach to framing questions, with a mind-set of innovation to deal with the gendered context of research (Fonow & Cook, 1991, p. 5).

ACTION ORIENTATION

The orientation of feminist research is toward social change. This can be accomplished by participating with people in an examination of positions and options, by historically analyzing the past for the purpose of future social change, or by focusing on the policy implications of research findings. "A personal commitment to feminism and to caring as a standard for professional nursing practice can only lead to the demand for major changes in the structure and provision of health care service to all human beings" (Gaut, 1991, p. 6). This change can be accomplished by attention to research with an action orientation.

ATTENTION TO THE AFFECTIVE COMPONENTS OF THE RESEARCH ACT

Feminist research recognizes the affective dimension and sees emotion as a source of insight. This can be connected to the notion of reciprocity between researcher and the researched manifested either in friendship or in negative interactions.

USE OF THE SITUATION AT HAND

This use of everyday, existing situations is particularly important for nursing research because nursing's major interest is the experiences of people in health and illness situations.

Conclusion

Professionalism has failed to bring nursing the power and prestige that were anticipated by nursing's early leaders. Professionalism is a patriarchal invention and by its very nature is alienating to women. By accepting the liberal tradition of knowledge development embodied in professionalism, nurses have not appreciated their own knowledge acquired through their caring experience. Rather than joining with other women to change the dominant social order to one that values women's unique differences, nurses have focused primarily on attaining professional status. Only recently have nurses begun to recognize that the received view of knowledge development is not sufficient for addressing the complex concerns of nursing as a human science. This realization has resulted in nursing seeking alternate approaches.

Feminism offers much to nursing through its focus on praxis. The liberalist feminist tradition of seeking equality is not sufficient to meet the challenges facing nursing. The socialist feminist perspective offers more direction. It suggests that nursing knowledge development should be directed toward creating a social order in which women are not subordinate to men. This means that our efforts should not be geared to maintaining the status quo within our field of practice but rather should be focusing on ways to alter public policy. Socialist feminism suggests that women as a social group have the more valid perspective because they have no vested interest in maintaining the status quo in society. Applying this view to nursing, nurses in practice have a more legitimate perspective of nursing than nurse leaders and educators. Thus, the distinctive experience of nursing practice should guide nursing research and the outcomes of research should be tested within the reality of practicing nurses because that reality may be quite different to that of the nurse researcher. The actual process of research should itself be dialectical, thus effecting some change in those participating. This approach may help to reduce the current chasm between nursing practice and research. Jean Watson urged nursing to "question its old dogmas, transcend its existing paradigms, and refocus its scientific attention to human phenomena that are consistent with the nature of nursing and preservation of humanity" (1988, p. 22). Feminism, particularly socialist feminism, has the potential to help nurses to meet this challenge and to make a significant contribution to changing the existing social order of health care and gender relations.

References

Anderson, J. (1991). Current directions in nursing research: Toward a poststructuralist and feminist epistemology. *The Canadian Journal of Nursing Research, 23*(3), 1–3.

Ashley, J. (1976). *Hospitals, paternalism, and the role of the nurse.* New York: Teachers College Press.

Aydelotte, M. (1990). The evolving profession: The role of the professional organization. In N. Chaska (Ed.), *The nursing profession: Turning points* (pp. 9–15). St. Louis: Mosby.

Baer, E. (1987). 'A cooperative venture' in pursuit of professional nursing status: A research journal for nursing. *Nursing Research, 36,* 18–25.

Baines, C. (1991). The professions and the ethic of care. In C. Baines, P. Evans, and S. Neysmith (Eds.), *Women's caring: Feminist perspectives on social welfare* (pp. 36–72). Toronto, Canada: McClelland & Stewart.

Belenky, M., Clinchy, B., Goldberger, N., & Tarule, J. (1986). *Women's ways of knowing.* New York: Basic Books.

Bolaria, B. S. (1988). Sociology, medicine, health, and illness: An overview. In B. S. Bolaria & H. Dickinson (Eds.). *Sociology of health care in Canada* (pp. 1–14). Toronto, Canada: Harcourt Brace Jovanovich.

Chinn, P. (1987). Response: Revision and passion. *Scholarly Inquiry for Nursing Practice, 1*(1), 21–24.

Church, O. (1990). Nursing's history: What it was and what it was not. In N. Chaska (Ed.), *The nursing profession: Turning points* (pp. 3–8). St. Louis: Mosby.

Coburn, J. (1987). I see and am silent. In D. Coburn, C. D'Arcy, G. Torrance, & P. New (Eds.), *Health care and Canadian society: Sociological perspectives* (pp. 441–462). Markham: Fitzhenry and Whiteside.

Cott, N. (1987). *The grounding of modern feminism.* New Haven, CT: Yale University Press.

Farganis, S. (1989). Feminism and the reconstruction of social science. In A. Jaggar & S. Bordo (Eds.), *Gender/Body/Knowledge: Feminist reconstructions of being and knowing* (pp. 207–223). New Brunswick, NJ: Rutgers.

Fawcett, J. (1992). Conceptual models and nursing practice: The reciprocal relationship. *Journal of Advanced Nursing, 17*, 224–228.

Flexner, A. (1915). Is social work a profession? *School Soc, 1*, 901–911.

Fonow, M., & Cook, J. (1991). Back to the future: A look at the second wave of feminist epistemology and methodology. In M. Fonow & J. Cook (Eds.), *Beyond method: Feminist scholarship as lived research* (pp. 1–15). Bloomington: Indiana University Press.

Gaut, D. (1991). Caring and nursing: Explorations in feminist perspectives—Introductory remarks. In R. Neil & R. Watts (Eds.), *Caring and nursing: Explorations in feminist perspectives* (pp. 5–8). New York: National League of Nursing.

Glazer, P., & Slater, M. (1987). *Unequal colleagues.* New Brunswick, NJ: Rutgers.

Harding, S. (1986). *The science question in feminism.* Ithaca, NY: Cornell University Press.

Hughes, L. (1990). Professionalizing domesticity: A selected synthesis of nursing historiography. *Advances in Nursing Science, 12*(4), 25–31.

Jaggar, A. (1983). *Feminist politics and human nature.* Totowa, NJ: Rowman & Allenhead.

Jaggar, A., & Bordo, S. (1989). *Gender/body/knowledge: Feminist reconstructions of being and knowing.* New Brunswick, NJ: Rutgers.

Kirkwood, R. (1991). Discipline discrimination and gender discrimination: The case of nursing in Canadian universities, 1920–1950. *Atlantis, 16*(2), 52–63.

Lyon, B. (1990). Getting back on track: Nursing's autonomous scope of practice. In N. Chaska (Ed.), *The nursing profession: Turning points* (pp. 267–274). St. Louis: Mosby.

MacPherson, K. (1991). Looking at caring and nursing through a feminist lens. In R. Neil & R. Watts (Eds.), *Caring and nursing: Explorations in feminist perspectives* (pp. 25–43). New York: NLN.

Melosh, B. (1982). *The physician's hand: Work culture and conflict in American nursing.* Philadelphia: Temple University Press.

Miller, K. (1991). A study of nursing's feminist ideology. In R. Neil & R. Watts (Eds.), *Caring and nursing: Explorations in feminist perspectives* (pp. 43–56). New York: NLN.

Nagle, L., & Mitchell, G. (1991). Paradigmatic issues in research and practice. *Advances in Nursing Science, 14*(1), 17–25.

Nolan, M., & Grant, G. (1992). Mid-range theory building and the nursing theory-practice gap: A respite care case study. *Journal of Advanced Nursing, 17*, 217–223.

O'Brien, P. (1986). 'All a woman's life can bring': The domestic roots of nursing in Philadelphia, 1830–1885. *Nursing Research, 36*, 12–17.

Parse, R. (1981). *Man-living-health: A theory of nursing.* New York: Wiley.

Parsons, M. (1986). The profession in a class by itself. *Nursing Outlook, 34*, 270–275.

Reverby, S. (1987). A caring dilemma: Womanhood and nursing in historical perspective. *Nursing Research, 36*, 5–11.

Roberts, S. J. (1984). Oppressed group behavior: Implications for nursing. *Advances in Nursing Science, 5*(4), 21–30.

Rose, H. (1988). Beyond masculine realities. In R. Bleier (Ed.), *Feminist approaches to science* (pp. 57–76). New York: Pergammon.

Silva, M. C., & Rothbart, D. (1983). An analysis of changing trends in philosophies of science on nursing theory development and testing. *Advances in Nursing Science, 6*(3), 1–13.

Smith, D. (1990). *The conceptual practices of power: A feminist sociology of knowledge.* Toronto, Canada: University of Toronto Press.

Stainton, M. C. (1982). *The birth of nursing science. Canadian Nurse, 78*, 24–28.

Thompson, J. (1987). Critical scholarship: The critique of domination in nursing. *Advances in Nursing Science, 10*(1), 27–38.

Torrance, G. (1987). Socio-historical overview. In D. Coburn, C. D'Archy, G. Torrance, & P. New (Eds.), *Health care and Canadian society: Sociological perspectives* (pp. 6–32). Markham: Fitzhenry and Whiteside.

Watson, J. (1988). *Nursing: Human science and human care: A theory of nursing.* National League of Nursing.

Webster, G., & Jacox, A. (1985). The liberation of nursing theory. In J. McCloskey & H. Grace (Eds.), *Current issues in nursing* (pp. 20–29). Boston, MA: Blackwell.

Chapter 11

Nursing Science in the Global Community

Shaké Ketefian,
RN, EdD, FAAN

Richard W. Redman,
RN, PhD

Knowledge development and research are generally embedded in cultural values and perspectives. This article examines the development of knowledge in nursing in a global context and addresses the degree to which Western values and the social environment in the United States shape nursing theory development. Three perspectives illustrate the influence of U.S. values and contextual factors. Questions are raised about the relevance of knowledge to other cultural or national contexts. Recommendations are made for nursing inquiry that makes knowledge more applicable to the global community. Keywords: knowledge development, international nursing.

For many years, nurses from other countries have been enrolled in U.S. graduate programs. Colling and Liu (1995) report a 10% increase in international students attending U.S. graduate programs in nursing in the past decade. In their survey of international students, these authors identified 239 students from 49 countries. In many parts of the world, U.S. nursing appears to be highly regarded.

As the diversity and ethnic mix of the U.S. population has increased, global awareness has also increased. In the past decade, many institutions and nurses have become involved in international activities such as consultation, collaborative research, and exchange visitor arrangements.

Source: Ketefian, S., Redman, R. (1997). Nursing Science in the Global Community. *Journal of Nursing Scholarship,* 29(1):11–15. Reprinted with permission by Sigma Theta Tau International.

Yet, despite the increase in international activities, the nature of nursing theory, research, education, and practice has not changed appreciably to be globally relevant. The degree to which parochialism may have played a role in explaining the slow pace of change in this regard has not been fully examined.

Boyacigiller and Adler (1991) examined the degree to which Western parochialism and ethnocentrism are embedded in the concepts of organizational theory. These authors reviewed the research literature in management science from three perspectives: (a) the influence of post World War II America and its environment on organizational theory development (b) the volume of international articles published in American management journals and (c) the degree to which American beliefs and values have shaped organizational theory development. Their assessment, overall, was that organizational theories are parochial and many do not acknowledge awareness of non-U.S. contexts, models, or values. Many Americans have shaped theories central to organizational and human behavior with the assumption that these beliefs have universal applicability. Free will (versus determinism) and individualism (versus collectivism) are just two examples of how Western values have shaped research and theory in organizational science. The authors call for the development of organizational sciences in which universal, intercultural theories are clearly explicit.

Following the approach taken by Boyacigiller and Adler (1991), we describe three perspectives in our examination: (a) contextual—the influence of the U.S. social environment on nursing theory development (b) quantitative—the rapid expansion of U.S. doctoral programs in nursing, the shaping of nursing journals by U.S. nurse scientists, and the degree of international scientific representation in these journals and (c) qualitative—the degree to which U.S. values have shaped nursing theory development. The status of multicultural knowledge development in the United States is then presented followed by selected recommendations. Given the magnitude of the topic, no attempt is made to be comprehensive. Rather, the ideas presented represent select perspectives and observations of the authors who are educators in the United States, but who have had extensive international experience. The views presented here are intended to serve as catalysts for further discussion.

Perspectives

Contextual Perspective

The influence of social forces on American nursing can be examined from several perspectives. These include (a) social trends and values and how they shape nursing knowledge development, (b) the influence of technology and reimbursement systems on nomenclature in nursing,

and (c) the development of nursing education and research infrastructures as social phenomena. Each is described briefly to illustrate the contextual influences.

Many recent U.S. social movements have had considerable effect on nursing theory. One example is the emphasis on health promotion and risk reduction. The social emphasis on behavior related to diet, exercise, and other types of health-promoting behaviors have influenced the shaping of public policy as well as the education of health professionals. To a considerable degree, they have also shaped the direction of nursing science and research. Another example is the way in which the emergence of the women's movement has shaped the thinking of a whole generation of women and has led to the development of new public policies in education, employment, health, and other domains. Recognition that women's health problems should be given priority has led to research by health professionals, including nurses, resulting in a body of scientific knowledge in this domain.

The Nursing Interventions Classification (NIC) work at Iowa (McCloskey & Bulechek, 1994) is another example of a social force influencing nursing knowledge development. NIC has been developed as a comprehensive classification of treatments that nurses perform in an attempt to create a standardized language of both nurse- and physician-initiated nursing interventions. Interest in developing this taxonomy can be traced in part to the need for nurses to develop a universal language. Catalytic social forces such as the rapid technologic development of literature data bases, clinical information systems in practice settings, and the need for taxonomies that are compatible with reimbursement systems have resulted in the need for standardized nursing nomenclature. This development has profound implications for nursing practice and knowledge development internationally. The degree to which U.S. nursing interventions are shaping the rapid development of "universal" taxonomies and languages that reflect nursing practice throughout the world is a pressing question. In addition, there is considerable interest in using taxonomies such as NIC to redefine nursing knowledge inductively. Again, the degree to which U.S. nursing interventions and practices reflect nursing practice in other countries is a question of critical importance internationally.

Social values and contextual influence also relate to the quality of nursing care. Definitions of nursing care quality vary, ranging from using the proper amount of resources to accomplish nursing goals to meeting patients' requirements. Assessing the quality of nursing care, whether focused on the appropriateness of a given intervention to a patient's needs or the selection of alternatives as a function of resources available illustrates how context-dependent quality can be. The expectations of a client, the socially defined role of the nurse, and the technology available can vary considerably. Furthermore, the importance of each of these variables in the quality equation can vary, depending on the context, and in turn drive the research questions and methodologies. Thus, the manner in which the pressing questions of the discipline are framed are very likely to reflect the values, philosophy, and practices of the culture and society in which they are asked.

Explorations of theory in nursing began in the 1960s. Since then, in an effort to define what is distinctive about nursing science and theory, nurse scholars and theorists have widely debated their ideas. Many of these ideas have been characterized as metatheories or conceptual frameworks. In the past decade, the nursing literature has reflected a shift in thinking. Now many investigators favor working with propositions and theories characterized as middle-range theories rather than with conceptual frameworks because middle-range theories provide the basis for generating testable hypotheses related to particular nursing phenomena and to particular patient populations.

Expansion of doctoral programs along with the magnitude and refinement of nursing research over the past several decades has been impressive. Thus, it can be argued that such advances in U.S. nursing have rightfully placed it in an enviable position vis-à-vis international peers.

The scope and orientation of much of nursing research is American without global characteristics. Frequently, research findings are presented and received by international colleagues as though the work is applicable to other national and cultural contexts. In addressing such issues, Zwanger (1987) states that American nurses are recognized as leaders in doctoral education in the world and that

> *They are . . . the oracles of the international academic nursing community. As a consequence, in many instances, their ambiguous tendencies, unclarified ideas, and conceptions are accepted as bona fide facts. (pp. 33–34)*

Zwanger draws on the Israeli experience in stating that some of those who complete their degree in the United States wish to transplant American ideas to their native land. She then describes the inappropriateness of doing so, which in some cases results in failure to function effectively in one's home settings. She makes a case for U.S. doctoral faculty to "pay attention to global content and international nursing issues," emphasize comparative studies, and assist international students to gear their doctoral research to problems in their own countries.

Quantitative Perspective

The International Council of Nurses now represents 110 national associations as members, with a total of 1 million nurses (Splane & Splane, 1994). Of 110 schools worldwide offering doctoral degrees in nursing, 62 are in the United States and 48 in all other countries combined. Moreover, according to anecdotal data, an indeterminate number of non-U.S. educational programs are programs where nurses have the opportunity to obtain doctoral degrees in fields other than nursing.

A limited number of international exchanges of students and faculty have occurred over the years (Fenton, 1994), although exchange has gained momentum recently, yet such opportunities are not made available to students by many institutions further, international exchanges typically occur during undergraduate study rather than graduate study. At the doctoral level, during the 1970s, many institutions either abandoned a second language requirement altogether or began accepting a computer language in its stead. A recent American Academy of Nursing publication (1995) identifies five graduate programs in nursing in the United States with a cross-cultural focus, some of which include international nursing. Thus, in most cases, doctoral students' exposure to the world beyond the United States might come when they have the opportunity to study with international students as peers.

Examination of the growth in journal publication and in doctoral education gives readers another perspective on the growth in nursing knowledge and science. The major journal for reporting research in nursing, *Nursing Research*, was established in 1952 by the American Journal of Nursing Company later it was followed by the publication of *Research in Nursing and Health* in 1977 and *Advances in Nursing Science* in 1978. Since that time, many journals have been established that report research in nursing, nursing theory, and nursing practice. As specialty organizations grew, so did journals concerned with the practice and research of their clinical area of practice. In the early days of *Nursing Research*, it was not uncommon to see papers authored by social scientists, reporting on studies concerned with *nurses* rather than with *nursing*.

Ketefian and Redman (1994) reported that the first doctoral programs in nursing were established in 1933 (Teachers College, Columbia University) and 1934 (New York Univer-

sity), both offering the Doctor of Education degree. In the next 25 years, only two more programs were established. Growth in doctoral programs since then has been exponential. Of the 62 institutions in the United States offering doctoral degrees in nursing, 75% offer the PhD, the remainder offers a DNS, DNSc, or EdD. As to the nature of these programs, Grace (1978) and Murphy (1981) have described the development of doctoral programs in three phases: Phase I (inception to 1959) is characterized by focusing on education for nurses for functional roles; Phase II (1960–69) is characterized by a focus on education for nurses in a second discipline, referred to as nurse scientist training; Phase III (1970 to the present) is characterized by a focus on education in and of nursing.

A review of the content of U.S. journals suggests that many report on international issues, some have articles co-authored by nurses from overseas, and others have a regular international column, however, the effect of these developments, although significant, is not major. Many libraries now subscribe to international journals yet class assignments do not often include readings from these journals. A few journals now have international representatives on their review boards.

Qualitative Perspective

The Code for Nurses (American Nurses Association, 1985) represents embodiment of the values of American Nursing. The preamble reads, in part,

When making clinical judgments, nurses base their decisions on consideration of consequences and of universal moral principles, both of which prescribe and justify nursing actions. The most fundamental of these principles is respect for persons. Other principles stemming from this basic principle are autonomy (self-determination), beneficence (doing good), nonmaleficence (avoid-

ing harm), veracity (truth-telling), confiden-
tiality (respecting privileged information),
fidelity (keeping promises), and justice (treating
people fairly). (p. i)

The values in the code, and others emanating
from them, find expression in nursing theories
and conceptual frameworks developed by U.S.
scholars. Indeed, they permeate the nursing literature. These values are at times explicit and at
other times implicit.

Why are value assumptions important? Values have important effects on people, communities, and societies the primary concern of
nursing is people—individually or in the
aggregate. An understanding of behavior and
the values that underlie behavior becomes a
critical starting point for designing and implementing nursing interventions. Value assumptions underlying U.S. nursing are profoundly
influenced by American culture, social mores,
and the biases of the people who produce this
literature. Yet a reading of U.S. literature suggests that the ideas therein are claimed to be
either acultural or universal.

Most nursing theories and nursing research
are developed and implemented in the United
States and, therefore, can be said to be influenced by the social and cultural context of this
country. In the next section, we offer specific
examples of the influence of culturally specific
values and assumptions—and present comparisons or contrasts gleaned from the literature.

GRADUATE AND HIGHER EDUCATION IN NURSING

In the United States, it is assumed that academic study is "good" and necessary for nursing
education and that higher education (at college
and university level) is even better. However, in
many countries these are not assumptions; the
terms often have different meanings.

Hockey (1987) draws on her knowledge and
experience in European countries, and states

that in some countries "higher education" refers
to academic study beyond that required for
qualification for practice. In addition, she
explains that typically with higher education
come leadership positions, even though some
nurses do not wish to assume such positions.
Thus, she poses the dilemma in ethical terms: Is
"higher education" necessary for nursing? In
another poignant example from the Austrian
experience, she reveals that nurse training
begins at age 15 and notes that "nursing autonomy assumes a different meaning" under these
circumstances (p. 77).

Another author from the same conference
describes the experience of Norway and its
dilemmas that highlight value conflicts and
value differences of a significant magnitude for
that country. The main dilemma posed by Haugen Bunch (1987) is whether Norwegian nurses
should study in the United States or in Norway.
Each choice is described as having significant
consequences for Norwegian nursing. She
describes the choices as (a) studying social and
natural sciences, (b) developing nursing science,
or (c) blending the two. At the University of
Bergen (Norway), where an Institute of Caring
Sciences was established in 1979, many believe
that caring is not subject to scientific inquiry,
that nursing cannot be both holistic and scientific, that science may compromise the nursing
discipline, that nursing can use relevant scientific principles from other disciplines, and that
there is no need for a separate nursing science.
Thus, if nurses study in Norway, with its tuto-
rial educational model, their role models will
not be nurses and they will learn the traditions
of other disciplines rather than of nursing. If, on
the other hand, they study in the United States,
they will be socialized in nursing's scientific tradition and will have nurse role models. Haugen
Bunch warns that for those educated in the
United States there will be the danger of bringing back to Norway "undigested American

knowledge that is presented as 'Norwegian truisms'—forgetting the need for value clarification so that the knowledge will fit Norwegian culture and traditions" (p. 103). Throughout her presentation she emphasizes the importance of adapting and testing theories and concepts before, "being applied and integrated to the Norwegian culture" (p. 103).

NURSING SCIENCE AND JAPAN

According to a Japanese nurse who did graduate work in the United States, Japanese nurses have imported nursing knowledge and literature since the end of the 19th century. The works of many American authors and theorists have been translated into Japanese by exchange nurses and by those who came to the U.S. for master's and doctoral degrees (Minami, 1987). Minami claims that many of these nurses "were not aware of the differences between the Japanese and American cultures or social context" (p. 66) and claimed that nursing was universal. She describes fundamental differences in the cultural milieu of the two countries that make concepts developed in one country inapplicable or irrelevant in the other. She also describes dilemmas faced by American-educated Japanese nurses in functioning in their home settings. Communication differences, for example, exist in eight areas: physical proximity, self-disclosure, trust in words, boundary in human relationships, commitment, contract dependency, independence autonomy, independence, and confrontation (p. 70). She says that Americans communicate with language while Japanese communicate with empathy, and she provides examples. These differences are characterized by Boyacigiller and Adler (1991) as high-context or low-context cultures. The external environment, the situation, and nonverbal behavior determine communication in high-context cultures like the Japanese, and subtlety, facial expression, relationship, and timing are valued. In low-context cultures like the United States,

meaning comes from the spoken word and legal contracts are valued.

Multicultural Knowledge Development in the United States

Rapid change in the demographic composition of the U.S. population has occurred within the past several decades. Some demographers estimate that by the 21st century, one third to one half of the population will be other than Euro-Caucasian. Thus, a reversal is anticipated whereby groups that were minorities will collectively become the majority. The importance of a change of such magnitude is immense. An appreciation for diversity and for the varying needs of people who are different—with regard to any number of characteristics—is needed. Nowhere is this appreciation more compelling than in health care and nursing.

A small group of nurse investigators has been developing research and theory that is culturally sensitive. In a recent American Academy of Nursing monograph (AAN, 1995), a group of authors define culturally competent care as that which "takes into account issues related to diversity, marginalization, and vulnerability due to culture, race, gender, and sexual orientation" (p. 4). In their assessment of the state of knowledge development in this area, the authors identify the dearth of principles to guide selection of culturally sensitive research questions and selection of culturally appropriate methodologies. Many nursing programs do not offer content relevant to this area and fewer still require doctoral students to enroll in seminars about cross-cultural nursing.

The authors of the AAN monograph (1995) identify two metatheories and studies based on them that have shown promise of generating knowledge that is culturally sensitive. One theory is Leininger's (1985), wherein she posits that care, as the essence of nursing, is universal across cultures, although its forms and expressions may vary. The authors cite a number of nursing studies in which Leininger's theory helped researchers generate knowledge related to cultural care. The other metatheory cited is the "care deficit theory" (Orem, 1991). This theory enables study of self-care practices used by diverse social groups. Its relevance for populations in a number of European countries—as well as Mexico and Thailand—is being studied by a network of collaborators (AAN, 1995).

In addition to the two metatheories, others are being developed that are referred to as "situation-specific theories" (AAN, 1995). Examples are studies of Middle Eastern immigrants (Lipson, Reizian, & Meleis 1987 ; Meleis, 1981; Meleis & Jonsen, 1983), patterns of health-seeking behaviors among Arab children (May, 1985), and postpartum transition among Arab women (El Sayed, 1986). The authors contend that, collectively, such studies can be synthesized to provide conceptualizations of patterns of responses to health–illness transitions, thus enabling development of a situation-specific theory in a particular population (AAN, 1995, p. 10).

Methodological concerns in the conduct of research with ethnically and racially diverse groups have received increasing attention as well. The U.S. Department of Health and Human Services (1990) has recently stipulated that ethnically and racially different groups be included as research subjects. Porter and Villarruel (1993) provide a cogent analysis of research issues and propose a set of guidelines to be considered for the design of research. Consideration of appropriate sensitivity is reflected in conceptualizing and conducting research, including each step of the research process and investigator activities. It is implied that unless these design considerations are present and deliberatively addressed, the relevance and applicability of the outcome of the research to diverse populations would be questionable.

OTHER KNOWLEDGE DEVELOPMENT STRATEGIES

Over the years, nurses in many countries have identified their inability to describe nursing practice, client populations, or geographic areas as a serious constraint (Clark, 1994). To meet this need and to contribute to knowledge development for nursing, various classification systems have been developed. The Nursing Minimum Data Set was developed by Werley in the late 1960s (Werley & Lang, 1988) and in turn spurred other developments.

In the early 1980s, a classification of nursing diagnoses was proposed by the North American Nursing Diagnosis Association, where the phenomenon of concern is patient status (McLane, 1987). More recently, the Nursing Interventions Classification (NIC) project was developed. The use of nursing diagnoses and NIC is becoming widespread in the United States and internationally. Such standardization has many advantages: it helps expand nursing's knowledge base, provides a common language to communicate the functions of nursing, provides shared understanding of nursing practice across national and cultural boundaries, and highlights the distinctive contribution nursing makes toward solving health problems. The International Council of Nurses currently has a project in progress with these goals in mind (Clark, 1994). Although we do not know how the different knowledge development strategies will evolve, significant developments are providing the basis on which to build continuing work by nurse scholars in doctoral programs around the world.

Next Steps

Some authors discuss the urgent need to develop nursing knowledge relevant to the health of the global community (Meleis, 1993). A Western perspective generally pervades organizing concepts and frameworks in nursing and thus is a dominating influence in knowledge development and research. Meleis expressed concern that U.S. nursing doctoral programs may be producing nurse scientists who do not challenge Western perspectives, particularly in terms of definitions and assumptions related to nursing phenomena.

In 1997, we are at a critical juncture for American nursing science. Given the global society in which we live, nursing science now faces the challenge of moving to its next phase of development, which we call "becoming globally relevant." This movement entails a variety of activities and changes in the way we do science, a responsibility that should be shared by scientists in the U.S. and internationally. We need to test nursing models, propositions, and hypotheses in several countries, include relevant content in educational programs, provide opportunities for doctoral students to develop nursing research internships abroad, involve international scholars in editorial review boards, increase the representation of international authors in U.S. journals and vice versa, encourage international students to focus their dissertations on topics pertinent to their countries, integrate collaborative international research in the ongoing work of scientists in leading nursing institutions throughout the world, and expand the criteria for promotion and tenure to include such activity.

We hope the questions raised in this essay will be viewed as opportunities by the global nursing community. If future discussions result in recognition of the challenges facing nursing knowledge development and doctoral education throughout the world, then our purpose will have been served.

References

American Academy of Nursing. (1995). *Diversity, marginalization, and culturally-competent health care: Issues in knowledge development*. Washington, DC: Author.

American Nurses Association. (1985). *Code for nurses with interpretive statements*. Kansas City, MO: Author.

Boyacigiller, N. A., & Adler, N. J. (1991). The parochial dinosaur: Organizational science in a global context. *Academy of Management Science, 16*(2), 262–290.

Clark, J. (1994). The international classification of nursing. In J. McCloskey & H. K. Grace (Eds.). *Current issues in nursing* (4th ed.) (pp. 143–147). St. Louis: Mosby-Year Book.

Colling, J. C., & Liu, Y. C. (1995). International nurses' experiences seeking graduate education in the United States. *Journal of Nursing Education, 34*(4), 162–166.

El Sayed, Y. A. (1986). *The successive-unsettled transitions of migration and their impact on postpartum concerns of Arab immigrant women*. Unpublished doctoral dissertation, University of California, San Francisco.

Fenton, M. V. (1994). Development of models of international exchange to upgrade nursing education. In J. McCloskey & H. K. Grace (Eds.). *Current issues in nursing* (4th ed.) (pp. 202–206). St. Louis: Mosby-Year Book.

Grace, H. (1978). The development of doctoral education in nursing: An historical perspective. *Journal of Nursing Education, 17*(4), 17–27.

Haugen Bunch, E. (1987). International perspectives and implications for doctoral education in nursing: Norwegian perspective. In *International perspectives and implications for doctoral education in nursing* (pp. 97–105). Portland, OR: Oregon Health Sciences University School of Nursing.

Hockey, L. (1987). Ethical issues in higher education in nursing. In *International perspectives and implications for doctoral education in nursing* (pp. 75–85). Portland, OR: Oregon Health Sciences University School of Nursing.

Ketefian, S., & Redman, R. W. (1994). The changing face of graduate education. In J. McCloskey & H. K. Grace (Eds.). *Current issues in nursing* (4th ed.) (pp. 188–195). St. Louis: Mosby-Year Book.

Leininger, M. M. (1985). Ethnography and ethnonursing: Models and modes of qualitative data analysis. In M. M. Leininger (Ed.). *Qualitative methods in nursing*. New York: Grune & Stratton.

Lipson, J. G., Reizian, A., & Meleis, A. I. (1987). Arab-American patients: A medical record review. *Social Science and Medicine, 24*(2), 101–107.

May, K. M. (1985). *Arab-American immigrant parents' social networks and health care of children.* Unpublished doctoral dissertation, University of California, San Francisco.

McCloskey, J. C., & Bulechek, G. M. (1994). Standardizing the language for nursing treatments: An overview of the issues. *Nursing Outlook, 42*(2), 45–63.

McLane, A. M. (1987). *Classification of nursing diagnoses: Proceedings of the seventh conference.* St. Louis: Mosby-Year Book.

Meleis, A. I. (1981). The Arab-American in the Western health care system. *American Journal of Nursing, 6,* 1180–1183.

Meleis, A. I. (1993). A passion for substance revisited: Global transitions and international commitments. In *Proceedings of the 1993 Annual forum on doctoral nursing education* (pp. 5–22). St. Paul, MN: University of Minnesota School of Nursing.

Meleis, A. I., & Jonsen, A. (1983). Ethical crises and cultural differences. *Western Journal of Medicine, 138*(6), 889–893.

Minami, H. (1987). Reflections of the cultural and social milieu on the development of nursing science in Japan. In *International perspectives and implications for doctoral education in nursing* (pp. 63–74). Portland, OR: Oregon Health Sciences University School of Nursing.

Murphy, J. F. (1981). Doctoral education in, of, and for nursing: An historical analysis. *Nursing Outlook, 29*(11), 645–649.

Orem, D. E. (1991). *Nursing: Concepts of practice* (4th ed.). New York: McGraw-Hill.

Porter, C. P., & Villarruel, A. M. (1993). Nursing research with African American and Hispanic people: Guidelines for action. *Nursing Outlook, 41*(2), 59–67.

Splane, V. H., & Splane, R. B. (1994). International nursing leaders. In J. McCloskey & H. K. Grace (Eds.). *Current issues in nursing* (4th ed.) (pp. 49–56). St. Louis: Mosby-Year Book.

U.S. Department of Health and Human Services. (1990). *Healthy people 2000: National health promotion and disease prevention objectives.* Superintendent of documents. Washington, DC: U.S. Government Printing Office.

Werley, H. H., & Lang, N. M. (Eds.). (1988). *Identification of the nursing minimum data set.* New York: Springer.

Zwanger, L. (1987). International perspectives and implications for doctoral education in nursing: The Israeli case. In *International perspectives and implications for doctoral education in nursing* (pp. 17–43). Portland, OR: Oregon Health Sciences University School of Nursing.

Chapter 12

A Global Perspective on Domestic and International Tensions in Knowledge Development

Kim Lutzen, RN, PhD

Can over 7 million nurses in the world make a difference in the health and illness of the world's peoples? Nurses in many countries have achieved recognition as members of a scientific discipline, and they are in positions to make valuable contributions to health care. However, such achievement may not be a priority for all nurses. Examination of the domestic and international tensions from a global perspective is necessary to understand current barriers to the development and use of nursing knowledge.

Tensions and instability occur when nurses differ in their goals or in cultural or moral values. Nurses actively engaged in research are a minority compared to the majority of nurses who do not have access to nursing journals, advanced education, or the opportunity to attend international conferences. Researchers believe nursing knowledge is the core of professionalization, but many nurses engaged in the difficult, stressful work of direct nursing care have not seen significant improvements in

direct patient care as the result of nursing research. Comparing the issues nurses are struggling with in each of these "worlds" illustrates their differences. Some issues are practical, some theoretical, depending on the particular social and academic culture. For example, more nurses may be dealing with questions such as, "What methods can I use to prevent wound infections when I have no fresh water?" than the questions such as, "What paradigm should I use for this research?" Both problems indicate important issues in developing nursing knowledge, but they require different strategies.

Knowledge development in nursing can come from advancement of clinical knowledge, conceptual knowledge, or empirical knowledge (Schultz & Meleis, 1988). Meleis and colleagues (1994) said that scholarliness includes critical thinking, connections to practice, commitment to the discipline's mission, substantive mastery, philosophical analyses, rigorous investigations, and awareness of the relationship between knowledge development and its effects on society. From a global perspective, the progress and development of nursing science is most successful as an international endeavor, based on shared fundamental values and health-related goals.

Source: Lutzen, K. (2000). A global perspective on domestic and international tensions in knowledge development. *Journal of Nursing Scholarship, 32*(4): 335–337. © 2000 Sigma Theta Tau International. Reprinted with permission by Blackwell Publishing, Ltd.

Broad-based scholarly debate about nursing science is necessary to answer the most crucial question: "Is this science and, if so, what is it good for?"

Tensions in developing global nursing knowledge arise from many sources. A basic problem is language barriers. Participation in international scholarly debate requires good knowledge of the English language as well as the language of nursing. Further, the culture of international nursing conferences requires knowledge and experience. These difficulties are not insurmountable. Recognizing and addressing them are essential for collaboration that builds nursing science.

The most crucial tensions, however, are not the difficulties of language. They are attitudes and perceptions within nursing, as well as between nurses and colleagues in other professions, that are counterproductive to the progress of nursing globally. My focus in this analysis is the tensions within nursing, both within and among countries. Discussion of the situation in my country, Sweden, provides accounts of both domestic and international tensions and indicates how and why a global perspective of nursing knowledge can make a difference in health care.

Domestic Tensions

Nursing in Sweden, as in many other countries, has been influenced by American nursing. At about the same time nursing education in Sweden became part of the academic system in 1977, the United States already had 2,300 nurses with doctoral degrees. While a few nurses in Sweden were discussing how to define nursing and what type of nursing research should be conducted, nurse researchers in the United States were publishing textbooks and papers on nursing theory and research. Communicating across national boundaries, despite cultural and geographic distance, gave Swedish nurse researchers a push forward in providing evidence of the relevance and uniqueness of nursing science.

Today, almost 25 years later, approximately 300 of Sweden's 100,000 nurses have doctoral degrees in nursing or in health-related disciplines. Nursing theory and meta-theory are often integrated into the curriculum. The conceptual and methodologic developments pertaining to nursing in the United States and Canada are often referred to in journal publications by Swedish authors. However, these trends obscure the "political" tensions of a newly emerging field within a country.

One of the most important sources of political, as well as academic, tensions can be related to this question: If nursing science is an academic subject, then why does this subject belong to nurses? Whether nursing science should "belong" to the profession of nursing is a question that has not been resolved in a scholarly manner (Lutzen & Barbosa da Silva, 1995). An event illustrating this tension occurred shortly after the reform of nursing education in Sweden when the first professorships in nursing (or caring science) were appointed. Among the persons seeking a professorship in nursing was a (male) nonnurse psychologist. After a long and rigorous review process and based on good and acceptable qualifications, this person was appointed professor of nursing. Protests arose, especially among doctoral students who argued that they wanted a nurse to have this appointment. Many nurses who had taken courses in qualitative methods and nursing theory, under the leadership of prominent nurse-researchers from the United States, thought the psychologist received the chair mainly because he used quantitative research methods. The gap between qualitative and quantitative researchers widened.

Because most doctoral students are completing their doctoral studies with medical faculty, the question of "methods" is fraught with tensions. Compromises are made to compete for funds. Doctoral students who pursue qualitative studies need more time for data collection and analysis, and they fear they are lagging behind students who use quantitative methods and conduct randomized studies. Thus, a researcher may be tempted to construct an instrument to "get the data" rather than to reflect on the epistemology of the research question. This tension is perpetuated by the perception of methods as inherently good or bad, including among nurse researchers who now are in the position of mentoring doctoral students.

Such a claim of methodologic superiority, made in the name of a paradigm shift, creates distance among scholars instead of promoting agreement that a diversity of methods can exist in the same space and time. Such an approach places more emphasis on ideology than on knowledge. The tendency for a specific paradigm to become an "action plan" (Powers & Knapp, 1995) that does not take into account the diversity of perspectives, theories, and methods is not constructive to the development of nursing globally.

Because Sweden is a small country, with few professors of nursing on major research funding committees, integrity, objectivity, and fairness in judging applications for funds are especially important. Even if measures are taken to guarantee that each application receives a fair and competent review, tensions and mistrust occur when a proposal for a project with a qualitative design is rejected. The applicant may believe that it was tuned down because of its method, not because the proposal was weak. A qualitative study, because of the language within the paradigm, may be poorly understood by reviewers and therefore may be judged as poorly written, but it also may lack the rigor and clarity necessary to persuade readers of its importance.

Another source of domestic tension in the development of nursing in Sweden is that "nursing" and "nursing research" were defined by the Board of Medical Research (MFR) in 1983, not by the professional nursing organization. The definition is broad, focused on "care" rather than "nursing." Accordingly, the domain of research is not specific to nursing. Most significant is that care and nursing are viewed as comple-

ments to medicine, thus complicating the argument of a unique domain of knowledge. Moreover, this definition divides Swedish nurses; as many applaud it as reject it. Some argue that a definition of nursing should evolve when new knowledge relevant to the discipline is generated. Others say definitions are created by formal decisions that give direction and focus.

Before the MFR definition of nursing/caring in Sweden, the American Nurses Association (1980) made a public statement in which nursing was defined as the "diagnosis and treatment of human responses to actual or potential health problems." Neither the Swedish nor the American definition included the word "knowledge." The focus on "what nurses do" rather than on "what nurses know" may be part of the reason nurses lack authority over their own domain. The act of doing can be defined and controlled by others, but "knowing"—having theoretical and practical knowledge—is personal and cannot be controlled by others. Perhaps defining nursing and nursing research in Sweden in 1983, while nursing research in Sweden was in its infancy, was a step taken too early.

International Tensions in Nursing Knowledge

Two different scenarios illustrate in the development of nursing knowledge. At a recent international conference, a nurse from an Eastern European country was delivering her paper about children with chronic illness. Her English was halting, for which she apologized; her face flushed with embarrassment as she mispronounced important concepts in the paper someone had translated into English for her. The transparencies she used were simple but clear, and they contained essential information, but they could not compare to the PowerPoint slide presentation of the previous speaker. During the discussion following her paper, she could not answer many questions because of language barriers. The references in her paper were all from English-speaking countries, including her own work that had been published in an American nursing journal.

In the next room was a nurse researcher from an English-speaking country. She had poise and humor, was relaxed in her presentation that also was focused on children with chronic illness. Her face was flushed with excitement, not embarrassment. She began the PowerPoint slide presentation with pictures of her university and the children's hospital in which she conducted the research. She wrote her own paper; no translation was necessary, and she did not need to apologize for mispronunciations. The references in her paper were also exclusively from English-speaking countries. The work of the nurse-researcher next door was not cited.

The two nurse researchers were attending the same conference; they had the same area of interest. They cited the same references from Anglo-Saxon countries. They had colleagues who listened to their presentations. Yet a cultural bias may have precluded a global interest in uniting these nurses' technology, but from a gap between countries. The only real factor separating the two researchers was the wall between them, but their access to future international collaboration was different.

A Global Perspective

Ketefian and Redman (1997) pointed out that knowledge development and research are generally embedded in cultural values and perspectives. The authors questioned to what extent Western values and the social environment in the United States shape nursing theory development, but Parse (1992) called for an "international commitment from nurses of all nations to use extant nursing theories and frameworks, rather than the biomedical model" as a way to enhance the devel-

opment of nursing. The juxtaposition of these two statements is significant. The first statement "reaches out" over the continents and invites nurses to take part in scholarly efforts; the second statement invites us to stay where we are in our scholarly endeavor. Although Parse is right that the biomedical model is inadequate in answering the questions of nursing practice, one wonders whether the nursing theories that Parse mentioned are those theories generated only in the American context. In Sweden, probably every school of nursing has at some time included American nursing theories in its curriculum.

What then does a global perspective mean? Why is it necessary, and how can it be achieved? The term global is used to mean that the whole world is included in the acceptance of the main ideas, values, and goals of something essential for future development. Examples include the United Nations and the World Health Organization; the International Council of Nurses comes close, but it is not yet a global organization because not all countries are represented. These and other global organizations show the necessity of concerted efforts to achieve agreement on policies, such as equality and human rights, that affect all people.

For nurses to achieve a global perspective in knowledge development, the following key issues must be addressed. First, a closer critical analysis of the meaning of nursing development is necessary. What should be developed, how, and why? Does development refer to an idea, theory, practice, or research? Because research can never be value free, identifying and comparing values internationally is necessary for gaining insight about how different values influence the development of nursing.

Second, values pertaining to nursing as a profession and the value of good health, although related, should be distinct from each other. Common values in nursing may exist, such as the

ICN's code of ethics, but professional values may be enmeshed in social and cultural values. The moral values underpinning health-related goals also vary according to social, political, and economic conditions and policies. In one country, health may be seen as a commodity, something a person privately pays for. In another country access to health care is constitutionally regulated, a basic social value everyone is entitled to, and in many more countries, health is incidental or nonexistent.

Third, comparison of moral and cultural values is necessary, not to come to an agreement, but to create meta-perspectives that integrate and include these values.

Fourth, finding ways to overcome some language barriers, such as at international conferences, should be facilitated by modern technology, but the real barrier to achieving a global perspective is not simply that a nurse cannot speak English. The nursing language itself can be a barrier because it consists of terms, conceptualizations, and metaphors that are used to communicate social and cultural values. Between the researcher and the practitioner, status and position are also communicated if the practitioner does not understand what is being said.

Fifth, creating ways to open up the methodologic discussion to what strategies can facilitate inclusion is necessary. The qualitative versus quantitative debate has not been constructive, and it should be replaced by discussion of what methods would be most effective in addressing particular problems in particular contexts. For example, a "life-world" perspective would place an emphasis on the person and his or her unique experience, while an "epidemiological" perspective is necessary to find out how many people are affected in a similar way and what factors correlate.

Sixth, the purpose of nursing research is to generate theory, and the purpose of theory is to build knowledge that can be applied to improve nursing practice. This assumption, found in most nursing research texts, indicates that research questions originate in practice. If so, then nurses also must address whether theories imported from one country are applicable in another cultural context.

Conclusions

Differences exist both within and between countries, as illustrated in the domestic and international tensions related to the development of nursing knowledge. True scholarship, especially in such a diverse field as nursing, should reflect a profound sense of intellectual integrity, exchange of ideas, and fairness in evaluation of the accomplishments of others. Only then will the vision become a reality that the 7 million nurses of the world make a difference in health of the world's peoples.

References

American Nurses Association. (1980). *Nursing: A social policy statement*. Kansas City: American Nurses Association.

Ketefian, S., & Redman, R. W. (1997). Nursing science in the global community. *Image: Journal of Nursing Scholarship, 29*, 11–15.

Lutzen, K., & Barbosa da Silva, A. (1995). Delineating the domain of nursing science in Sweden: Some relevant issues. *Journal of Nordic Science, 15*, 4–7.

Meleis, A. I., Hall, J. M., & Stevens, P. E. (1994). Scholarly caring in doctoral nursing education: Promoting diversity and collaborative mentorship. *Image: Journal of Nursing Scholarship, 26*, 177–180.

Parse, R. R. (1992). Nursing knowledge for the 21st century: An international commitment. *Nursing Science Quarterly, 5*(1), 8–12.

Powers, B. A., & Knapp, T. R. (1995). *A dictionary of nursing theory and research* (2nd ed.). London: Sage.

Schultz, P. R., & Meleis, A. J. (1998). Nursing epistemology: Traditions, insights, questions. *Image: Journal of Nursing Scholarship, 20*, 217–224.

Part Three

NURSING'S METAPARADIGM: CONCEPTUALIZATIONS OF NURSING AND HEALTH

In the late 1970s and early 1980s, Fawcett (1984) and others explicated the notion of a nursing metaparadigm. A metaparadigm represents the broadest consensus of the general parameters of a discipline, the fundamental orientation within which nearly all scholars within the discipline work. Fawcett (1984) and others have long maintained that the metaparadigm of nursing is comprised of four main concepts—person, health, environment, and nursing—together with their broad definitions and some general propositions about their interrelationships. Agreement on a nursing metaparadigm, thus defined, is far from unanimous within the discipline, but the utility establishing some parameters for a far-ranging discipline that often seems to have none at all is hardly debatable.

In this section, six scholars present various perspectives on nursing and health. In the metaparadigm, "nursing" is commonly construed as *nursing actions*. For our purposes in this part of the book, I have taken the license to broaden that conceptualization somewhat to address nursing practice as *praxis* and nursing as a discipline. In Chapter 13 (written by this author in 1994), I assert that the realization of nursing theory-guided practice is perhaps the greatest challenge that nursing as a scholarly discipline has ever faced. In light of the many challenges faced by nursing in many contexts, this is quite a claim, and it was not made lightly. I offer what I believe to be a useful definition of *nursing theory*. I also call for a more explicit acknowledgment of the fact that values, above all, guide practice.

In Chapter 14, Reed explicates the ontology of the discipline of nursing in a unique way in which nursing is "an inherent human process of well-being." This construct can be related to the notion of nursing as a basic human science. Reed speaks of nursing as a way of knowing, a way of doing, and a way of being.

In Chapter 15, Johnson, in a philosophical study, examines nursing practice as an art. Parse (1998) regards nursing as a performing art, a characterization that is generally compatible with Johnson's explication here. Johnson makes several provocative claims, such as her assertion that the capacity of the nurse to grasp meaning in patient situations is not affected by the intellect and not based in reflection or reasoning. Ironically, there follows a lengthy section on the nurse's ability to determine rationally an appropriate course of action in which the meaning of the situation for the patient is not mentioned. Could the introduction of the overarching constructs of *values-based practice* and *evidence-based care* offer a coherent logical and humane alternative interpretation?

In Chapter 16, Pender explicates old and new views of health along with nursing's contribution to nurturing new conceptualizations. Although nursing's contributions to paradigmatic shifts in views of health in society have gone largely unrecognized, nurse scholars can certainly point to works in our literature from 1970 onward that offered a vision of health as experiential and unitary, and patterned rather than normed. These views from the nursing literature largely predated similar paradigmatic shifts now occurring at the cultural and societal levels.

In Chapter 17, continuing the theme of emerging views of health, Cowling describes a reconceptualization of healing in a new paradigm as the process of appreciating wholeness. Cowling links this theory-based practice explicitly to transformational praxis and describes in detail how one can practice fundamentally from a theoretical perspective *and* from one's values in moment-to-moment relating with a client.

In Chapter 18, Gadow discusses what is required to constitute the "ethical cornerstone" of nursing. She argues that in our contemporary world, premodern, modern, and postmodern conceptualizations coexist in a dialectical relationship. The premodern is represented as communitarian subjective immersion; the modern is represented as universalist objective detachment; and the postmodern is represented as relational engagement between particular selves.

Gadow's description of the multidimensionality of ethical discourse relates to the complexity and unpredictability with which we are confronted in *praxis*. Premodern, modern, and postmodern perspectives all represent values, albeit diverse values, and values guide practice. In the example given in Gadow's article, several different nurses behave very differently in different situations based on their individual values.

Collectively, these six chapters offer readers a chance to reflect on the nature of nursing itself, what constitutes nursing, and what constitutes health. All six chapters are oriented toward *praxis* in some way. It is incumbent on the advanced practice nurse, holding a graduate degree in nursing, to be able to explicate the nature of the discipline and its practice and to discuss with considerable depth the nature of health, generally construed as nursing's goal. The diversity of the chapters illustrates that there is no one correct, monolithic view. Many views coexist and interact continually to make up the discourse of the discipline that the practitioner must master.

References

Fawcett, J. (1984). The metaparadigm of nursing: Present status and future refinements. *Image, 16*(3), 84–87.

Parse, R. R. (1998). *The human becoming school of thought: A perspective for nurses and other health professionals.* Thousand Oaks, CA: Sage.

Chapter 13

Nursing Theory-Guided Practice: What It Is and What It Is Not

William K. Cody, RN, PhD

The full realization of nursing theory-guided practice is perhaps the greatest challenge that nursing as a scholarly discipline has ever faced. There may be multiple theories guiding practice within the discipline, but it is imperative that these be nursing theories. There is not space here to explicate the many benefits to humanity that emanate from true nursing theory-guided practice. Rather it is the intention of this column to elucidate the proposition that it is essential to the advancement of nursing science and the future of the discipline to seek greater clarity as to what constitutes nursing theory-guided practice. This phrase is often heard in the halls and classrooms of schools of nursing, but not everyone using the term "nursing theory" means the same thing.

Sometimes the term "theory" is used in nursing to refer any knowledge that is useful in general health care or the care of a particular population—as in the content of most undergraduate courses, for example. For many nurses, including some advanced practitioners and faculty, all of this knowledge may be called "nurs-

ing theory." For others, the term "nursing theory" is used to refer only to the particular knowledge that has to do directly with planning and implementing conventional nursing care, as in the steps of the generic "nursing process." Nurses using the term in this way are more selective as to what they admit as "nursing theory," yet they do not see the necessity of using a specific nursing framework to guide practice. Another assertion often heard is that "most nursing theories haven't been tested yet." Such a use of the term "theory" is closely related to the legacy of positivism, in which a "theory" must be empirically verifiable on the basis of objective measurement. This belief system also gives rise to the term "research-based practice," which reflects the belief that it is appropriate to take empirical findings directly into practice.

A distinct use of the term "nursing theory" and one with which readers of *Nursing Science Quarterly* are, no doubt, familiar, refers specifically to a distinct and well-articulated system of concepts and propositions rooted explicitly in a philosophy of nursing and intended solely to guide nursing practice and research. These attributes are the minimal criteria for any conceptual system to be called a nursing theory. Merely to have been written by a nurse or used

Source: Cody, W. K. (1994). Nursing theory-guided practice: What it is and what it is not. *Nursing Science Quarterly*, 7(4):144–145.

by nurses does not and cannot turn knowledge into nursing theory. This use of the term is not original with the author it is simply commensurate with the use of the term "theory" in all other academic disciplines. Of course, all knowledge is open to anyone to learn and use, but members of a discipline have the obligation to concern themselves specifically with the knowledge base of their discipline, to participate in its development, to guide its use, and to evaluate the work of their colleagues on the basis of the work's relation to the extant theory base of that discipline.

In Nightingale's time, and for years thereafter, nurses were the nutritionists, the sanitarians, the physical therapists, and the respiratory therapists in Wald's time, they were the social workers and health educators. All of these roles have evolved into distinct professions, and nowhere is the nurse considered the chief expert in any of these fields today. To expect contemporary nurses to have extensive knowledge in such nonnursing areas is unfair and impractical. To call such knowledge nursing knowledge is plainly retrogressive and antithetical to the advancement of nursing science. The same is true of medical knowledge, but medicine still dominates nursing politically, and many nurses actually value having the medical tasks delegated to them. The resulting interdisciplinary dynamic creates the impression among many nurses that mastery of much of the medical canon is the chief requisite to practice nursing. It is important for contemporary nurses to understand that what is merely delegated from another (more powerful) discipline can also be taken away. As more and more nurses recognize the distinction between the knowledge base and goals of medicine and nursing, nursing will be free to progress more rapidly toward full standing as an autonomous discipline.

The notion that research findings do or should guide practice is quite prevalent in contemporary nursing. This idea, as mentioned previously, is associated with the interpretation of the term "theory," which holds that any theory must be testable in a quantitative manner. Thus, the idea that research findings guide practice is linked to the objectivistic, reductionistic legacy of logical positivism, but even under logical positivism, it was not the empirical findings that were said to provide direction for future practice but rather the theory as supported through empirical testing. Theory was believed to guide research and practice. The research findings were to feed back into the theory, which would then (continue to) guide research and practice. This was the dominant model of the theory-research-practice triad throughout the much-heralded yet largely disastrous era of "value-free science" (Jacox & Webster, 1986).

More recently, it has been widely acknowledged that all scientific endeavors are value laden. Especially in the social or human sciences, it has become increasingly clear that values, above all, guide practice. Theory must be rethought for the postmodern age to explicitly address the question of values—not only what values but whose. For example, if any discipline within the human sciences is to be norm based, then who determines those norms and why should they be valued by others? In nursing science, if human health is conceptualized within a framework of norms, then what value is demonstrated for persons whose health is judged to be outside the norm—for what purpose, and with what consequences?

A nursing theory that explicitly posits a value for the human, regardless of societal norms and expectations, guides the nurse to practice in a wholly respectful way that precludes labeling and trying to change the person (Parse, 1992). It is true, as Habermas (1974) and others have charged, that the theories of a bygone era, falsely purged of values, are now and always were incapable of meaningfully guiding practice in human affairs, but theories that incorporate and explicate their proponents' values certainly have the capacity to guide practice. It is always, essentially, values that guide practice of any kind.

There is a kind of investigation frequently published in nursing literature that has to do with problem solving in the practice arena. These investigations address practical problems of hands-on health care practice, such as dressings, positioning, and pulmonary toilet, sometimes comparing two techniques. Surely the time has come for nursing as a scholarly discipline to realize that these investigations constitute practical problem solving and do not constitute scholarly research undertaken to advance the knowledge of the discipline. Scholarly research is guided by and develops, expands, or tests theory. This is one of its defining characteristics. Much of the nursing problem-solving literature is like testing two methods of slicing onions: you will favor the method that makes your eyes tear less. Certainly it can be said that if a nurse tested two ways of promoting decubitus healing and the decubiti treated one way healed faster, without untoward consequences, then that way could be tentatively recommended for future use. This is not nursing research per se it is problem solving. Neither does such a procedure really guide practice. What guides practice here is the value for promoting healing and the desire to do so while avoiding harm to the person.

Nursing theory-guided practice is based on theory that is specific to the discipline of nursing, explicitly rooted in a philosophy of nursing, and intended solely to guide nursing practice and research. True theory-guided practice is far more comprehensive and complex than mere application of the results of problem-solving investigations. Only when nurses everywhere are guided in their practice by a theory base specific to nursing will nursing have achieved parity with other scholarly disciplines. As a discipline coming of age in the late 20th-century dawning of the postmodern era, nursing is poised to make a remarkable contribution to 21st-century human science and practice. Nursing as a scholarly discipline comprises not only what it is and has been, but also what it can become. History tells us plainly that nursing not guided by nursing theory becomes something else!

References

Habermas, J. (1974). *Theory and practice* (J. Viertel, Trans.). Boston: Beacon. (Original work, 4th ed., published in German in 1971)

Jacox, A., & Webster, G. (1986). Competing theories of science. In L. Nicoll (Ed.), *Perspectives on nursing theory* (pp. 333–341). Boston: Little, Brown.

Parse, R. R. (1992). Human becoming: Parse's theory of nursing. *Nursing Science Quarterly, 5*, 35–42.

Chapter 14

Nursing: The Ontology of the Discipline

Pamela G. Reed,
RN, PhD, FAAN

The purpose of this article is to contribute to clarifying the ontology of the discipline by extending existing meanings of the term nursing to propose a substantive definition. In this definition, nursing is viewed as an inherent human process of well-being, manifested by complexity and integration in human systems. The nature of this process and theoretical implications of the new nursing are presented. Nurses are invited to continue the dialogue about the meaning of the term and explore the implications of nursing, substantively defined, for their practice and science. Keywords: deconstruction, knowledge development, metaparadigm, ontology, postmodernism.

Distinguishing the term *nursing* as a noun from its use as a verb was put forth most profoundly by Rogers (1970), whose vision extended the scholarship of earlier nursing theorists to thrust nursing forward to be recognized as both a scientific discipline as well as a professional practice. It is time, however, to push back the frontier once again, beyond these two important understandings of nursing, by proposing a new meaning of nursing. With this new meaning, the term itself represents the nature and substance of the discipline. In other words, *nursing* is the ontology of the discipline.

The ideas put forth here are done so in the spirit of accepting Watson's (1995) "postmodern challenge" to exploit the climate of deconstruction of nursing (see Rampragus, 1995

Reed, 1995) to extend and, by some degree, reconstruct current understandings of nursing. Smith's (1988a) article outlined the ongoing dialogue about two meanings of nursing, as a verb and a noun. This dialogue is revisited here for the purpose of further clarifying what is the ontology of the discipline, long considered a crucial question by seminal thinkers in nursing (Ellis, 1982; Rogers, 1970; Roy, 1995).

Continuing the Dialogue: Nursing as a Process of Well-Being

It is proposed here that there exists a third and perhaps most basic definition of nursing in which nursing represents the *substantive* focus of the discipline. Disciplines are characterized by their substantive focus: archaeology is the study

Source: Reed, P. (1997). Nursing: The ontology of the discipline. *Nursing Science Quarterly. 10*(2):76–79.

of the archaeo, or what is ancient and primitive. Astronomy is the study of the astro, astronomical phenomena such as the motion and constitution of celestial bodies. Biology is a branch of knowledge about biol, or living matter. Chemistry deals with the processes and properties of chemical substances. Physics is the study of physical properties and processes. Psychology is the study of the psyche, referring to mental processes and activities associated with human behavior, and nursing, the discipline, is proposed here to be the study of nursing processes of well-being, inherent among human systems.

This meaning of nursing, as an inherent process of well-being, derives in part from the root word, nurse, defined as a process of nourishing, of promoting the development or progress of something. The meaning also derives from synonyms of nurse meaning to heal, to foster, to sustain (Laird, 1971; *Webster's New Collegiate Dictionary*, 1979). These descriptions signify that nursing involves a process that is developmental, progressive, and sustaining, and by which well-being occurs.

The Inherent Nursing Process

The theme of human beings' inherent nursing processes as the substantive focus of the discipline is supported in nursing theorists' works from Nightingale in 1859, to the mid 20th century writings of Henderson, to the contemporary turn-of-the-century ideas of Schlotfeldt. Nightingale (1859/1969) wrote about the person's "innate power" and the inner "reparative process." Henderson (1964) eloquently symbolized the power of the nurse within, describing nursing as "the consciousness of the unconscious, the love of life of the suicidal . . . the eyes of the newly blind, a means of locomotion for the infant . . . the voice for those too weak or withdrawn to speak" (p. 63). Watson (1985) referred to "self-healing processes," and Schlotfeldt (1994) stressed human beings' "inherent

ability and propensity to seek and attain health." In addition, this nursing process is not necessarily based upon a reversal of a disease process, but more upon a moving forward, to gain a sense of well-being in the absence or presence of disease.

The discipline's understanding of how a nursing process is manifested is shifting away from the mid 20th century mechanistic conception of nursing as a process external to patients and conducted by the nurse, that is, the old nursing process. The process of nursing is viewed now more from a relational perspective, congruent with contextual and transformative conceptions of the world (see Newman, 1992; Pepper, 1942). Nursing is a participatory process that transcends the boundary between patient and nurse and derives from a valuing of what Rogers (1980, 1992) described as human systems' inherent propensity for "innovation and creative change."

"Human systems" refers to an individual or a group of human beings (Rogers, 1992, p. 30). As such, human systems, whether in the form of individuals, dyads, groups, or communities, emanate and participate in nursing processes. Nursing processes may be manifested, for example, in the grieving that an individual experiences, in the caring that occurs among people and their families and nurses, in the healing practices shared by a culture, or in many other as yet undiscovered patterns of nursing. Today, these patterns may be described as intentional or unconscious, automatic or contemplative, relational or chemical, or simply unknown. Nevertheless, with continued nursing research, education, and practice, nursing processes can be learned and knowingly deployed to facilitate well-being. Murphy's (1992) visionary book, for example, addresses some of these possibilities. He proposes a future wherein people are more aware of their innate healing potential and employ it to more purposefully enhance health. Nightingale did not invent nursing, described here in terms of an inherent propensity for well-being. Just as earthquakes existed before geologists and photosynthesis before botanists, nursing processes existed in human beings, ultimately described by Nightingale (1859/1969) as that which nurses were to facilitate by placing the patient in the best situation possible. It follows, then, that nursing does not belong exclusively to certain groups of people, such as "well" persons or professional nurses it belongs to human nature.

Defining the substance of the discipline of nursing in terms of a well-being process inherent among human beings does not negate the importance of knowledge of factors that interface with nursing to influence well-being and healing. Examples of these factors, often the focus of study in ancillary professions and disciplines, include the environmental, financial, cultural, surgical, and pharmacological. However, any sense of well-being involves, most basically, a nursing process. The quest for nursing is to understand the nature of and to facilitate nursing processes in diverse contexts of health experiences.

The Nature of Nursing Processes

What is the nature of nursing processes that distinguishes them from other human processes? It is proposed that the intersection of at least three characteristics—complexity, integration, well-being—distinguishes human processes as nursing specifically, nursing processes are manifested by changes in complexity and integration that generate well-being. Importantly, other distinguishing characteristics of nursing processes may be identified as the dialogue continues beyond this article.

This new understanding of the nature of nursing processes derived from various theorists' work, such as von Bertalanffy's (1981) systems view of human beings Rogers' (1970, 1992) science of unitary human beings Lerner's (1986)

developmental contextualism and complexity theory (see Kauffman, 1995; Waldrop, 1992). Although the translation of these theorists' ideas may not be entirely congruent with those presented here, their ideas nonetheless can help inform development of a new nursing ontology.

Human beings are viewed as open, living systems and not as passive but intrinsically active and innovative. As an open system, human systems are capable of self-organizing, where *self* refers to the system as a whole. Self-organization is an inherent capacity for generating qualitative change out of ongoing events in the life of a system and its environment.

In his seminal work on development, Werner (1957) explained this process of qualitative change as his "orthogenetic principle," which posits that living organisms change over time from lower to higher levels of differentiation and integration. Werner (1957) called this change "development," in contrast to mechanistic processes of change, which are not developmental.

Similarly, Rogers' (1980) principles of homeodynamics describe the inherent innovative patterning of change that occurs in open systems, both environmental and human. Her three principles of helicy, resonancy, and integrality together depict the nature of qualitative change in human beings in terms of ongoing movement from lower to higher levels of diversity.

Complexity theorists (e.g., Kauffman, 1995 Waldrop, 1992) and developmentalists (e.g., Lerner, 1986; Werner, 1957) in particular have clarified a distinction between quantitative and qualitative change, both of which are necessary for development contrasting terms such as complexity and order and differentiation and organization depict this distinction. Similarly, two distinct forms of change can be identified in Rogers' (1980, 1992) works, namely diversity and innovation (Reed, 1997).

Because of the articulation between quantitative and qualitative change, human systems are not simply complex systems (SCS) but rather are complex innovative systems (CIS) (see Stites, 1994). In the context of nursing, then, nursing processes entail at least two forms of change, complexity and integration.

COMPLEXITY

Complexity refers to the number of different types of variables that can be identified in a given situation. A variable is simply something that varies (Webster's, 1979). Complexity occurs when human systems experience or express variables (e.g., life events, physiologic events) as parts, separated from the whole, rather than as patterns of the whole. Thus, for example, complexity is evident when loss of a loved one or chronic illness introduces many new and seemingly disconnected variables into an individual's life, on various levels of awareness. Increasing complexity means change in quantity (size or number) not change in quality of the whole this would become chaotic were it not accompanied by corresponding changes in integration.

INTEGRATION

Integration refers to a synthesizing and organizing of variables such that there is a change in form, not just change in size or number of events. A certain level of complexity is needed for integration to occur. Integration is evident, for example, when people construct meaning or identify a pattern in the variables or events experienced. Integration may also occur on levels of awareness that are not yet so readily apparent. Integration is trans*form*ative, involving qualitative change in form.

Well-Being

While changes in complexity and integration may be used to explain many facets of human development and systems' changes, this process may also be used to understand health, healing, and well-being. The rhythm between complexity and integration is proposed here to be a means by which innovative change occurs, as a manifestation of the underlying process called nursing. Thus, well-being may be explained in part by changes in complexity that are tempered by changes in integration. Complexity provides life with diversity, specialization, and depth in experiences, whereas integration provides organization, coherence, and breadth.

Examples of nursing processes are abundant. For example, groups incorporate new attachments or children into an organization called family. Persons with spinal cord injuries develop different pathways that link together shattered parts of life and bodily functions. Premature infants' behaviors become more innovative as they organize the complexity of their environment. Adults reminisce to integrate past life events and inevitable death. Healing after the loss of a loved one or the occurrence of chronic illness requires an integration of what seem like disjointed events and experiences, including memories of the past, future dreams, altered rhythms and routines, physical pain and other bodily symptoms, sadness, anguish, and self-doubt. Further, Sachs (1995) depicted what can be called nursing processes through his stories about people with various maladies, such as a colorblind painter and a surgeon with Tourette's syndrome. These people were able to create a new organization that fit with their altered needs and world. These health events, in all their initial complexity and heartbreak, gave way to metamorphoses and innovation. Regardless of whether there is a "cure" that can reverse a particular ailment, well-being occurs when the particulars of a life experience are brought together and synthesized in a coherent way. Any less, and people risk feeling dis-integrated, dis-associated, dis-organized.

While the centrality of well-being as a focus in nursing has been established, other disciplines also may be concerned with well-being and its correlates. However, promoting well-being based on a perspective of the inherent process of complexity and integration is distinctly nursing.

Challenging the Status Quo: Nursing Reconstructed

The definition of nursing proposed here is that of an inherent process of well-being, characterized by manifestations of complexity and integration in human systems. The substantive focus of the discipline, then, is not how nurses per se facilitate well-being but, rather, how *nursing processes* function in human systems to facilitate well-being. The focus is, in a very basic sense, how nurses can facilitate nursing.

Refocusing the Lens

This new construction of nursing provides another lens of focus for nursing researchers and practitioners. Smith (1988b) wrote metaphorically about three different camera lenses used to view human wholeness. One in particular, the motion lens, focuses on process and rhythmic flow and requires a "creative leap" to identify this process. Nurses typically encounter people in motion, in dynamic flow with their environment, whether in life-threatening experiences or perceived memory loss, chronic illness or acute pain.

The creative leap necessary for formulating the motion lens of nursing inquiry may be to address the rhythmic processes of complexity and integration that enhance well-being across these health experiences. From premature infants to dying adults and their families and communities, it is proposed that human systems have nursing processes, that is, inherent resources for well-being based on a capacity to integrate their complexities.

Debates on holism and on what represents the critical focus of nursing may be enlivened by including a new ontology of nursing—an ontology that transcends debates about part versus whole, person versus environment. Nursing processes are not necessarily bound by dimensions such as biologic, environmental, or social. Instead, the lens is focused on any human process that manifests complexity and integration related to well-being. Looking through this new lens, researchers and practitioners may identify a myriad of human manifestations of wholeness, whether they be labeled physiologic, phylogenic, or philosophic, that are integral to well-being.

Nursing as a Metaparadigm Concept

Given this reconstructed view of nursing, as a substantive focus of the discipline, the term *nursing* should be a central concept in the nursing metaparadigm. In the past, for good reason, some have suggested the elimination of the term nursing from the metaparadigm (Conway, 1985). However, rather than remove the term nursing from the metaparadigm, this fin-de-siècle may be the time in nursing history to consider renaming the discipline to something other than a verb, to better distinguish the disciplinary label from the substantive focus of the science and practice.

To help clarify this distinction, a term such as Paterson and Zderad's (1976) "nursology," or another disciplinary label with the "nurs" prefix could be developed, while reserving the term *nursing* as the process word and verb that it is, for the metaparadigm. By identifying nursing as a substantive, metaparadigm concept, nurses can better claim their unique focus and clarify the ontology of their discipline.

Approaching the Frontier

Rogers (1992) explained that one could not push back the frontier of knowledge until one approached it. This article has not been about maintaining the status quo but about approaching a frontier so that others might join in a dialogue that pushes back the frontier a bit more. In this era of healthcare reform, the discipline must define nursing as nurses truly envision it and not necessarily as others would have it be defined. Nurses may decide against renaming the discipline as was suggested here. Nevertheless, within a broadened and partially reconstructed view of the discipline that embraces nursing at its most fundamental meaning, new understandings that blend with the old can emerge to present a fuller picture of the discipline.

Nursing (as practice and praxis) is a way of doing that creates good actions that facilitate well-being. Nursing (as syntax and science) is a way of knowing that creates goods in the form of knowledge, and nursing (the substance and ontology) is a way of being that creates patterns of changing complexity and integration experienced as well-being in human systems.

Nurses are invited to try on the substantive definition of nursing to see how it fits within the context of their practice and science. Ongoing philosophic dialogue about the ontology of the discipline will help ensure that nurse theorists are theorists of nursing in its fullest sense and, likewise, that nurse researchers are researchers of nursing and that nurse practitioners are practitioners of nursing.

References

Conway, M. E. (1985). Toward greater specificity in defining nursing's metaparadigm. *Advances in Nursing Science, 7*(4), 73–81.

Ellis, R. (1982). Conceptual issues in nursing. *Nursing Outlook, 30*(7), 406–410.

Henderson, V. (1964). The nature of nursing. *American Journal of Nursing, 64*(8), 62–68.

Kauffman, S. (1995). *At home in the universe: The search for laws of self-organization and complexity.* New York: Oxford University Press.

Laird, C. (1971). *Webster's new world thesaurus* (rev. ed.). New York: Simon and Schuster.

Lerner, R. M. (1986). *Concepts and theories of human development* (2nd ed.). New York: Random House.

Murphy, M. (1992). *The future of the body: Explorations into the further evolution of human nature.* New York: J.P. Tarcher.

Newman, M. (1992). Prevailing paradigms in nursing. *Nursing Outlook, 40,* 10–13.

Nightingale, F. (1969). *Notes on nursing: What it is and what it is not.* New York: Dover. (Original work published 1859)

Paterson, J. G., & Zderad, L. T. (1976). *Humanistic nursing.* New York: Wiley.

Pepper, S. P. (1942). *World hypotheses: A study in evidence.* Berkeley: University of California Press.

Rampragus, V. (1995). *The deconstruction of nursing.* Brookfield, VT: Ashgate.

Reed, P. G. (1995). A treatise on nursing knowledge development for the 21st century: Beyond postmodernism. *Advances in Nursing Science, 17*(3), 70–84.

Reed, P. G. (1997). The place of transcendence in nursing's science of unitary human beings. In M. Madrid (Ed.), *Patterns of Rogerian knowing* (pp. 187–196). New York: National League for Nursing Press.

Rogers, M. E. (1970). *Introduction to the theoretical basis of nursing.* Philadelphia: F. A. Davis.

Rogers, M. E. (1980). A science of unitary man. In J. P. Riehl & C. Roy (Eds.), *Conceptual models for nursing practice* (2nd ed., pp. 329–337). New York: Appleton-Century-Crofts.

Rogers, M. E. (1992). Nursing science and the space age. *Nursing Science Quarterly, 5,* 27–34.

Roy, C. L. (1995). Developing nursing knowledge: Practice issues raised from four philosophical perspectives. *Nursing Science Quarterly, 8,* 79–85.

Sachs, O. (1995). *An anthropologist on Mars: Seven paradoxical tales.* New York: A. Knopf.

Schlotfeldt, R. (1994). Resolving opposing viewpoints: Is it desirable? Is it practicable? In J. F. Kikuchi & H. Simmons (Eds.), *Developing a philosophy of nursing* (pp. 67–74). Thousand Oaks, CA: Sage.

Smith, M. J. (1988a). Nursing: What's in a name? *Nursing Science Quarterly, 1,* 142–143.

Smith, M. J. (1988b). Perspectives of wholeness: The lens makes a difference. *Nursing Science Quarterly, 1,* 94–95.

Stites, J. (1994). Complexity research on complex systems and complex adaptive systems. *Omni, 16*(8), 42–50.

von Bertalanffy, L. (1981). *A systems view of man* (P. A. La Violette, Ed.). Boulder, CO: Westview Press.

Waldrop, M. M. (1992). *Complexity: The emerging science at the edge of order and chaos.* New York: Simon and Schuster.

Watson, J. (1985). *Nursing: Human science and human care.* Norwalk, CT: Appleton-Century-Crofts.

Watson, J. (1995). Postmodernism and knowledge development in nursing. *Nursing Science Quarterly, 8,* 60–64.

Webster's new collegiate dictionary. (1979). Springfield, MA: G. & C. Merriam Co.

Werner, H. (1957). The concept of development from a comparative and organismic point of view. In D. B. Harris (Ed.), *The concept of development* (pp. 125–148). Minneapolis: University of Minnesota Press.

Chapter 15

A Dialectical Examination of Nursing Art

Joy L. Johnson,
RN, PhD

Literature relevant to the art of nursing is immensely diverse and fragmented. This state is problematic in that progress in understanding nursing art cannot be made until the subject of nursing art is clearly delineated. In light of the need for conceptual clarity regarding nursing art, a dialectical study was undertaken to identify the distinct conceptions of nursing art that are represented in the nursing literature. The examined discourse was that contained in the works of 41 nursing scholars published between 1860 and 1992. The analysis revealed five distinct conceptualizations that can be identified as the art of (1) grasping meaning in patient encounters, (2) establishing a meaningful connection with the patient, (3) skillfully performing nursing activities, (4) rationally determining an appropriate course of nursing action, and (5) morally conducting one's nursing practice.

It is often said that nursing is an art and a science. Unfortunately, what is meant by the term *nursing art* is not well delineated or understood. In examining the theoretical issues nurses have concerned themselves with, it is clear that the majority of time and effort has been spent considering the nature of nursing science. Although numerous descriptions and definitions of nursing art have been suggested, little effort has been expended to analyze those definitions or to enter into a dialogue regarding the nature of nursing art.

Science alone will not solve all of the problems of nursing. Nursing is, after all, a practice discipline. Guidance regarding the use or application of scientific findings does not emanate from nursing science itself. As Ellis indicated, nursing

is much more than the application of scientific findings. The practitioner cannot just "select from a rack of ready-to-wear theories."[1(p. 1434)] It is therefore essential that the manner in which knowledge, judgment, and skill are used in the clinical setting be carefully considered. These phenomena fall generally under the rubric of the art of nursing. Ultimately, an understanding of nursing art will further an understanding of how excellence can best be pursued and achieved in nursing practice.

The characterization of nursing as an art is not a recent development, and the literature relevant to the art of nursing is immensely diverse. It includes works such as Nightingale's[2] *Notes on Nursing* and Benner's[3] *From Novice to Expert*. Despite the abundance of writings on the topic of the art of nursing, there have been few instances in which nursing scholars have

Source: Johnson J. L. (1994). A dialectical examination of nursing art. *ANS, 17*(1):1–14.

addressed one another's positions. This failure is due in part to the fact that nursing scholars have tended to pursue their conceptions of nursing art in isolation and have not considered other conceptions. Nursing scholars have not confronted one another in light of their differences, resulting in the current situation in which a plethora of diverse views concerning the art of nursing are relatively unquestioned and unexplored.

Schlotfeldt[4] pointed out that the future of the nursing profession depends on the ability of its members to identify and resolve issues. Yet nurses will be unable to resolve issues related to the art of nursing unless the subject at issue is clearly set forth. Walker identified the need for such an analysis when she argued that the controversy regarding the art of nursing "has been difficult to resolve for the point of contention has not been clearly set forth."[5(p. 118)] The tremendous diversity of ideas regarding the art of nursing expressed in the nursing literature will remain a source of confusion unless the diversities are put in order and rendered intelligible. When differences of opinion remain implicit, or even concealed, as in the nursing discourse relevant to the art of nursing, they cannot serve as the basis for the collective effort required to further thought.

In light of the state of fragmentation that characterizes the nursing literature relevant to the subject of nursing art, a philosophic study was undertaken to discover the common ground that underlies the differences of opinion regarding the art of nursing and to transmute the current diversity into rational and intelligible controversy. This study sought to render the existing diversity more intelligible so that a rational debate of fundamental issues can proceed and a better understanding of nursing art can be attained.

Method

The approach that was taken for this study was a critical examination and systematic analysis of the nursing discourse concerning the art of nursing. The method is one developed by Adler[6] and

his colleagues at the Institute for Philosophical Research in Chicago to examine the controversies that surround such philosophic ideas as freedom, love, and equality. The aim of this method, which Adler[6] referred to as a *dialectical approach*, is to outline and clarify the structure of a controversy, and it involves a process of constructive interpretation. The goal of this philosophic method is to explicitly formulate patterns of agreement and disagreement. The challenge of the dialectical method is to achieve a nonpartisan treatment of positions or views. The dialectical task, therefore, involves rendering an objective, impartial, and neutral report of a many-sided discussion. Using this approach, the dialectician examines and clarifies what is implicit in the discourse. By way of constructive interpretation, the researcher attempts to find similarities and dissimilarities among the various conceptions.

Although the works examined in this study are historical in the sense that they date to a specific time and place, the intent of this study was to examine the ideas contained in them apart from their historical context. The study was in no way historical in its aim or its method. Therefore, for the purpose of this study, it was assumed that the authors concerned with the art of nursing are engaged in a continuing dialogue, even though they belong to different historical periods.

The point of departure for this study was the manifold and often confusing diversity that exists on the subject of nursing art. The general subject of nursing art includes a broad field of discourse and covers a variety of themes. Rather than seeking to include the work of every nursing author who has written on the subject of nursing art, a sample of works was required that was representative of the existing diversity of views regarding the art of nursing. Literature that was broadly related to the topic of nursing art was included in the study. In total, the works of 41 authors composed the examined discourse. The findings reported here are part of a larger study[7] that examined the issues and controversies that exist regarding nursing art.

Distinct Conceptualizations of Nursing Art

Based on an examination of the nursing litera-ture related to the art of nursing, it was conclud-ed that there are diverse answers to the question "what is the art of nursing?" The use of the term *art of nursing* in no way ensures that those involved in the discourse refer to the same sub-ject. Part of the dialectical task involved deter-mining whether there are distinct conceptions of the subject within the examined discourse. The questions that guided this determination includ-ed "is *art* being used in the same sense?" and "does the discussion involve one subject or sever-al distinct subjects?" To identify the distinct conceptualizations of nursing art, each work was carefully read, and relevant passages believed to be germane to the topic were noted. Ties of rele-vance that connected the various authors were sought, and points of agreement were estab-lished. These points of agreement served to delineate each distinct conceptualization.

In examining the discourse, it was found that there were five separate senses of "nursing art." They can be described as

1. The nurse's ability to grasp meaning in patient encounters
2. The nurse's ability to establish a meaning-ful connection with the patient
3. The nurse's ability to skillfully perform nursing activities
4. The nurse's ability to rationally determine an appropriate course of nursing action
5. The nurse's ability to morally conduct his or her nursing practice

It should be pointed out that although the authors who have written about nursing art pro-vide evidence for the construction of these con-ceptions, the identification of these conceptions is not theirs per se. It should also be noted that although these subjects are mutually exclusive,

most authors have conceptualized nursing art as consisting of more than one ability therefore, these authors are viewed as addressing more than one conception of nursing art. Finally, it cannot be concluded that an author's apparent silence on a particular conceptualization of nursing art indicates a denial of that conceptualization. The descriptions that follow focus primarily on the similarities of thought regarding each concep-tion, rather than the issues, or points of disagree-ment, that exist regarding these conceptions.

Ability to Grasp Meaning in Patient Encounters

The situations that confront nurses are often characterized by uncertainty, ambiguity, and indeterminacy.[8] This is due in part to the fact that nursing practice situations are complex. The complexity of a patient's situation can be further compounded when patients are unable to articu-late their needs, either because they are unaware of the needs or because they are incapacitated.[9] Consequently, the nurse must grasp the meaning of each particular patient situation and deter-mine what in the situation is relevant. For select authors,[3,8–33] nursing art involves the ability to grasp meaning in patient encounters. According to these authors, the artful nurse, as compared with the nurse who lacks art, can grasp what is significant in a particular patient situation. The term grasping meaning is used here to describe the process of attaching significance to those things that can be felt, observed, heard, touched, tasted, smelled, or imagined, including emo-tions, objects, gestures, and sounds.

Although marked variation can be found among the descriptions of the authors who have been construed to conceptualize nursing art as the grasping of meaning, several points of agree-ment can be found. First, nursing art is seen as based in an immediate perceptual capacity and is not affected by the intellect. This capacity to grasp meaning is often referred to as intuition. Rather than being based in reflection, or reasoning, the art of nursing according to this view is based in an immediate perceptual capacity that is more integrated than simple sensation and more concrete than intellection it is based in a capacity that involves the external senses as well as the imagination.

Using this capacity, the artful nurse attributes meaning to things that are felt, observed, or imagined. It is the artful nurse who can *sense* the meaning or significance of a situation, such as when a patient is distraught, *perceive* patterns, such as the set of signs and symptoms that indicate when a patient is going into cardiogenic shock, have a *feel* for what he or she is doing or sense what should be done, such as *knowing* when to use humor to help relieve the tension of a situation. Thus, Chinn and Kramer stated, "Esthetic knowing is what makes possible knowing what to do with the moment, instantly, without conscious deliberation."[14(p. 10)] Nursing art is thought to involve the direct apprehension of what is to be done, or what is the case, and is unmediated by concepts. The immediacy of the art of grasping meaning was emphasized by Benner and Wrubel, who argued that "the person does not assign meanings to the situation once it is apprehended because the very act of apprehension is based on taken-for-granted meanings embedded in skills, practices, and language."[9(p. 42)]

A second point of agreement is that the art of grasping meaning results in a form of understanding that defies accurate or complete description. The insights gained by this perceptual ability are thought to be tacit, nonpropositional, personal, and as such incommunicable. Carper, for example, argued that esthetic knowing is gained by "subjective acquaintance, the direct feeling of an experience"[13(p. 149)] and that this knowing defies discursive formulation. The meanings that the artful nurse grasps are concrete and individual, pertaining to a particular patient situation (e.g., this particular patient that I am nursing and can observe in front of me

who happens to have had an appendectomy), rather than abstract, pertaining to patients in general (e.g., appendectomy patients). Orlando emphasized this distinction when she stated that the nurse must distinguish between general principles and "the meanings which she must discover in the immediate nursing situation in order to help the patient."[25(p. 1)]

A third point of agreement to be found is that the art of grasping meaning is a perceptual ability that can be honed and developed over time. Rew,[31] for example, argued that the nurse can learn to become sensitive to the signals and feelings that he or she experiences and, over time, can learn to understand their significance. Similarly, Newman[21] argued that nurses can learn to attend to and trust their inner experiences. Benner[3] contended that perceptual abilities are formed by previous experiences and by immersion in the present perceptual environment. Consequently, the information taken in by the senses is endowed with meaning. According to Benner,[3] it is through experience that the nurse learns to immediately focus on what is relevant in a patient situation and to grasp its meaning. Using past experiences, or foreknowledge, the artful nurse has the ability to recognize patterns and can therefore make sense of ambiguous, unstructured situations. According to Benner, "Past concrete experience . . . guides the expert's perceptions and actions and allows for a rapid perceptual grasp of the situation."[3(pp. 8–9)]

Finally, according to those who affirm this first conception of nursing art, the art of nursing is a holistic capacity. The nurse's perceptual ability allows him or her to immediately grasp the meaning of a situation, instead of piecing together an understanding of what is happening. In contrast, the nurse who is not artful must assess every minute detail, breaking down a situation into its component parts to discover what is of significance. Benner and Wrubel described the artful capacity as "a perceptual awareness that singles out relevant information from irrelevant, grasps a situation as a whole rather than as a series of tasks, and accomplishes this rapidly and without incremental deliberative analysis of isolated facts or bits of information."[10(p. 13)]

Ability to Establish a Meaningful Connection with the Patient

The connection between the nurse and the patient is considered by many authors[13–18, 21–24,26–30,34–43] to be of particular importance, particularly in the current era of increasing technology. Many emphasize that it is the artful nurse's interactions that can bridge the gap introduced by technology and that such interactions can promote "wholeness and integrity in the personal encounter, the achievement of engagement rather than detachment, and . . . [denial of] the manipulative impersonal orientation."[13(p. 156)] *Connection*, as it is used here, refers to an attachment, or union, that occurs between patients and their nurses. The term *connection* is used because, unlike the term *relationship*, it encompasses short-term or fleeting encounters as well as long-term associations. According to these authors, a meaningful connection between the nurse and the patient is central to the provision of nursing care, as it is through this connection that services such as physical and emotional support are offered and accepted. Kim,[39] for example, pointed out that the core of nursing resides in human-to-human actions. Similarly, Gadow suggested that the central question in nursing is not "how can we help them [patients] to recover?" but, instead, "how can we recover them [and] overcome the distance between us?"[16(p. 12)]

The second conception of nursing art is distinguished by four major points. First, it is contended that nursing art is nondiscursive that is, it is expressed in the nurse's actions or behaviors. According to those who hold this second conception of nursing art, the art of nursing is "unmediated by conceptual categories."[13(p. 154)] It cannot be expressed through words instead, it is expressed in the concrete actions and gestures of the artful nurse in response to a particular patient. Paterson and Zderad argued that "nursing is an experience lived between human beings"[28(p. 3)] and that nursing art is evident in the synchronicity between the nurse and the patient.

Second, it is contended that its expressive nature constitutes an essential characteristic of nursing art. Chinn and Kramer maintained that this expression takes the form of "human actions—words, behaviors, and other symbols—that give communicable form to what we know."[14(p. 6)] Although it is agreed that nursing art is expressive, there is little agreement regarding what exactly is expressed in nursing art. For some authors, emotions play an important role in the origin of art. For example, Watson[41] argued that through their art, nurses express emotions or feelings. The work of Pep lau[29] suggested that the expression of nursing art is appropriately limited to the expression of sentiments such as concern, compassion, and caring. Paterson and Zderad,[28] on the other hand, suggested that nursing art involves the expression of the nurse's state of being.

Third, it is argued that the art of nursing occurs in relation to another human being. The ideas of philosopher Martin Buber[44] are echoed frequently in the works of authors who have conceptualized nursing art as the ability to establish a meaningful connection. Buber[44] posited that relationships are of two kinds. The first is a subject-to-subject, or "I–Thou," relationship, which is a relationship of connectedness and affirmation of another person's being. The second type of relationship is subject to object, or "I–It," which arises out of a stance of separation and detachment, in which the individual is differentiated over and against a world of objects. Authors who hold that nursing art is establishing a meaningful connection with the patient contend that nursing art can only occur when the nurse stands in a subject-to-subject relationship with the patient. For example, Paterson and Zderad stated, "If she enters into genuine relation with the patient (I–Thou) her effective power (caring, nursing skills, hope) brings forth form (well-being, more-being, comfort, growth)."[28(p. 92)]

Finally, the authors who support the view that nursing art is the ability to establish a meaningful connection are in agreement regarding the necessity of authenticity on the part of the nurse. Bishop and Scudder argued that "the inauthentic nurse merely plays the role of nurse rather than really being a nurse."[34(p. 102)] It is held that the artful nurse must be genuine, any attempt to mask or hide feelings will serve only to distance the nurse from the patient, thereby threatening the relationship between the nurse and the patient. Parse[26] referred to this authenticity as genuine or true presence. Similarly, Watson asserted that "the degree of transpersonal caring (in this sense of unity of feeling) is increased by the degree of genuineness and sincerity of the nurse."[41(p. 69)]

Ability to Skillfully Perform Nursing Activities

The conceptualization of nursing art as the skillful performance of nursing activities is one of the earliest conceptions of nursing art found in the nursing discourse.[2,3,5,9–12,45–59] It is from this view that we see in early nursing curricula the attainment of nursing skills being referred to generally as the "nursing arts." Price contended that nursing art involves the ability to "recognize the nursing needs of the patient and to develop skill, through practice, in various procedures designed to answer those needs."[54(p. 19)] According to the authors who hold the view that nursing art is the ability to skillfully perform nursing activities, the artful nurse is one who has a demonstrable capacity to effectively carry

out nursing procedures and techniques. *Skill*, as it is used here, refers to a developed proficiency or dexterity. *Nursing activities* are all those tasks, procedures, and techniques that a nurse carries out in his or her practice.

The focus of these authors' conceptualizations of nursing art is an array of activities both manual and verbal in nature. For example, we see in the work of Nightingale[50] a list of behaviors that the good nurse must demonstrate. These behaviors include such things as moving silently through the sickroom, keeping constant watch over the sick, and airing out the sickroom on a regular basis. Nightingale[50] expected the artful nurse to do more than understand these edicts. She expected these behaviors to be instantiated in the nurse's practice the artful nurse knows more than what is to be done, she knows "how to do it."[50(p. 1)] Wiedenbach[58] numbered among the skills the nurse must possess the ability to perform back rubs, to take a pulse, and to help a patient walk as well as the ability to handle necessary equipment, such as a cardiac pacemaker and the circular–electric bed: "These skills involve manipulations and techniques—executed with finesse to achieve desired results."[58(p. 28)]

Those who hold this third conception of nursing art were found to be in agreement regarding three central points. First, according to the authors, the art of nursing is primarily a behavioral ability that is, it involves observable actions and focuses on the process of doing, rather than the process of knowing. As such, it is concerned with the nurse's demonstrable ability, not his or her knowledge per se. Heidgerken made this distinction clear when she stated, "The principles, procedures, and technics, or science, of nursing are learned in the classroom. The art, or skill, of nursing is learned on the ward."[48(p. 9)] Although there is agreement among the authors who hold this third conception that nursing art is ultimately a behavioral ability, there is no consensus regarding the role that one's intellectual capacity plays in the art of nursing. Some theorists argue that the activities must be intelligently performed. Montag,[49] for example, contended that skill without understanding is mere imitation. Similarly, Heidgerken[48] contended that the memorization and demonstration of step-by-step procedures will not produce an artful nurse. Tracy, on the other hand, contended that "the nurse should have so mastered her procedures that the minimum of thought is needed for their use."[57(p. 29)] Similarly, Benner and Wrubel[9] argued that nurse's everyday actions are effective not because they think about them, or base them on theory, but because they have a sophisticated repertoire of reactions.

Second, those who conceptualize nursing art as skillful performance of nursing activities are in agreement about the claim that nursing art can be learned. Key to learning the art of nursing are persistent practice and repetition. Goodrich maintained that practical experience for student nurses should be "sufficiently long to allow of a constant repetition of procedures."[47(p. 42)] Heidgerken, however, warned that practice alone is not enough and that "the attitude of the learner, the will to improve, and eradication of mistakes are all equally as important as practice."[48(p. 54)]

Finally, there is also evidence of agreement regarding the fact that certain criteria can be used to judge the art of nursing. When discussing the art of nursing, these theorists inevitably use descriptors such as fluidity of movement, adroitness, coordination, and efficiency. Stewart indicated that nursing art involves "manual dexterity, lightness, steadiness, quickness of movement, strength, endurance, and that complete coordination of head and muscle which cannot be acquired except by long, directed training."[55(pp. 324–325)] Similarly, Heidgerken[48] argued that the artful nurse's activities must have the appropriate form, elimination of excess movements, appropriate timing, force, and coordination are among the qualities that characterize the activities of the artful nurse.

Ability to Determine Rationally an Appropriate Course of Nursing Action

For those[2,4,5,25,39,40,45,46,48–53,55,56,58–78] who support the fourth conception of nursing art, intellectual activity is essential to the performance of nursing care. According to this fourth conception, nursing art refers to the nurse's ability to rationally determine an appropriate course of nursing action. The term rational ability, as it is used here, refers to the intellectual ability to effectively draw valid conclusions from existing knowledge.

This fourth conception of nursing art is characterized by five points of agreement. First, it is argued that nursing art is practical in nature. According to these authors, the aim of this ability is the determination of an appropriate course of action. Nursing art, it is argued, is action oriented and not simply aimed at understanding. Beckstrand,[60] for example, contended that the aim of nursing art is the control of practice. Dickoff and James[62] concluded that nursing art is concerned ultimately with producing nursing situations. Similarly, Orlando contended that nursing art is a rational capacity that is aimed at "helping the patient."[25(p. 70)]

Second, it is contended that there is an underlying discipline on which nursing art rests. All of the authors who contend that nursing art is a rational ability emphasize the importance of knowledge, specifically scientific knowledge, to nursing art. Orem stated, "The art of nursing is the nurse's quality or habit of reasoning and judging correctly about the design and production of the kind and amount of nursing needed according to the principles or laws of nursing itself. Science and technique are 'the first necessary conditions for honest art.' The point of view of nursing as art therefore encompasses the point of view of *nursing as knowledge*."[52(p. 24)]

Arguments about the importance of knowledge for nursing art are often tied to the claim that nursing is a profession. Abdellah and colleagues, for example, argued, "Professionalization of nursing requires that nurses identify those nursing problems that depend for their solution upon the nurse's use of her capacities to conceptualize events and make judgments about them. Nurses need to become skilled in recognizing both overt and covert nursing problems, in analyzing them in terms of relevant principles and in working out courses of action by applying nursing principles."[45(p. 11)] It was assumed by Abdellah et al.,[45] as it was by all of the authors who support this fourth conceptualization of nursing art, that the nursing profession possesses a distinct body of knowledge and that this body of knowledge provides the foundation for nursing practice.

Leininger[73] also contended that nursing art is based on scientific knowledge. She believed that nurses must, if they are to be effective, "scientifically care" for their patients. *Scientific caring*, according to Leininger, "refers to those judgments and acts of helping others based upon tested or verified knowledge."[73(p. 46)] The importance of knowledge to artful practice is echoed by all of the authors. Kim stated, "Knowledge is antecedent to action."[39(p. 146)] Diers contended that "nursing practice is done consciously, if not always with a formal plan, that it is not done mindlessly."[65(p. 31)] Finally, Rogers claimed that "the art of nursing develops only as it incorporates more and more of science unto itself. The nature of its art lies in the core of scientific knowledge it embodies."[75(p. 32)]

The third point of agreement regarding the art of rationally determining an appropriate course of nursing action is that it presupposes that nurses possess a thorough understanding of what is before them and the actions they should take. According to this perspective, the artful nurse solves problems by selecting the intervention that is best suited to the intended end. This process of instrumental problem solving involves a thorough consideration of the facts of

a situation and is made rigorous by the application of scientific theory. For example, Johnson[70] argued that an artful nurse thinks "logically, soundly, and searchingly" about the causes and effects in a given nursing situation. The key point is that the artful nurse's actions are not "automatic" or "blind" but instead are grounded in an intellectual activity, in which knowledge or information of certain kinds is considered to determine which actions will result in the best possible patient outcome.

Fourth, it is contended that the art of rationally determining an appropriate course of nursing action involves a process of logical reasoning in which scientific principles and theories are applied to problems identified in practice. According to this view, the artful nurse uses evidence to reason through the best course of action to be followed. Beckstrand described this process in the following manner:

> *Once the conditions requiring changes in the client's situation are determined, a practitioner examines the situation to identify the possibility of making the changes desired. First, a practitioner uses scientific knowledge of necessary and sufficient conditions to determine if desired changes are realizable. Next, a practitioner examines the situation to determine whether conditions for achieving the desired changes exist. . . . As a result, the set of realizable outcomes in practice is determined by what is scientifically possible within the exigencies of the practice situation.*[61(p. 177)]

The steps of the nursing process (assessment, planning, implementation, and evaluation) are seen as the steps that an artful nurse takes to ensure quality patient care. The emphasis of this approach is on deliberate, systematic, and scientifically based care.

Finally, it is contended by those who hold the fourth conception of nursing art that the art of nursing can be judged according to certain standards. They agree that the appropriateness of a nursing action can be judged on the basis of whether the identified course of action enabled the practitioner to attain his or her identified goals or standards. For example, Henderson[37] contended that a nurse's art can be evaluated according to the degree to which the patient has reestablished independence. Some authors have suggested additional criteria for evaluation. Dickoff, James, and Wiedenbach,[63] for example, suggested that nursing art can be evaluated using the criteria of coherency, palatability, and feasibility.

Ability to Conduct One's Nursing Practice Morally

For a final group of authors,[2,3,9,11,15–18,34,38,47,50–53,60,61,67,68,79–81] nursing art involves the ability of the nurse to practice morally: The nurse is obligated to practice in such a way that seeks to avoid harm and to benefit the patient. The term moral, as it is used here, refers to that which is good, or desirable, for human beings. These authors are in agreement regarding four central points. First, it is held that good or excellent nursing practice is, by necessity, moral in that it is directed toward the good of the patient. As Goodrich stated, "So much is nursing of the essence of ethics that it is consistent to assert that the terms good and ethical as applied to nursing practice are synonymous."[47(p. 5)] Conversely, the view that nursing art can under any circumstances be amoral or immoral is antithetical to this position. Indeed, for these authors, the moral aspect of nursing cannot be separated from the notion of excellence in nursing, either existentially or analytically. This is the case, it is argued, because unlike the fine arts, nursing is an art that deals directly with human beings. Artful nursing, Curtin[79] asserted, is inextricably entwined with human life and the achievement of particular human ends.

According to those who hold that nursing is a moral art, a nurse may be technically competent and knowledgeable, yet if he or she does not make moral choices in the performance of patient care, he or she is not artful. Lanara[81] argued that values and ideals must guide the nurse's care. In a similar fashion, Gadow[17] posited that good nursing is more than a cluster of techniques in that it involves a commitment to a moral end and is directed and judged by that end. This position is also supported by Bishop and Scudder, who argued that the artful nurse's ability consists in more than the ability to efficiently complete tasks: "[The] technician uses techniques which are evaluated by efficiency whereas, the professional makes decisions which are evaluated by the good."[34(p. 69)]

Second, it is held that the possession of skill and knowledge are necessary, but not sufficient, conditions for the moral conduct of nursing practice. Indeed, it is presupposed by many of these authors that the artful nurse must be competent in his or her practice. As Curtin[80] pointed out, the license to practice nursing does not include permission to practice poorly. In stating that one is a professional, one is claiming a certain level of competence.

Third, it is argued by those who hold that nursing art is the ability to morally conduct one's practice that nursing art involves a commitment to care competently for patients. Curtin stated that "although knowledge and skill are integral to the practice of a profession, the foundation consists of the performative declarations professed by its practitioners and the fidelity of the practitioner to these promises."[80(pp. 101–102)] The moral responsibility to nurse well involves a commitment not only to nurse a patient competently, but to "sustain excellent practice in the face of unreasonable demands and lack of appreciation on the part of patients."[35(p. 37)] The artful nurse not only must be competent, but must also consistently demonstrate competence in his or her practice, no matter how arduous the circumstances.

Finally, the notion that the artful nurse must possess moral virtues is reiterated in various forms by all of the authors who ascribe to the notion that the art of nursing is of a moral nature. Expressed in all of their works is the belief that the artful nurse must be properly motivated in his or her action. Rather than being motivated by self-aggrandizement or expediency, the artful nurse is motivated by care and concern for others. Benner and Wrubel suggested that the same act done in a caring and uncaring way may have different effects and that only a nurse who cares about his or her patients will notice small differences in their behaviors and create unique solutions to patient problems: "Caring makes the nurse notice which interventions help, and this concern guides subsequent caregiving. Caring causes the nurse to notice subtle signs of improvement or deterioration in the patient. In fact, caring . . . is required for expert human practice."[9(p. 4)]

Accordingly, the nurse who does not care about his or her patient cannot nurse well. Lanara[81] argued that the ability to care about patients rests on the nurse's capacity to love others and that nurses, inspired by the ideal of love, will care not only for, but about, their patients. It is love, according to Lanara,[81] that allows the nurse to transcend obstacles and become heroic in his or her nursing practice.

Conclusion

Through the identification of these five conceptions of nursing art, nurses can begin to understand the structure of the discourse regarding nursing art. After one goes beyond the description of the five conceptions identified, differences of opinion can be found among the authors who affirm a particular conception of nursing art. Indeed, each of the five conceptions is a subject of controversy in that each comprises numerous conceptual, existential, and normative issues.

It is evident that although nursing scholars have written about the subject of nursing art, few have acknowledged one another's conceptions. Indeed, to date, there has been little recognition that different conceptions of nursing art exist. When one examines the discourse regarding the art of nursing, it is clear that not all of the authors agree about the nature of nursing art. This state of affairs is consistent with the state of the nursing discourse in general. Kikuchi and Simmons accurately characterized this state of affairs when they stated

> *Although nursing scholars are prone to speak or write on the same topic, use the same words, or express a common interest in knowledge development, there is very little in their productions to indicate that they share to any great degree a common understanding, a coming-to-terms, that would allow for the minimal topical agreement required before questions can be commonly interpreted, controversies identified, issues debated, and answers commonly agreed upon.*[82(p. 3)]

It is hoped that the identification of distinct conceptions of nursing art will facilitate productive debate and analysis among nursing's scholars.

The method employed in this research is limited in that it does not answer the question "what is nursing art?" The next step must be taken: to examine each of these conceptualizations in detail to determine which conceptualization or group of conceptualizations is sound. The findings of this study provide the groundwork for future philosophic analyses, thereby bringing nursing one step closer toward a sound conception of nursing art. It is only when a sound conception of nursing art is developed that nursing will be able to answer questions regarding how nursing art should be pursued and developed. It is hoped that nursing scholars in the future will dispute the nature of nursing art more explicitly and extensively.

References

1. Ellis R. The practitioner as theorist. *Am J Nurs.* 1969;69:1434–1438.

2. Nightingale F. *Notes on Nursing: What It Is, and What It Is Not.* New York: Dover; 1969.

3. Benner P. *From Novice to Expert: Excellence and Power in Clinical Nursing Practice.* Menlo Park, CA: Addison-Wesley; 1984.

4. Schlotfeldt RM. Resolution of issues: An imperative for creating nursing's future. *J Prof Nurs.* 1987;3: 136–142.

5. Walker LO. *Nursing as a Discipline.* Bloomington, IN: Indiana University; 1971. Dissertation.

6. Adler MJ. *The Idea of Freedom, I: A Dialectical Examination of the Conceptions of Freedom.* Garden City, NY: Doubleday; 1958.

7. Johnson JL. *Toward a Clearer Understanding of the Art of Nursing.* Edmonton, Alberta, Canada: University of Alberta; 1993. Dissertation.

8. Tanner C. Curriculum revolution: The practice mandate. In: *Curriculum Revolution: Mandate for Change.* New York: National League for Nursing; 1988:201–216.

9. Benner P, Wrubel J. *The Primacy of Caring: Stress and Coping in Health and Illness.* Menlo Park, CA: Addison-Wesley; 1989.

10. ———. Skilled clinical knowledge: The value of perceptual awareness. *Nurs Educ.* 1982;7(3):11–17.

11. Benner P. The role of experience, narrative, and community in skilled ethical comportment. *ANS.* 1991;14(2):1–21.

12. Benner P, Tanner C, Chesla C. From beginner to expert: Gaining a differentiated clinical world in critical care nursing. *ANS.* 1992;14(3):13–28.

13. Carper BA. *Fundamental Patterns of Knowing in Nursing.* New York: Teachers College, Columbia University; 1975.

14. Chinn PL, Kramer MK. *Theory and Nursing: A Systematic Approach,* 3rd ed. St. Louis: Mosby–Yearbook; 1991.

15. Gadow S. Clinical subjectivity: Advocacy with silent patients. *Nurs Clin North Am.* 1989;24:535–541.

16. ———. *Beyond Dualism: The Dialectic of Caring and Knowing.* Presented at the conference "The Care-Justice Puzzle: Education for Ethical Nursing Practice" at the University of Minnesota; October 13, 1990; Minneapolis, MN.

17. ———. Nurse and patient: The caring relationship. In: Bishop AH, Scudder JR, eds. *Caring, Curing, Coping: Nurse, Physician, Patient Relationships.* Tuscaloosa, AL: University of Alabama Press; 1985:31–43.

18. ———. Body and self: A dialectic. *J Med Philos.* 1980;5:172–185.

19. Moccia PA. A critique of compromise: Beyond the methods debate. *ANS.* 1988;10(4):1–9.

20. ———. *A Study of the Theory-Practice Dialectic: Towards a Critique of the Science of Man.* New York: New York University; 1980. Dissertation.

21. Newman MA. The spirit of nursing. *Holistic Nurs Pract.* 1989;3(3):1–6.

22. ———. *Health as Expanding Consciousness.* St. Louis: Mosby; 1986.

23. ———. Newman's theory of health as praxis. *Nurs Sci Q.* 1990;3:37–41.

24. ———, Sime AM, Corcoran-Perry SA. The focus of the discipline of nursing. *ANS.* 1991;14(1):1–6.

25. Orlando IJ. *The Dynamic Nurse-Patient Relationship: Function, Process and Principles.* New York: G.P. Putnam's Sons; 1961.

26. Parse RR. Human becoming: Parse's theory of nursing. *Nurs Sci Q.* 1992;5:35–42.

27. ———. *Man-Living-Health: A Theory of Nursing.* New York: Wiley; 1981.

28. Paterson JG, Zderad LT. *Humanistic Nursing.* New York: National League for Nursing; 1988.

29. Peplau HE. The art and science of nursing: Similarities, differences, and relations. *Nurs Sci Q.* 1988;1:8–15.

30. ———. *Interpersonal Relations in Nursing: A Conceptual Frame of Reference for Psychodynamic Nursing.* New York: G.P. Putnam's Sons; 1952.

31. Rew L. Nurses' intuition. *Appl Nurs Res.* 1988;1:27–31.

32. ———. Intuition in decision-making. *Image J Nurs Schol.* 1988;20:150–153.

33. Tanner CA. The nursing care plan as an instructional method: Ritual or reason? *Nurs Educ.* 1968;11(4): 8–10.

34. Bishop AH, Scudder JR. *The Practical, Moral, and Personal Sense of Nursing: A Phenomenological Philosophy of Practice.* Albany, NY: State University of New York Press; 1990.

35. ———. Nursing ethics in an age of controversy. *ANS.* 1987;9(3):34–43.

36. ———. *Nursing: The Practice of Caring.* New York: National League for Nursing Press; 1991.

37. Henderson V. The nature of nursing. *Am J Nurs.* 1964;64(8):62–28.

38. ———. Excellence in nursing. *Am J Nurs.* 1969;69:2133–2137.

39. Kim HS. *The Nature of Theoretical Thinking in Nursing.* Norwalk, CN: Appleton-Century-Crofts; 1983.

40. ———. Structuring the nursing knowledge system: A typology of four domains. *Schol Inq Nurs Pract.* 1987;1:99–114.

41. Watson J. *Nursing: Human Science and Human Care: A Theory of Nursing*. New York: National League for Nursing; 1988.

42. ———. The lost art of nursing. *Nurs Forum*. 1981;20:244–249.

43. ———. Caring knowledge and informed moral passion. *ANS*. 1990;13(1):15–24.

44. Buber M; Smith RG, trans. *I and Thou*, 2nd ed. New York: Charles Scribner's Sons; 1958.

45. Abdellah FG, Martin A, Beland IL, Matheney RV. *Patient-Centered Approaches to Nursing*. New York: Macmillan, 1960.

46. Abdellah FG, Levine E. *Better Patient Care Through Nursing Research*. New York: Macmillan; 1965.

47. Goodrich AW. *The Social and Ethical Significance of Nursing: A Series of Addresses*. New York: Macmillan; 1932.

48. Heidgerken LE. *Teaching in Schools of Nursing: Principles and Methods*. Philadelphia: Lippincott; 1946.

49. Montag MI. *The Education of Nursing Technicians*. New York: G.P. Putnam's Sons; 1951.

50. Nightingale F. *Training of Nurses and Nursing the Sick* [Microfiche, Adelaide Nutting Historical Nursing Collection]. London, UK: Spottiswoode; 1899.

51. ———. *Suggestions for Thought to the Searchers After Truth Among the Artizans of England* [Microfiche, Adelaide Nutting Historical Nursing Collection]. London, UK: George E. Eyre & William Spottiswoode; 1860.

52. Orem DE. *Nursing: Concepts of Practice*, 4th ed. St. Louis: Mosby-Yearbook; 1991.

53. ———. The form of nursing science. *Nurs Sci Q*. 1988;1:75–79.

54. Price AL. *The Art, Science and Spirit of Nursing*, 2nd ed. Philadelphia: W.B. Saunders; 1960.

55. Stewart IM. The aims of the training school for nurses. *Am J Nurs*. 1916;16:319-327.

56. ———. Practical objectives in nursing education. *Am J Nurs*. 1924;24:557–564.

57. Tracy MA. *Nursing: An Art and a Science*. St. Louis: Mosby; 1938.

58. Wiedenbach E. *Clinical Nursing: A Helping Art*. New York: Springer; 1964.

59. ———. The helping art of nursing. *Am J Nurs*. 1963;63:54–57.

60. Beckstrand J. The notion of a practice theory and the relationship of scientific and ethical knowledge to practice. *Res Nurs Health*. 1978;1:131–136.

61. ———. The need for a practice theory as indicated by the knowledge used in the conduct of practice. *Res Nurs Health*. 1978;1:175–179.

62. Dickoff J, James P. A theory of theories: A position paper. *Nurs Res*. 1968;17:197–203.

63. Dickoff J, James P, Wiedenbach E. Theory in a practice discipline: Part II. Practice oriented research. *Nurs Res*. 1968;17:545–554.

64. Dickoff J, James P. Taking concepts as guides to action: Exploring kinds of know-how. In: Nicoll LH, ed. *Perspectives on Nursing Theory*, 2nd ed. Philadelphia: Lippincott; 1992:576–580.

65. Diers D. *Research in Nursing Practice*. Philadelphia: Lippincott; 1979.

66. ———. Learning the art and craft of nursing. *Am J Nurs*. 1990;90:65–66.

67. Dock LL. *Short Papers on Nursing Subjects*. New York: M. Louise Longeway; 1900.

68. Dock LL, Steward IM. *A Short History of Nursing: From the Earliest Times to the Present Day*, 3rd ed., rev. New York: G.P. Putnam's Sons; 1937.

69. Donaldson SK, Crowley DM. The discipline of nursing. *Nurs Outlook*. 1978;26:113–120.

70. Johnson DE. A philosophy of nursing. *Nurs Outlook*. 1959;7:198–200.

71. ———. The nature of a science of nursing. *Nurs Outlook*. 1959;7:291–294.

72. ———. Theory in nursing: Borrowed and unique. *Nurs Res*. 1968;17:206–209.

73. Leininger M. Caring: A central focus of nursing and health care services. In: Leininger MM, ed. *Care: The Essence of Nursing and Health*. Thorofare, NJ: Slack; 1984:45–59.

74. ———. *Care, Discovery and Uses in Clinical and Community Nursing*. Detroit, MI: Wayne State University Press; 1988.

75. Rogers ME. *Reveille in Nursing*. Philadelphia: F.A. Davis; 1964.

76. ———. *An Introduction to the Theoretical Basis of Nursing*. Philadelphia: F.A. Davis; 1970.

77. ———. Nursing science and art: A prospective. *Nurs Sci Q*. 1988;1:99–102.

78. Schlotfeldt RM. Structuring nursing knowledge: A priority for creating nursing's future. *Nurs Sci Q*. 1988;1:35–38.

79. Curtin LL. The nurse as advocate: A philosophical foundation for nursing. *ANS*. 1979;1(3):1–10.

80. Curtin L. The commitment of nursing. In: Curtin LL, Flaherty MJ, eds. *Nursing Ethics: Theories and Pragmatics*. Bowie, MD: Robert J. Brady; 1982:97–102.

81. Lanara, VA. *Heroism as a Nursing Value: A Philosophical Perspective*. Athens, Greece: Sisterhood Evniki; 1981.

82. Kikuchi JF, Simmons H. Prologue: An invitation to philosophize. In: Kikuchi JF, Simmons H, eds. *Philosophic Inquiry in Nursing*. Newbury Park, CA: Sage; 1992:1–4.

Chapter 16

Expressing Health through Lifestyle Patterns

Nola J. Pender,
RN, PhD, FAAN

Few concepts have received more attention from health professionals and the public during the last decade than health. This is largely due to the emergence of disease prevention and health promotion as global priorities. Unfortunately, the nature of health as a positive life process is poorly understood. Theoretical formulations of health often lack specificity and existing measures almost without exception reflect a narrow clinical perspective of health as the absence of disease. The purpose of this chapter is to propose a system for classifying expressions of health of persons in their entirety and to suggest related indicators of high-level health.

During the last decade, nursing, as well as other health disciplines, has recognized the limitations of medical and technological approaches for improving the quality of life and health of the world's population. Major changes in social, political, and environmental conditions of living and the life ways of large segments of society are necessary, if significant improvements in health are to occur during the next century. Thus, disease prevention and health promotion have become global agendas with the potential for achieving health goals unattainable previously through curative interventions. The escalating commitment to health promotion among nations raises important questions concerning the nature of health. What is the *critical essence* of that which is to be promoted? A review of relevant scientific literature confirms that health as a human life span process is poorly understood.

Historically, illness, not health, has been the primary concern of the health professions and mortality and morbidity the indicators of "health" used most frequently (Smith, 1981). Therefore, it is not surprising that in reviewing studies of health, Terris (1975) identified the following illness-related approaches to health assessment: measurement of impairment, assessment of physiological systems in relation to established norms, and measurement of performance in the context of potential decrements. The concept of health has not fared much better in nursing. Although health along with person, environment, and nursing constitute the commonly accepted metaparadigm of the discipline (Fawcett, 1984), the concept of health seems to elude clear theoretical descriptions and, to an even greater extent, useful empirical specifications. Reynolds (1988), in reviewing the measures of health used in reports of nursing research, found that, despite articulation of a holistic concept of health in dominant theoreti-

Source: Pender, N. J. (1990). Expressing health through lifestyle patterns. *Nursing Science Quarterly, 3*(3): 115–122. Reprinted by permission of and copyright © 2002 Sage Publications, Inc.

cal views within the discipline, nurse scientists tended to use indicators derived from a clinical model as the absence of disease.

Is health such a complex human process that it cannot be studied qualitatively or quantitatively? Is high-level health a utopian state, a mirage to be fantasized but never achieved (Dubos, 1965)? On the other hand, if health can be the object of systematic investigation, can it *only* be defined by negation, that is as the absence of disease? Unwilling to settle for such a narrow definition, various health disciplines have attempted to define health from fragmented perspectives placing primary emphasis on psychological, sociological, cultural, or spiritual dimensions. Some attempts have been made to synthesize these perspectives to achieve a complete view of health. Parse (1987) refers to this approach as the totality paradigm, in which persons are considered as biopsychosocial spiritual beings responding and adapting to their environment. A major question about this additive approach is whether the whole is equal to or greater than the sum of the parts.

Person and Health: New Views of Old Concepts

Within the past two decades in nursing, there has been a significant conceptual shift toward viewing persons as unified wholes possessing integrity and manifesting characteristics that are more than and different from the sum of the parts. According to Rogers (1970),

> The unity of man is a reality. Man interacts with his environment in his totality. Only as man's wholeness is perceived does the study of man begin to yield meaningful concepts and theories. Only as man's oneness is apprehended is it possible to identify man's distinctive attributes. (p. 44)

This shift in nursing toward a unitary view of human beings has resulted in increasing reliance

on the tenets of human science in addition to the reductionistic paradigm of traditional science for understanding health. How do individuals *experience* health, and what *meanings* do they give these experiences that have emerged as central questions within the discipline? Tripp-Reimer (1984) suggested that within nursing health be reconceptualized to incorporate both etic and emic perspectives. In the etic perspective, objective observations without input from those observed are used to determine health. In the emic perspective, the meaning of health to individuals within their particular culture is ascertained. Concerns relevant in the latter perspective include these: How is health expressed? Is the expression of health universal or culture specific? Are expressions of health qualitatively different at various developmental phases throughout the life span?

In contrast to the totality paradigm based primarily on the etic perspective, the simultaneity paradigm (Parse, Coyne, & Smith, 1985) captures the emic perspective. Within the latter paradigm each person is viewed as a synergistic being in open, mutual, and simultaneous interchange with the environment. In this context, health is a wholistic unfolding of humans in interaction with the environment in which all the elements or dimensions of health are experienced as a unitary phenomenon. Based on Rogers's theory of unitary human beings, Newman (1979) defined health as the totality of the life process evolving toward expanded consciousness. Parse et al. (1985), also in the Rogerian tradition, described health as a "process of becoming uniquely lived by each individual . . . a nonlinear entity that cannot be qualified by terms such as *good*, *bad*, *more*, or *less*. Unitary man's health is a synthesis of values, a way of living . . . a continuously changing process that man cocreates" (pp. 9–10). Definitions with similar themes have been offered by Pender (1982), who described health as the actualization of inherent and acquired human potential, and Watson (1988), who defined health as harmony with self and environment. A new approach for combining objective (etic) and subjective (emic) health perspectives is needed to avoid a conception of health in which observable physical and behavioral aspects are viewed as separate or in oppositional relationship to experiential aspects. It is the author's belief that both perspectives are valuable and can coexist within the discipline of nursing.

Along with acceptance of a unitary view of health, there is an increasing tendency in nursing to reject the health–illness continuum that Newman (1979) criticized on the grounds that it maintains a false dichotomy by polarizing health at one end of the continuum and illness at the other end. If nursing is to facilitate a client's movement toward health on the health–illness continuum, this must always be away from illness. An "either–or" dichotomy precludes the existence of high levels of health in the presence of a disability or chronic illness. This belief, if carried to its logical conclusion, would imply that health promotion efforts are futile for millions of Americans young and old who have a chronic disease incurable by existing medical means. Health promotion would only be considered appropriate for the favored few without any evidence of disease, thus disenfranchising the poor, the old, and the disabled of services directed toward optimizing their health. To address this dilemma, Newman (1979) suggested a synthesis of the concepts of diseases and nondisease into an integrative concept of health.

Taking another theoretical approach to the problem posed by the health–illness continuum, Pender (1987) described health as the primary life experience with illness superimposed on health. Health can exist without illness, but illness never exists without health as its context. When illness occurs, it is synthesized as part of the ongoing health experience modifying it in varying ways—changing the quality of the experience and *decreasing* or *increasing* overall feelings and perceptions of health. Unlike Parse (1981), who rejects the idea of health as existing to varying degrees, Smith (1981) views health as a comparative term. It has long been recognized that all persons free of disease are not equally healthy. It is the degree to which health is present from both objective and subjective points of view that should be mutually assessed by nurse and client. It is only on the basis of both perspectives that effective efforts can be directed toward appropriate health enhancement activities.

The dominant definition of health espoused by a society has profound political and economic implications because the dimensions of that definition and their associated measures often become major social concerns. Frequently, programs of national and international scope are established to bring about positive changes in the identified indicators of health (McDowell & Newell, 1987). Thus, the discipline of nursing faces one of its biggest challenges in decades—how to best articulate the dimensions of health of persons in their entirety and develop valid and reliable indicators of health as a unitary phenomenon. Such indicators must be articulated with a level of conceptual clarity that permits communication of this perspective to other health disciplines and the public. The clinical view of health as the absence of disease has been the dominant definition in the United States for decades. It is time for a paradigmatic shift to a unitary conception of health that will enable society to deal capably with the multiplicity of factors now known to have an impact on health status.

As nursing moves forward in developing a unitary concept of health, strongly influenced by the tenets of human science, the discipline should not lose sight of empiricism as a viable approach to health-related research. Some questions asked about health are best addressed within a traditional science paradigm. For example, health processes outside of conscious awareness may be observable using highly sophisticated methods and techniques (Norbeck, 1987). Nursing can provide leadership to the health disciplines in blending the approaches of traditional and human sciences. Differences between the two paradigms should not be interpreted as conflict but as integrative tension that promotes creativity in scientific endeavors (Kritek, 1989).

Health as Pattern

Rogers (1970) identified the energy field as the fundamental unit of the universe for the science of nursing. The human and environmental fields are coextensive and in an intimate relationship. Pattern is the distinguishing characteristic of an energy field, which becomes more complex throughout the life span. Persons shape their own health experiences to a considerable extent as they make choices from the options available to them (Parse, 1981). Innate to energy fields are generative powers that can facilitate positive patterning and repatterning, resulting in progressively healthier conditions of being, as objectively measured and subjectively reported.

There is no single, universal health pattern that all human beings share. Health when viewed as a lived experience, that is, within the emic perspective, represents many alternative realities. Only individuals can reveal the hidden meanings that they create for health. Although health has many different shades of meaning, there are recurring themes or commonalities that persons report as expressions of health when queried as to what health means to them. The critical question is this: What are the varying human patterns most indicative of health?

Dimensions of the Health Experience

In 1981, Smith proposed a model of health with four dimensions reflective of existing literature: the clinical dimension defining health as the absence of disease, the role performance dimension describing health as competent performance of socially defined roles, the adaptive dimension characterizing health as flexible adjustment to changing life situations, and the eudaimonistic dimension viewing health as exuberant well-being. Laffrey (1986) operationalized Smith's model in a scale intended to determine the extent to which individuals viewed health along each of these dimensions. In further research, Woods and colleagues (1988) supported the health conception model of Smith in a study of 528 women who were asked, "What do you mean when you say you are in good health?" Their work contributed to the further elaboration of the eudaimonistic view of health identifying nine images consistent with this dimension: actualizing self, practicing healthy life ways, positive self-concept, positive body image, social involvement, fitness, effective cognitive function, positive mood, and harmony.

Parse et al. (1985) conducted a phenomenological study of 400 men and women who were asked to write descriptions of a personal situation in which a feeling of health was experienced. Recurring themes were identified for persons of differing ages. As an example, the recurring themes for persons between 20 and 45 years of age as expressed within the theoretical framework of man–living–health were spirited intensity, fulfilling inventiveness, and symphonic integrity.

Classifying Expressions of Health

In this section, a system for classifying human expressions of health is proposed. Five dimensions of human health expression are organized further into 15 subcategories as shown in **Table 16-1**. This framework for studying health has emerged as a result of discussions with colleagues, review of the literature, and reflection on 5 years of quantitative and qualitative research conducted by a health promotion research team (S. N. Walker, K. R. Sechrist, M. F. Stromborg, & N. J. Pender) in which the health and health practices of approximately 2,000 adults were studied. The following assumptions undergird the proposed classification:

1. Integration of the views of clients as well as health professionals is essential to derive a useful definition of health.
2. Health is a manifestation of person/environment interactional patterns that become increasingly complex throughout the life span.
3. Some human health patterns can be directly observed, others must be self-reported.

The five dimensions within the classification are expressed in common language and the alliteration, although originally unintended, may be useful. Each of the five dimensions of health expression—affect, attitudes, activity, aspirations, and accomplishments—should be assessed in terms of daily fluctuations as well as evolving patterns over time. The five dimensions are proposed as culture free, whereas some of the 15 subcategories and potential indicators may be culture specific. Tools already exist to measure some of the suggested indicators; for others, approaches to description and/or measurement remain undeveloped. Consistent with a unitary view of human beings, a comprehensive assessment tool could be constructed to assess all of the dimensions simultaneously.

Affect

Sensation and emotion are fundamental attributes of humanness that are expressions of wholeness or unity (Rogers, 1970). *Affect* as used here is intended to denote emotions and feelings as subjectively experienced. Affect can be assessed best through personal report, but facial expressions, body positions, or gestures, as well as an increasing array of technologic measures (biofeedback, electromagnetic resonance imaging), can provide some indication of internal emotional states. The link between emotions and illness has been suspected for centuries, but little has been known about feelings as an expression of health. Recent research in psychoneuroimmunology indicates that person/environment interactions and accompanying emotional responses may moderate immune function (Kiecolt-Glaser & Glaser, 1987). Certain emotional patterns such as serenity and harmony may enhance immune competence; their polar opposites may impair immune capabilities. There is also considerable evidence that physiological changes related to activity have an impact on emotions. For example, production of endogenous opiates or internal tranquilizers can contribute to emotional experiences of comfort and calm (Watkins & Mayer, 1982).

Feelings and emotions have a direct effect on the quality of the lived experience of health. The emotions identified in Table 16-1 are those frequently reported as expressions of high-level health. *Serenity* is a sense of tranquility, a peaceful inner state, amid life's ebb and flow. *Harmony* emanates from feelings of relatedness to God and/or the universe and is sometimes described as a feeling of being at peace with nature and fellow humans. *Vitality* is a sense of energy and power. *Sensitivity* is intense knowing of self and others. Feelings of serenity, harmony, vitality, and sensitivity at any moment reflect much more than the current life situation. Human beings have the unique ability to evoke emotions in response to remembered events from the past or anticipated events in the future. This capacity provides persons with the power to transcend current situations—to be unbound by time and space. Persons may be calm, content, or even joyous in the face of difficult situations because of their vision of a greater good to be attained in the future.

Exploration of emotions as important expressions of health presents many exciting challenges to the research community. Current research on the connections between emotions and illness need to be recast in a positive perspective. Research questions from this viewpoint might be these: What person/environment interaction patterns encourage positive emotions? Which emotional patterns or fluctuations in patterns are healthful, which are unhealthful, and are these

Table 16–1   CLASSIFICATION SYSTEM FOR EXPRESSIONS OF HEALTH

AFFECT

Serenity	Harmony	Vitality	Sensitivity
Calm	Close to God	Energetic	Aware
Relaxed	Contemplative	Vigorous	Connected
Peaceful Content	At one with the universe	Zestful	Intimate
Comfortable		Alert	Loving
Glowing		Fit	
Happy		Buoyant	
Joyous		Exhilarated	
Pleasant		Powerful	
Satisfied		Courageous	

ATTITUDES

Optimism	Relevancy	Competency
Hopeful	Useful	Purposive
Enthusiastic	Contributing	Initiating
Open	Valued	Self-motivating
Reverent	Caring	Self-affirming
Trustful	Committed	Innovative
	Involved	Masterful
	Challenged	

ACTIVITY

Positive Life Pattern	Meaningful Work	Invigorating Pay
Eating a healthy diet	Setting realistic goals	Having meaningful hobbies
Exercising regularly	Varying activities	Engaging in satisfying leisure activities
Managing stress	Undertaking challenging tasks	Planning energizing diversions
Obtaining adequate rest	Assuming responsibility for self	
Avoiding harmful substances	Collaborating with coworkers	
Building positive relationships	Receiving intrinsic or extrinsic rewards	
Seeking and using health information		
Monitoring health		
Coping constructively		
Maintaining a health-strengthening environment		

ASPIRATIONS

Self-Actualization	Social Contribution
Growth or emergence	Enhancement of global harmony and interdependence
Personal effectiveness	Preservation of the environment
Organismic efficiency	

ACCOMPLISHMENTS

Enjoyment	Creativity	Transcendence
Pleasure from daily living	Maximum use of capacities	Freedom
Sense of achievement	Innovative contribution	Expansion of consciousness
		Optimized harmony between man and environment

effects general or person-specific? Are different emotional profiles expressive of health at different points in the life span? What interventions on the part of health professionals assist clients in achieving positive emotional patterns? What self-care strategies can increase the frequency of positive emotions? Do emotions perceived as negative detract from or at times promote health?

Emotions can be a positive integrative force (Rogers, 1970). It is the richness of emotional experience that is uniquely human. Research approaches must be used that capture this richness as well as rhythms and fluctuations in emotional patterns. Recent scientific breakthroughs in understanding emotions will fuel increased interest and expanded research efforts in this area in the next decades.

Attitudes

Language, thought, and the ability to form attitudes and beliefs characterize unitary human beings and result from innate capacities to abstract and image features or person/environment interaction. Humans not only think in concepts and relationships but also give meanings to such abstractions. According to Rogers (1970), persons seek to organize the world of experience and make sense of it and can do so because of the capacity for rational thought. Attitudes structure the way persons see their world and, like emotions, express persons' values and priorities.

Attitudes can be developed in relation to specific situations, events, or actions. Life in its entirety can be viewed as an event. As such, persons develop attitudes or beliefs about their own personal lived situation as well as the life process as a shared experience with others. It is these general attitudes or beliefs that are proposed to profoundly influence health.

Attitudes expressive of high-level health are presented in **Table 16–1**. These are recurring cognitive themes in the literature and in more than 75 in-depth interviews conducted by the author and her colleagues with persons considered to have stellar health behaviors. Three subcategories of attitudes have been proposed: optimism, relevancy, and competency.

Attitudes toward life, its value, meaning, and ultimate worth are reflected in the subcategory of *optimism*. Beliefs that all will end well despite life's changing circumstances and that there are possibilities for personal growth even in difficult situations is expressed through an optimistic outlook. Optimism is enhanced by reverence for life and trust in God or the orderliness of the universe. Optimism expands openness to creative possibilities in life patterns.

Relevancy is grasping one's place in the world with an appreciation for unique, personal contributions. Relevancy is expressed through self-respect and a feeling of acceptance by others as a useful and contributing member of society. Persons experiencing a sense of relevance are caring, committed, and involved in life. Relevancy also has an eternal time frame by which persons come to appreciate the importance of their personal existence within infinite time and space.

Competency is expressed in personal clarity about actual and potential capabilities and belief in the power to channel capabilities into meaningful patterns of work and play. Competent persons actively initiate challenging life situations. They are interactive rather than passive, challenged rather than threatened, and self-affirming rather than self-debasing. Perceptions of personal competency are transferred to fellow humans with resultant appreciation of their unique patterns and emergent potential.

Positive attitudes and beliefs express high-level wellness. They are an integral part of health as a lived experience.

Activity

Movement is an alternative to language for communicating thought (Engle, 1984). Activity reflects patterns of energy distribution as well as person/environment rhythmicity. Movement is a means whereby space and time become experienced reality (Newman, 1979). Movement augments awareness of human and environmental fields. According to Newman, the total pattern of movement reflects the organization or disorganization of the thought and feeling processes of the individual. Activity expressive of health facilitates the fuller emergence of personal potential. Three dimensions of activity considered expressive of health are positive life patterns, meaningful work, and invigorating play (see **Table 16–1**).

Positive life patterns go beyond isolated health practices to action patterns that are an integral part of life ways. Thoughtful patterning and repatterning of daily routines and rhythms through informed decision making based on an awareness of options enhance human capacity for optimal well-being. Clusters of behaviors with empirical support for their health-enhancing properties are the backbone of positive life patterns. Eating well, exercising regularly, obtaining adequate rest, and managing stress represent behavioral clusters comprising positive life patterns. Such patterns must be sustained over time to optimize health. Exercise as one behavioral cluster expressive of health is a good example of unitary characteristics. If exercise is to be maintained, it must be of appropriate rhythmicity, periodicity, complexity, and intensity for a given human field. Human and environmental fields must have compatible activity rhythms and patterns to optimize health.

Health is also expressed through *meaningful* work. More energy is expended on work than on any other human activity. Work that is health promoting has been characterized as challenging, varied, well directed, interpersonally satis-fying, and both intrinsically and extrinsically rewarding. In recent years, attempts have been made to achieve greater harmony between human fields and work patterns. Child care, flexible time, job sharing, and the use of home as a satellite work site are only a few of the examples of greater awareness of the need for compatibility between person/environment patterning and work.

The rhythm between work and *invigorating play* changes throughout life. For most children, play constitutes the major activity in which they engage. In fact, meaningful work as an expression of health may not be relevant until the preschool or school years when confronted by the "tasks" of learning. The harmonious integration of work and play often becomes disrupted in young, middle aged, and older adult years. Young and middle-aged adults, in striving to be successful, to achieve adequate pay, and to contribute meaningfully to society, may neglect play. Some compensate for this imbalance by focusing on enjoyable aspects of work and reinterpreting work as play. Older adults often have considerable discretionary time for play but lament lack of resources for recreational pursuits or the absence of meaningful work. It is predicted that leisure time will expand for many persons in the United States in the future as efforts are made to maximize the employment rate in a large and diverse population (Bezold, Carlson, & Peck, 1986). For both younger adults on shortened work weeks and the aging population in part-time employment, meaningful hobbies, satisfying leisure activities, and energizing diversions will be increasingly important as expressions of personal health.

Aspirations

Human beings are inherently purposeful. Life is not a random series of events, but an organized unfolding of each individual in light of personal aspirations and choices. Persons choose the directions in which they evolve in light of the range of options within awareness. Unfortunately, for persons in disadvantaged groups such as the poor and some ethnic/racial minorities, the range of choices is often constricted, limiting options for self-realization. Unnecessary limitations on self-expression is dehumanizing as well as detrimental to the continuing viability and vitality of a society.

The capacity of human beings to bring about changes in human and environmental fields is important for achievement of aspirations and goals. By modifying the nature of person/environment interactions, individuals can maximize available choices. Although persons usually have considerable freedom of choice concerning the goals they will pursue, the goals selected must be compatible with those of society. Social and cultural values as well as the needs of significant others provide a context for setting goals. Inherent in humanness is the moral responsibility for the ethical selection of goals and the means used to accomplish them.

Aspirations within a society often reflect normative patterns—the usual rather than the unusual, the average rather than the exception. Fitting in to societal norms rather than exceeding them is often condoned and encouraged to the detriment of creative change. Individuals possess unique capabilities for self-transcendence (Sarter, 1988). It is only as society encourages people to achieve their uniqueness unconstrained by normative expectations that we will have instances of maximized human health potential for systematic study.

Self-actualization and social contribution are proposed as two subcategories of aspirations needing further clarification and study in relation to human health patterns. Self-actualization is not a new term. Maslow (1970) popularized the concept in his writings as a high-level need for human organisms. Self-actualization is predicated on fulfilling a more basic need for self-preservation. Suggested empirical indicators for self-actualization

are growth or self-emergence, personal effectiveness, and organismic efficiency. *Self-actualization* is an orientation toward being all one can be and fulfilling one's personal potential.

Social contribution enhances global harmony, creates health interdependence, and promotes an ecologically balanced environment for present and future generations. The community in which we live is a world community in which annihilation is an ever present threat. Social contribution as an expression of health is a sensitivity to the needs and potentials of all people, which results in responsible social actions within a particular life situation. It is through shared aspirations of aggregates that social changes supportive of health are realized.

Accomplishments

Accomplishments as expressions of health can be identified as the payoffs for a life well lived. They are unencumbered by time and space and may be viewed as daily achievements, life attainments, or states to be experienced only after death. Regardless of the time frame, persons need bench marks to measure their progress, their emergence as unique human beings. Accomplishments confirm a person's selfhood as well as his or her oneness with the evolving universe.

In modern society, accomplishments are often viewed as measures of worth rather than as expressions of health. Too frequently, being and becoming are sacrificed to doing, thus destroying the balance among affect, attitudes, activity, aspirations, and accomplishments. When kept in proper perspective, accomplishments contribute to the richness of human experience. Creative achievements of human beings throughout history have markedly enhanced the quality of life for others.

Enjoyment, creativity, and transcendence are accomplishments proposed as expressive of health (see **Table 16–1**). *Enjoyment* is a condition in which there is heightened aesthetic awareness of the multiple dimensions of human and environmental fields. Positive emotions and thoughts predominate. Daily experiences are sources of joy. Human unfolding, its challenges and exigencies as well as successive stages of development, provide continuing sources of pleasure.

The capacity for *creativity* is inherent in all human beings. It is expressed through envisioning new configurations within human and environmental fields and restructuring reality or abstractions consistent with these envisioned patterns. Creativity is experienced as performing at one's optimum, maximizing human capabilities, and accelerating diversity and complexity.

Transcendence is stretching beyond the realm of human experience toward new options and possibilities (Parse, 1981). It is experienced as freedom from constraint and expansion of human consciousness to encompass infinite time and space. It is the experience of optimum mutuality and harmony between person and environment.

Accomplishments are the expression of life purpose and thus the expression of health. Their pursuit directs human patterning and evolutionary emergence.

Concluding Comments

Health is a life span process, a largely subjective and private experience, only partially observable by traditional scientific methods. Although defining health only in terms of negation, that is, as the absence of disease, has been common practice for more than a century, this approach will no longer suffice in an era of increasing concern about the promotion of health and the quality of life for human populations. Health as an experience is not fragmented, it only becomes fragmented in the minds of health professionals with differing perspectives. A new view of health is needed that is positive, comprehensive, unifying, and humanistic. This article represents one attempt to move toward that goal. It is imperative that an increasing number of nurse scientists direct their efforts toward expanding our under-standing of human health processes and the personal, social, political, and environmental factors affecting the health of differing populations if significant progress is to be made in optimizing health for a larger segment of the world population in the years ahead.

References

Bezold, C., Carlson, R., & Peck, J. (1986). *The future of work and health*. Dover, MA: Auburn House.

Dubos, R. (1965). *Man adapting*. New Haven, CT: Yale University Press.

Engle, V. F. (1984). Newman's conceptual framework and the measurement of older adults' health. *Advances in Nursing Science, 7*(1), 24–36.

Fawcett, J. (1984). *Analysis and evaluation of conceptual models of nursing*. Philadelphia: Davis.

Kiecolt-Glaser, J., & Glaser, R. (1987). Psychosocial moderators of immune function. *Annals of Behavioral Medicine, 9*, 16–20.

Kritek, P. (1989, April). *Nursing research enterprise in clinical practice: An agenda for the future*. Paper presented at Northern Illinois University Annual Research Conference, DeKalb, IL.

Laffrey, S. C. (1986). Development of a health conception scale. *Research in Nursing and Health, 9*, 107–113.

Maslow, A. H. (1970). *Motivation and personality* (2nd ed.). New York: Harper & Row.

McDowell, I., & Newell, C. (1987). *Measuring health: A guide to rating scales and questionnaires*. New York: Oxford.

Newman, M. (1979). *Theory development in nursing*. Philadelphia: Davis.

Norbeck, J. S. (1987). Empiricism and health promotion research. In M. E. Duffy & N. J. Pender (Eds.), *Conceptual issues in health promotion: Report of proceedings of a Wingspread Conference* (pp. 110–120). Indianapolis, IN: Sigma Theta Tau International.

Parse, R. R. (1981). *Man-living-health: A theory of nursing*. New York: Wiley.

Parse, R. R. (1987). *Nursing science: Major paradigms, theories, and critiques*. Philadelphia: Saunders.

Parse, R. R., Coyne, A. B., & Smith, M. J. (1985). *Nursing research: Qualitative methods*. Bowie, MD: Brady.

Pender, N. J. (1982). *Health promotion in nursing practice*. Norwalk, CT: Appleton-Century-Crofts.

Pender, N. J. (1987). *Health promotion in nursing practice* (2nd ed.). Norwalk, CT: Appleton & Lange.

Reynolds, C. L. (1988). The measurement of health in nursing research. *Advances in Nursing Science, 10*(4), 23–31.

Rogers, M. E. (1970). *An introduction to the theoretical basis of nursing.* Philadelphia: Davis.

Sarter, B. (1988). *The stream of becoming: A study of Martha Roger's theory.* New York: National League for Nursing.

Smith, J. A. (1981). The idea of health: A philosophic inquiry. *Advances in Nursing Science, 3*(3), 43–50.

Terris, M. (1975). Approaches to an epidemiology of health. *American Journal of Public Health, 65*, 1037–1045.

Tripp-Reimer, R. (1984). Reconceptualizing the construct of health: Integrating emic and etic perspectives. *Research in Nursing and Health, 7*, 101–109.

Watkins, L. R., & Mayer, D. J. (1982). Organization of endogenous opiate and monopiate pain control systems. *Science, 216*, 1185–1192.

Watson, J. (1988). *Nursing, human science, and human care.* New York: National League for Nursing.

Woods, N. F., Laffrey, S., Duffy, M., Lentz, N. J., Mitchell, E. S., Taylor, D., & Cowan, K. A. (1988). Being healthy: Women's images. *Advances in Nursing Science, 11*(1), 36–46.

Chapter 17

Healing as Appreciating Wholeness

W. Richard Cowling, III, RN, PhD

The "clinicalization" of human experience by the health care disciplines has been instrumental in denying important facets of human life and not fully accounting for the essence and wholeness of experience. A unitary conceptualization of healing as appreciating wholeness is proposed. Appreciating is actualized through a praxis approach used for research and practice—unitary pattern appreciation—created to bring the theoretical principles of unitary science into practical reality. It is essentially a praxis for exploration of the wholeness within human/environmental pattern. Healing is conceptualized as the realization, knowledge, and appreciation of the inherent wholeness in life that elucidates prospects of clarified understanding and opportunities for action. The essential features of the process of pattern appreciation are a synoptic stance toward pattern information, a participatory engagement with people in the exploration of wholeness, and the transformative nature of the process that illuminates the possibilities in wholeness. A case demonstrates the nature of the unitary pattern appreciation process and its healing qualities. Keywords: healing, nursing practice, nursing science, nursing theory, Rogers' science of unitary human being, transformation, unitary theory

As nursing has moved to assume an expanded role in the clinical care of patients, nurses have participated in the creation of "clinicalization" of human experience that has been instrumental in denying important facets of human experience. The clinicalization of human experience takes the form of an overemphasis on diagnostic representations that do not fully account for the essence and wholeness of the experience. This clinicalization is expressed in empirical, conceptual, and theoretical approaches that yield partial, and sometimes erroneous, accounts that miss the essential wholeness, unity, and uniqueness of human existence, similar to the androcentric bias in science noted by feminist scholars.[1] This occurs in spite of our claimed holistic perspective that has embraced spiritual care and complementary healing modalities. Related manifestations of this phenomenon are an overemphasis on clinical specialization, client interventions shaped by economics rather than need, educating natural healing tendencies out of students, general subjugation of our spiritual consciousness to economics of health care, treatment protocols that do not consider wholeness of human existence, and overreliance on physical/material conceptions and models of human health and illness. A recent study[2] comparing

Source: Cowling, WR. Healing as Appreciating Wholeness. *Advances in Nursing Science* 2000;22(3):16–32.

alternative healers and nurses described healers as creating a sacredness and reverence around their work in contrast with the clinical structures and techniques of nursing. An alternative to the clinicalization perspective is the focus of healing with its attendant concern for wholeness.

A Differentiated Healing Conceptualization

It is acknowledged that there is a range of potential meanings given to healing that is extensive and diverse.[3] Kritek[3] points out that healing is a gerund derived from heal, which means whole. A gerund is a term originating from a verb but used as a noun. Consequently, the foundational meaning of the term is directly derived from the notion "to heal" or the activity of becoming whole. Therefore, healing is a process that becomes an object. Kritek's[3] comprehensive essay on the construct of healing and her reflections on the multiple meanings of the construct provide an opening and an invitation for articulating a unitary perspective of healing. She forcefully demonstrates the depth, richness, specificity, and focus that context brings to the meaning assigned to healing by persons and groups. She warns of "the anomalous situation where a sought-after wholeness is conceptualized and pursued in a manner that implicitly or explicitly denies or ignores dimensions of the human condition that are essential to achieving that wholeness."[3(pp. 11–12)] Furthermore, Kritek sheds light on the situation in which nurses are educated to attend to the subjective and objective meanings associated with wholeness and healing and to devise responses based on those meanings, yet "the ambitiousness of this intention is only superficially acknowledged, and the skills and the knowledge necessary to excel in such an effort are not yet delineated."[3(p. 14)] A unitary conceptualization of healing as appreciating wholeness responds to Kritek's concerns and cautions.

A unitary conceptualization of healing as appreciating wholeness differentiated from the synthesized view in the current literature provides an alternative to be considered as a framework for a healing science and practice. The synthesized view of healing as a nursing construct is elaborated by Kritek.[3] In spite of the variety of meanings, there is an overarching idea of wholeness inherent in healing stemming from what Kritek refers to as "some admixture of complementary conceptualizations," as seeking or reaching for a desired wholeness. There is an understanding that wholeness is an ideal rather than a reality, "since no human is actually whole."[3(p. 14)] A goal or destination toward this ideal is implied. It also is understood that dissonant definitions of wholeness are differentiated, more or less, by their potential as confining and limiting in viewpoint and by the degree of complexity and robustness.

A unitary conceptualization of wholeness,[4] which is at the heart of healing, is clearly a departure from this synthesized view of healing. A unitary view posits that human beings are irreducible wholes and that the unitary nature of the environment also is irreducible. The concept of field is central to the unitary perspective and "provides a means of perceiving people and their respective environments as irreducible wholes."[4(p. 29)] Although Rogers did not explicate a conceptualization of healing, it is clear that a unitary conceptualization of healing, grounded in wholeness, would require an understanding of human being/environmental wholeness as unitary. Practice and science through a unitary lens would accept the reality of wholeness not as an ideal, but as a given. Human beings and their environments would be approached as integral fields within fields that could not be extracted into parts, or more specifically, in theoretical terms as unitary energy fields. Newman puts it more succinctly and directly, "unbroken wholeness is what is real—not the fragments we devise with our way of describing things."[5(p. 37)]

While I have a deep respect for the theoretical language of the science of unitary human beings, I have an even greater reverence for the experiential nature of wholeness that supports this theoretical language. That is, my experience of being human engaged in practicing nursing with other human beings suggests a reality of wholeness. Newman aptly points out that we are embedded in what we want to study, and the nature of nursing requires that we engage in the experience of it to understand it fully.[5] My own view is that the nature of nursing is one of responding to the wholeness of human experience, I have used the practice and research enterprises simultaneously in an attempt to engage in nursing with a reverence for the wholeness humans bring to that engagement and to prepare myself for knowing and appreciating that wholeness. I have spent a considerable portion of my career developing this praxis that gives attention to the wholeness of humans and their environments and opens the possibilities for participatory, transformative change.[6–9] The approach has been refined to serve both the purposes of research and practice or can be used for either individually. I could not have sought this reverence for human wholeness or created an approach that attends to this wholeness without the conceptual system of unitary science. This is an example of what Wheeler and Chinn describe as praxis, "thoughtful reflection and action that occurs in synchrony."[10(p. 2)] Thus, it is for me theory and experience that create the synchronous context for reflection and action and provide the grounds for the perspective I have adopted of healing as appreciating wholeness.

The Appreciating Context

The appreciating context is based on the common understanding of the meaning of appreciation and the unitary perspective of pattern. In the dominant view of healing there is a seeking to understand desired wholeness through attention to the parts and the interrelationship of the parts to one another. In the practice of healing the focus is "on establishing, achieving, or regaining a sense of cohesion" among the parts.[3(p.17)] In the unitary view of healing as appreciating wholeness, the attention is on the pattern that emerges in human experiences, perceptions, and expressions occurring in unity and arising from human and environment mutual process. In the practice of healing, the focus is on appreciating the wholeness within this pattern. Pattern, in unitary terms, is the distinguishing characteristic of a field and gives identity to the field.[4] Each unitary human field pattern is considered to be unique along with its own unique environmental field pattern. In human terms, the pattern gives identity to and distinguished one person from another. It is the essence of being who you are; thus, pattern appreciation is reaching for this essence in each individual and seeing the wholeness within pattern. In summary, rather than knowing the parts to know wholeness, the unitary scientist/practitioner seeks knowing the pattern to know wholeness.

The elemental characteristics of appreciation were derived from reviewing the *Oxford English Dictionary* definitions of appreciation: perception of the full force; sensitive to and sensible of delicate impression and distinction; perception, recognition, and intelligent notice; expression of one's estimate; sympathetic recognition of excellence; and gratefulness, enjoyment, and understanding.[11] Appreciating means "perceiving, being aware of, sensitive to, and expressing the full force and delicate distinctions of something while sympathetically recognizing its excellence as experienced in gratefulness, enjoyment, and understanding."[7(p. 130)] The something in unitary healing science and practice terms is the wholeness inherent in field pattern as manifest in human experiences, perceptions, and expressions, or in simpler terms, the wholeness inherent in human life.

Unitary pattern appreciation reaches for the wholeness within pattern in the following six ways:[7]

1. It seeks a perception of the full force of pattern.
2. It requires sensitivity to and sensibility of the manifestations that give identity to each person's unique pattern.
3. It involves perception, recognition, and intelligent notice of human expressions that reflect pattern.
4. It takes the form of an estimate of unitary energy field pattern as a meaningful representation of the pattern called a profile (often emerges as story, metaphor, and music).
5. It implies sympathetic recognition of excellence of energy field pattern meaning that pattern is significant regardless of characteristics.
6. It is approached with gratefulness, enjoyment, and understanding that reaching for the essence of pattern has potential for a deepening understanding in service to the individual and knowledge development for practice and science, and ultimately transformation of participants.

These characteristics or features provide the context for establishing an appreciating endeavor with clients or participants.

The Appreciating Process

Unitary pattern appreciation was developed for the purpose of creating a unitary art and science that would bring theoretical principles into practical reality.[6,7] It consists of a process, orientation, and approach that can be used for research, practice, or combined research and practice intentions (praxis). Through its use over the past 2.5 years with participants in a praxis enterprise, I became aware of the healing nature of appreciation turned toward wholeness. Three critical features of pattern appreciation

create the conditions for healing: synoptic, participatory, and transformative.

Synoptic

The synoptic orientation provides an alternative to the process of analysis for understanding information. Murphy[12] employed an approach to his research on transformation known as synoptic empiricism. It was use in unitary pattern appreciation. According to Broad, "Synopsis is the deliberate viewing together of aspects of human experience which for one reason or another, are generally kept apart by the plain man and even by the professional scientist or scholar. The object of synopsis is to try to find out how various aspects are interrelated."[13(p. 8)] In the practice of appreciation, there is shift away from the attention on the interrelatedness of aspects and a focus on sensing an emerging pattern that reflects the wholeness of human life. Thus, aspects of human life, namely the experiences, perceptions, and expressions associated with living, are viewed together in an inclusive way to reveal the fullest picture of the inherent wholeness.

The scientist/practitioner may look for themes and commonalities in the pattern information or may use an assortment of ways of knowing that reveal a compelling sense of wholeness amidst the variety of phenomena of life. The synoptic process requires and inclusive view of what counts as pattern information. Pattern manifestations or phenomena that are labeled by participants as physical, emotional, mental, social, and spiritual are included as pattern information. They are understood contextually as arising from wholeness, not reflective of parts that do not exist in the unitary perspective. Observations by the scientist/practitioner of physical phenomena also are included as pattern information.

Ensemble is a useful concept to consider when thinking about the process of synopsis as a way of appreciating wholeness. Phenomena or features of human life are viewed as an ensemble that reflects pattern and wholeness. The definition of ensemble is "all the parts of anything taken together so that each part is considered only in relation to the whole."[11] In the case of unitary pattern appreciation, the term *facets* is substituted for *parts* since facet implies an aspect of something that is whole rather than something that is divisible into separate entities. The ensemble of phenomena of human life represents the facets of a pattern reflecting wholeness. As in the musical notion of ensemble, which means "the united performance of all voices or instruments in a piece of concerted music,"[11] the scientist/practitioner of pattern appreciation listens for the united concert of voices in the phenomena conveying the essence of the pattern and thus the wholeness, of human living. "The multiple, and sometimes seemingly disparate, manifestations of the field pattern form an ensemble of information that conveys a singularity of expression."[6(p. 140)] Developing one's ability to sense the pattern and wholeness is the goal of the synoptic process that supports healing.

Participatory

Appreciative inquiry and practice are fundamentally participatory inquiry and practice. People seek to participate in the research or practice based on an invitation and/or knowledge of the work of the nurse. Although my work has been primarily in the community and participants come to engage in the appreciating process from knowing about my research/practice, it is possible that clients of health care institutions might have access to this type of engagement through expert nurses who have developed the requisite knowledge and skills. Regardless of setting, it is critical that there be mutual understanding between the nurse and the participant from the beginning as to the nature of the appreciating process, the egalitarian ideal inherent in the relationship, the openness to emergent discovery in the work, the potential for negotiation, and the fact that potential outcomes are not predicted or prescribed.

The participatory orientation capitalizes on one of the major tenets of the science of unitary human beings: the capacity of humans to knowingly participate in change and in patterning.[4] It is this capacity that provides the opportunity for mutual discovery of possible avenues of action. The actions chosen emerge from the knowledge of wholeness that comes from exploration of one's pattern. The exploration and discovery mode of the process is created through a partnership. In this partnership, the nurse provides a contextual process of appreciating pattern, which is open to modification depending on the desires of the participant. The participant is viewed as an expert on his or her own life and the source of his or her own power and knowledge. Each encounter in the appreciating process is primarily in the form of a dialogue with content focused on life experiences, perceptions, and expressions. However, the use of music, imagery, or movement also might serve the dialogue and the emergence of useful pattern information to understand the person's wholeness.

The appreciative inquiry aspect has been developed over time using knowledge of participatory modes of inquiry.[14] Recently, I discovered a field of participatory inquiry in organizational life known as appreciative inquiry,[15] which has features similar to unitary pattern appreciation. In relation to the organizational context, "more than a method or technique, the appreciative mode of inquiry is a way of living with, and directly participating in, the varieties of social organization we are compelled to study."[15(p. 131)] Likewise, unitary pattern appreciation is a way of participating in the varieties of human life experiences that reflects the wholeness of human existence. It aims to use this participation as a way of bettering the lives of human beings and to grasp a deeper understanding for developing knowledge of human wholeness and healing.

The life process system practice model described by Schaef[16] has served to inform the refinement and development of aspects of the unitary pattern appreciation practice approach. This model of practice advocates for practitioner receptivity to the client's life process, embraces honoring this process, and acclaims the inherent healing capacity of the client. Likewise, in unitary pattern appreciation praxis the scientist/practitioner is receptive to the person's life experiences, perceptions, and expressions and honors the uniqueness of each individual life. The healing capacity is acclaimed through respect for the client's ability to participate knowingly in change. In the life process system model, as in unitary pattern appreciation, "Diagnosis is not the foundation for practice; wisdom arising from participation with clients is the foundation. In its denial of the primacy of diagnosis, the model implies a rejection of a dualistic view of illness (ill and not-ill) and of judgment as a critical attribute for the potential of healing."[7(pp. 139–140)] The ideal of control is inconsistent with the notions of unitary science predicated on acausality and unpredictability. Thus participation becomes central to the appreciating process of healing.

Transformative

The transformative potential of unitary pattern appreciation is the cornerstone of healing. By giving attention to the wholeness of human existence through appreciating pattern, phenomena are seen in a new context. For example, my praxis involves helping individuals who are experiencing despair. When the experiences of despair, the perceptions of despair, and the ways in which despair are expressed in one's life are placed in the context of the wholeness of one's life there are revelations that go beyond the tendency to treat and/or understand the despair as a symptom of a disease or a single condition. Returning to the organizational brand of appreciative inquiry, there is a similar perspective that relates to healing. In organizational appreciative inquiry "serious consideration and reflection on the ultimate

mystery of being engender a reverence for life that draws the researcher to inquire beyond superficial appearances to . . . the life generating essentials and potentials of social existence."[15(p. 131)] Likewise, in the case of unitary pattern appreciation, the inquirer/practitioner reaches for the essentials and potentials within the wholeness of human life, and like the organizational appreciative inquirer who is "drawn to affirm, and thereby illuminate, the factors and forces involved in organizing that serve to nourish the human spirit," the unitary nurse is drawn to affirm and illuminate the factors and forces that nourish awareness of the richness and potentialities in the wholeness of human life.[15(p. 131)] This creates a condition and context ripe with possibilities for transformation.

Unitary pattern appreciation also invites participants to consider the possibilities of seeing change within the consciousness of pandimensionality, which is a unitary view of time, space, and movement. However, this is a concept introduced in the context of the participant's life concerns and not imposed as the only way of viewing the realities of change. Thus, it is provided as one way of viewing change amidst many others. Ultimately, the participant's choice of viewing change is acknowledged and embraced as an aspect of the participatory and exploratory nature of unitary pattern appreciation. Pandimensional consciousness, a complex and abstract concept, is akin to Moss' spiritual concept of "unitive consciousness."[17] Unitive consciousness occurs when individuals become referent to infinity, meaning that they realize infinite potential and infinite time–space–movement–change. Moss[17] described unitive consciousness in ways similar to those Martha Rogers[4] used to conceptualize a pandimensional universe. Two descriptors best convey this pandimensional or unitive consciousness where we are "in a great sea of being infinite in all directions."[17(p. 65)] The first descriptor is "where feeling, sensation, and thinking are a unified continuum that is not limited by the boundaries of the body."[17(p. 65)] The second is "every moment is a new birth and what is being born is not merely the product of the past, not merely the cause of some earlier effect, but rather part of a ceaseless cosmos of revelation."[17(p. 66)] The transformation potential of pandimensional awareness is the same as that of unitive consciousness as Moss described it—that is, "to become referent to infinity is to not have our identity located in any finite notion of ourselves. We are movement and flow. Our careers, our health, our families and possessions may temporarily represent a harbor of our sense of self, but ultimately we are always far more."[17(p. 67)]

Finally, the transformative potential for scientists/practitioners rests within the way in which they learn to use themselves as instruments for pattern appreciation. Because the quest for pattern knowledge requires attention to all realms of data, one must develop data acquisition skills that allow the data to reveal themselves. This is very similar to the quest for data acquisition and verification in religious life described by Wilber.[18] A person must be developmentally adequate to a disclosure or the data will not reveal themselves. In meditative knowing, injunctive tools of Zen are used for this disclosure. Injunctive tools also are used for the disclosure. Injunctive tools also are emerging from the quest for understanding unitary pattern. The inquiry process associated with unitary pattern appreciation calls for a willingness to use injunctive devices that will open one to the revelation of unitary pattern data. Likewise, this inquiry process calls for the scientist/practitioner to use these data in ways that are responsive to the unique pattern of the individual in designing unitary nursing practice strategies. For most nurses, this would mean at least a relative transformation toward being a more sensitive instrument of awareness.

In summary, the healing potential of appreciating wholeness rests with these three foundational features of the process that are integrated within the context of an appreciating attitude. The nurse invites people to engage in a participatory exploration of the wholeness within life using a pattern lens that avoids the fragmentation of other ways of viewing experiences. By using a synoptic framework, all phenomena are considered relevant and are embraced as an ensemble of information that helps both the nurse and the participant see the wholeness within this pattern. Spiritual phenomena are considered along with physical, emotional, mental cultural, and social phenomena in an inclusive way. In contrast to the interpretative paradigm that seeks "to understand and derive meaning from the human experience,"[19(p. 71)] unitary pattern appreciation seeks to represent the wholeness within human experience by attending to pattern. In the unitary way of thinking, healing is not seeking a desired wholeness but rather is realizing, knowing and appreciating an inherent wholeness that illuminates potentials of understanding and possibilities of action.

A Case of Healing as Appreciating Wholeness

The following is a sketch of a case from my ongoing praxis project that demonstrates healing as appreciating wholeness. Karen, an early participant in the unitary pattern appreciation project, came in response to a flyer distributed in the community. She was in her early 50s, had three grown children, had been married and divorced twice, and was working as a legal secretary. She came to see me because of "ongoing despair." She said that when she saw the flyer she identified closely with the word despair. "I just feel like I'm in a lot of despair. I probably don't look it, but I am. I am broken spiritually. . . . It's not a psychological problem, but spiritually I need healing. . . . That's why I wanted to come—to heal that."

The process of pattern appreciation with Karen involved asking questions about the nature of her experiences, the perceptions she had of these experiences, and the ways in which despair was being expressed in her life. Some of the questions were contemplated in preparation, but most often they emerged from the content of the dialogue. The dialogue focused on past, present, and future, and it covered topics related to relationships, family, work, play, beliefs, spirituality, physical sensations, health, dreams, feelings, and aspirations, in addition to whatever topics Karen raised. During the dialogue, I attempted to position myself in a stance of openness to hear the wholeness within Karen's portrayal of life. My emphasis was not only on listening to the words but also on being sensitive to and sensible of the variety of information that came forth in dialogue—the ways in which words were stated, the expressions, the movements, and the posture as well as my own reactions. I did not take notes because I wanted to be fully present to the experience of the dialogue.

I have tried to capture the unitary pattern appreciation process by describing the experiential, perceptual, and expressive aspects of Karen's life phenomena and by explaining the ways in which the synoptic, participatory, and transformative features were integrated. It is important to clarify that experience, perception, and expression are sources of pattern information and are considered facets of pattern, not parts. A person experiences, perceives, and expresses all at once or contiguously. "Experience is the raw encounter of living loaded with sensation."[7(p. 133)] Experience involves sensing and being aware as a source of knowledge.[11] "Perceiving is the apprehending of experience or the ability to reflect while experiencing."[9(p. 202)] Experiencing and perceiving cannot be disentangled from one another. Perception is conscious knowing in the midst of experience. To express is to manifest.[11] Expression is manifesting the experience and perception of living that is the unique pattern of the individual. Expressions of pattern are the avenues to knowing pattern and thus wholeness. In the dialogue and the resulting text, the facets of experience, perception, and expression come forward in a unified way. They are disentangled here only as a simpler way of portraying the facets. There is a risk of violating the sense of wholeness involved in creating this representation of Karen's life as only excerpts can be portrayed from transcripts.

Experience

Karen recounted a childhood of instability and feelings of not being acknowledged. "I went to six schools by the time I was in the sixth grade. I mean there must have been a reason why we moved so much. I don't know what it was. It seemed like my father was under more and more stress and became more and more distant. . . . He was physically not available. His emotions weren't available. Then when my mother died, he remarried and became even more distant." After her mother died, her father never discussed the death.

Karen told of one incident in her childhood that for her symbolized the essence of being unacknowledged. She was in elementary school and was being chased and taunted by a little boy. She asked for help from the teacher, but the teacher told her not to worry. One day the little boy pushed her down on the playground, and she got a deep cut on her chin. When she went to the teacher, the teacher laughed and told her the little boy just liked her and that was his way of showing her. Karen's mother was called, and Karen was taken to the doctor. The doctor painted a big red Mercurochrome smile on her face, and her mother and the doctor laughed.

Karen married a man who was so involved with his career that he gave her very little attention. He criticized her appearance and what she chose to wear. He had to approve of her clothing purchases or he would not give her money to buy clothes. She married a second time and experienced a similar situation: "Both husbands . . . I kept hearing how much they loved me and yet it is not my definition of love or they're not available." She recounted a situation where as a young married woman she had a cat that had only one kitten. When she was away with her husband, her mother-in-law gave the kitten away without asking her even though the kitten was still nursing. When she became upset about it, her husband defended his mother. She portrayed this event as symbolic of this theme of not being acknowledged or recognized.

Karen went on to describe a recent time in her life after the end of the second marriage. She was being sexually harassed by a supervisor in a company for which she was working. This harassment went on for about 6 months. "He was married to a daughter of one of the founders, and he had a great deal of money." She finally had the courage to report him to her employers, and she was given a new assignment. Later she left the company because of the discomfort she felt.

Karen had read many self-help books and tried many alternative modes of healing, including workshops on energy, music, and color. She was making efforts at integrating exercise and diet changes in her lifestyle. She also was participating in a motherless daughter support group. None of these efforts had helped her in a deep way, but she expressed the feeling that the despair would have been worse if she had not done these things.

Perceptions

In relation to the death of her mother, Karen felt that no one ever recognized the pain she experienced. She brought this topic up in relation to parenting her own adult children. "I lost my mother when I was 19, so I'm real confused with what my role is. This has been a real issue for me. I don't know how an adult child relates to his or her parents." She went on to describe how she experienced parenting: "I do perceive them

as draining the life right out of me. I even say that to them. I do feel I don't get very much back. I wish someone would take care of me." Karen recounted the physical tiredness and physical constraints of her life experience.

Karen perceived her situation as spiritual in nature. Her biggest spiritual concern for the future was one of being punished for her involvement with the man who had sexually harassed her in the workplace. "Yes, even though I know there wasn't anything I could do. I understand how it happened and I didn't have any evil with him. Still, I think I participated—being weak or doing something so despicable." Shame was a dominant theme in her life and expressed itself in her feelings about herself and in her dreams. She described herself as invisible during the sexual harassment. "I left my body. I think of the experience just like children do. I felt very much like a child. Who could I tell? Nobody would listen to me. He had all the power. I felt just like a child. The one thing was that he knew me so well. We had known each other for a year before this started. I trusted him." She added, "I think the first person I told did shame me and that was like my worse fear."

During the second session with Karen, I asked her if she could identify any ongoing trend in her life. This was an attempt to reach for the essence of her life experience. She described feeling as if she were being punished and went on to clarify what she meant. "I guess there is a theme—people who should care about me, take care of me, or help me, letting me down or abandoning me—falling short." Karen perceived her life as lonely and lacking any sense of belonging. In this regard, she depicted this as searching for a home. She demonstrated it with the example of her mother's death and her sense of not belonging in her father and stepmother's home and then getting married and hoping to find safety and security with her husbands. "I think I was looking for that place where they have to take you when you come home. Home is where they have to let you come in when you come home. I don't have that." I asked here if it was like shelter, and she said, "If I draw it it's like a cave with a fire." She described the lack of a sense of belonging as an ongoing theme in her life and gave multiple examples from relationships with family members, spouses, and friends.

Expressions

There were multiple expressions of the underlying pattern and wholeness of Karen's life. These included her choices of words and phrases. It also included the tone of her voice; her posture; her reactions and responses to questions; the way she walked; her clothing; her affect; her likes and dislikes; her favorite activities, books, and movies; her behaviors; her personal belongings; and her home and work environments. Three examples of expressions were dreams, stories describing events, and drawings depicting her experiences and perceptions. She spoke about the relevance of her dreams in understanding her situation. "I do pay a lot of attention to my dreams. It's reflected in my dreams of futility, of working for how to accomplish something." Her dreams were filled with painful images of her futile efforts to clean herself or get out of entanglements or mires while surrounded by taunting and laughing groups of people. In one dream, Karen is in a bathtub that is in a room open to viewers. She is filthy and dirty, but the more she tries to clean herself, the more muddy she becomes and the more everyone laughs at her.

In another dream she is at a dance and the room is very cold. Everyone at the dance is wearing warm clothes. She is trying to put on a sweater when somehow her dress is pulled away. In another dream sequence she attempts to make a speech. While preparing her speech, the spiral of her notebook pops open and strikes her in the face. She went in front of the audience with a red, swollen cheek. "The man came in who was going to help me and I was so relieved.

I kept trying to turn it over to him, but whatever I did it just wasn't good enough, and I got really distressed about presenting myself to someone who was an expert and then not really following through—winging it. That's sort of how I'm looking at my life when I'm telling you that. I feel like I'm winging it and I should know better, but I don't. Yes, that's sort of how I feel about myself right now."

One of the stories she wrote expressed the experience and perceptions of the event in her childhood where she was harassed and pushed by the little boy. This is an excerpt:

> *Well, the little girl was very confused. She felt like she was falling down a deep dark hole, watching the tall teacher, laughing at her as she disappeared. Something was terribly wrong. She was really and truly afraid! She had asked for help but no one was listening. What she thought was frightening, apparently everyone else just thought was funny—very funny. What could she do? Her friends just disappeared and the only adult only laughed. So she convinced herself that she must be mistaken and decided she would just do her best to avoid the mean little boy.*
>
> *The next day at recess, the little boy seemed to know the teacher wasn't going to do anything to help the little girl, and he ran up to her when she was standing near the merry-go-round and pushed her so that she fell and got a deep cut on her chin. Her worst fears had been realized. Her mother was called and came to take her to the doctor. Certainly now someone would do something about this awful situation.*

But instead of comforting her and making plans to punish the mean little boy, the doctor started to laugh too and painted a big red circle on the little girl's face with Mercurochrome. Her mother started to laugh too, and the little girl felt herself falling down that hole again, watching people she loved and trusted laughing at her. Everything seemed topsy turvy and very, very scary. Who could she trust? Where was she really safe? What was the matter with her that she was terrified and everyone else seemed to be enjoying a good joke? Was she so worthless that her fear was laughable? Either they were wrong or she was. And this scared her the most.

Karen had drawn pictures as a child and teenager, but her father had told her to stop because there was no future in being an artist. She used drawings to express her life and supplement a journal that she kept as part of her recovery from the abuse of the sexual harassment experience. She shared her drawings with me. She described what the drawings meant as she displayed them. One image depicted a woman with a big hole in her chest and someone standing on her shoulders. Karen described the picture. "That was me. That was how I was feeling Sunday night. I feel like there is some protection, but I feel so empty. This is my heart. There is promise of good things, but I don't have any way of getting them. I am tired." One image showed her straining to pull herself out of a crack. Another image showed a figure on a hillside with a gleaming and glittering town in the distance. Karen said that this represented her being away from happiness and wanting to reach it but not being able to go that far. Still another image was a figure crouched in a cave with a fire. Karen explained that she was trying to stay warm in her dark spot of life.

Karen also had a drawing of a figure next to a door. She explained,

And this is pretty much despair. But then it gets better. And here I am and here I come. I'm all shaped up and I'm ready for things to get better. I'm all patched up. I'm trying to find a way out because the doorknob fell off. There is no way out. My only alternative is to bust down this door. I want to go, but it's not possible.

Karen described a series of drawings done when she was going through the problem with the sexual harassment: "[H]ere I am in the comforting arms. But then she walks away and leaves me. I will be dropped at any minute. Here

I am in a hollow again. The tip of my iceberg."

In explaining the essence of the drawings, Karen made the following remarks: "Yes, I'd like to feel, what you said, I'd like to feel my life is moving. I guess I'm tired of life . . . like that first drawing was about comforting arms dropping. The universe comes and gives me a hug and then forgets me. I feel forgotten. And I think I said before that we were talking about if Jesus came back and he would say, 'Hi, Richard. How are you? Who's that? Do I know you?'"

Synopsis, Participation, and Transformation

The synopsis, which replaces data analysis in conventional research, occurred in the unitary pattern appreciation process by looking at all facets of the data as a unit. In the beginning of my project I used a form that contained columns for experience, perceptions, and expressions and began looking across these facets for themes. I soon realized that disentangling the information was not necessary and as I read the transcripts and used a synoptic perspective the wholeness and pattern became evident. Synopsis also occurred in the unfolding dialogue that explored Karen's experience along with her perceptions and the ways in which these were expressed in her life. It was very important to acknowledge and honor the spiritual aspects of Karen's life in the process. The story that was written synthesizing the information was the most distinctive source of synopsis in the process.

Participation with Karen happened through setting the stage for the process to be negotiable and responsive to her needs, desires, and concerns. I talked with Karen about creating a partnership for this exploratory journey. Although I asked questions, Karen also asked my opinion, and I often shared my own experiences. There was a higher degree of freedom to share experiences, mutuality, and negotiation than in counseling sessions I had conducted using an interpersonal framework. When I presented the story that I created as Karen's profile, I asked her to consider whether or not it was an accurate representation of her life and to reject it, accept it, or alter it on her own terms. Throughout the entire process, Karen was viewed as the person who had the final decision on our process.

The transformation was experienced during the dialogues, at points of reflection on the process and content, in the creation of the story profile, and when I presented the story to Karen. In most cases, the dialogues led to deeper understanding of the nature of her experience in its fullest sense. She used a strategy that I suggested—to rewrite the endings of dreams. She adapted this strategy to rewrite the endings of actual events that had taken place in her life. These events were ones in which her pain or distress was not acknowledged and she was not supported. She reported that this activity created a greater sense of power that was useful to her in dealing with current life situations.

Story, Metaphor, and Music

After 3 weeks of dialogue I started to create a profile of Karen's pattern. I looked at the information from the transcripts and recalled my own experiences with her during our sessions. During my review of the transcripts I discovered that the most powerful metaphor in the text was the image of being in a cave with a fire, except Karen could not build a fire and often found trouble finding any shelter at all. I thought this image symbolized her life most clearly. The image of the cave and building fires became the source of inspiration for a story that I started writing as the pattern profile that would represent the wholeness of Karen's life. It took me approximately 3 weeks to develop the story. I also decided to include music as a way of conveying the themes within the story.

The story is a dream-like account of the life of a little girl as she grows up and becomes a woman. The girl starts out with a wonderful life with loving parents.

There was once a beautiful child . . . a bright and loving child . . . born into the world and belonging to the world . . . a world of love and of light and wonder...of stars and moons and playfulness . . . a world of laughter and joy. The child, a girl, was sheltered and cared for by two loving and adoring parents . . . parents of the universe with wisdom and compassion and with a deep understanding of children and what they needed to grow and blossom.

As the child grew older life became colder and harsher. Her parents became more preoccupied with life and preparing for changes in each season, but her mother had begun to teach the girl to build fires to keep herself warm. One day the child came home and her mother was gone and she never knew what happened. Her father did not want to talk about anything but his work, and he never had time to help the girl cultivate the building of fires. The father saw that she was growing up and thought she should be able to build her own fires.

Her father was working on one of his projects. He was always making things . . . interesting things . . . the girl wanted to know something about this, but she also sensed she could not interfere with her father's work. It was particularly cold that day and she decided to ask her father to build a fire. "Father," she said, "I am so cold. Would you build the fire?" The look in her father's eyes was more chilling than any cold air . . . or icy temperature she had ever felt before. Her father scolded her for asking. "It is time you learned to take care of yourself. You are old enough. If one is cold one finds warmth of his or her own will and action."

Her life after that became a series of attempts to find warmth in caves, to build fires, or to find someone to help her build fires. But after many disappointments she came to realize that there would be no help.

She built her own fires and it was easier this way—even if she was alone. The woman occasionally thought of her mother building fires and she missed that. No one ever built her a fire. They promised, but it never happened. She was alone except for her children. They needed many fires built because life was very cold.

At this point in her life, the woman meets a man who promises to build her fires. He tells her about a new kind of warmth that can be generated by the two of them being together. In the end, she suffers from her trust of this man.

The man taught her that she did not need fires to keep warm . . . he could give her warmth . . . and it would be better than fires . . . and she would not have give anything in return. The woman wanted to learn about this new warmth . . . she did . . . and she paid a heavy price for this new warmth. The man taught her how they could use each other to stay warm . . . how they could use the heat in their bodies . . . he didn't tell her the price. The price was a dear one . . . she must keep their warmth a secret . . . and if she told anyone she would suffer. The woman would have said no when she learned the price, but she was afraid of not being warm. You see the man had also found a way to take her fires away from her . . . and when she tried to build a fire there was no warmth.

This is where a song is introduced in the story. It conveys the sense of being trapped after being involved with the sexual harassment. The song is "Paralyzed" by Rosanne Cash. It conveys a sense of hopelessness that then leads to moving beyond the event. In fact, Karen had in her real life finally faced her abuser and brought charges against him. The words convey the story of a woman who is paralyzed by a relationship. It describes her running from the bedroom with her legs paralyzed. She attempts to carve out her future acknowledging that she is both a prophet and blind. She realizes that it is nobody's business and that no one is to blame. She believes

that she will meet the man sometime in the future with a new identity. She knows she has lifted the veil and walked through the flames and she will move on.[20]

In the story, after this experience, the woman learns that she has lost her power to build fires and finds herself at the mercy of her destiny. This experience is captured in a song by Nanci Griffith entitled "Southbound Train." This is the story of a woman who is riding a train headed south. She describes herself as staring at the sky and thinking about her childhood while she is holding back her tears. She says that a stranger is sleeping beside her and it feels to her as if she is his wife. It is probably her husband. She notices the towns and cities going by and thinks about them as passing like the pages in the story of her life. Most poignantly, she characterizes her heart as being on the baggage rack, very heavy, and she is yearning for someone to carry it for her. She longs to have someone pay attention to it and to handle it with care, noting that it has been damaged from being dropped and that it needs repair.[21]

As the woman pondered her situation she remembers the power she had as a child and the sense of belonging and she also becomes aware of angels. A song is introduced here, "Calling All Angels," sung by Jane Siberry. This song begins with some beautiful chanting of religious and spiritual incantations leading to the continuous chant of calling all angels. The singer describes her journey as full of tears and hurt and uncertainty. She yearns not to be left alone. She questions her life situation and why it exists. Yet at the same time, she notes the beauty of the sunset and nature, which brings love and intensity into life. The singer appears to have a revelation in understanding as she thinks about the beauty and realizes that even if she could crack the code that would explain her life, she would not give up the pain and suffering that goes with all the beauty. In other words, she knows that she needs to embrace all of life, including the harshness and the loveliness. The song ends with a chant about the features of life and the discovery of the reality of uncertainty.[22]

The last part of the story is about the girl awakening from the dream (the story) as a woman and realizing her own possibilities. This final part of the story was written to convey and portray the sense of hope and the woman's spiritual beliefs that are aspects of her life that keep her moving onward. In this sequence, she discovers a connection to a light and radiance that are sources of warmth. The light also takes the form of the presence of two beings who are guides and sources of support.

> *They both spoke simultaneously and said, "Sweet, perfect one . . . you are not alone . . . you belong to the universe . . . just like the stars and the plants and all the creatures. We are here to help you on your journey . . . you can count on us. Never again will you need to search for fires in caves . . . or build fires . . . for we will help you learn to keep the fire in you alive and strong . . . and you will always find warmth in this fire." And the woman knew . . . she belonged . . . and she would take her own journey and write her own story.*

The ending served two purposes: to suggest the possibilities inherent in realizing the wholeness of life and to acknowledge Karen's own power.

Karen was tearful after I presented the story and music. Excerpts from the transcripts that day capture her response: "Wonderful! Thank you. I loved it! The music was just great!" "I think you did a wonderful job! It's so wonderful. I hate for it to end. It's so great to be understood!" "This is such a gift." "This is so much better than being diagnosed." "I was thinking that while you were doing that. You make it so you validate my experience. That's something I've never had. It's always been wanting to change or what I did wrong. This felt a whole lot more about what went on instead of, 'Oh, Lord. I

have to change that now,' or 'If I would only. . . .'" A critical feature of the unitary pattern appreciation process, and also of healing through appreciating wholeness, is a willingness on the part of the scientist/practitioner to let go of expectation about change.

The story that was created represents a pattern profile specific to Karen. Karen was asked to review the story and determine if she thought it reflected her life experience and the underlying pattern of wholeness. One aspect of the participatory nature of pattern appreciation is to collaborate on the creation of the profile so that it represents the perspective of the participant. In some cases, an individual has created his or her own profile. In one case, it was a series of photographs with an essay about the person's philosophy. In other cases, individuals have altered aspects of the story profile to capture more accurately the wholeness of their life pattern. The profile becomes a referent point for considering one's life situation and possibilities for integration and/or change as well as a source for nursing knowledge arising from praxis.

Summary

It is difficult to convey the essence of the praxis of pattern appreciation and to portray the wholeness found in a human life pattern. The scientist/practitioner is not meant to capture this fully—this praxis is really about seeking to represent the wholeness within pattern as a healing project knowing that, at best, this is a representation of the wholeness and not the wholeness itself. It is my experience that as I reach with another for this representation of wholeness we are led to revelations that far exceed our current clinical diagnostic representations. The process itself—the actual engagements of participatory exploration—serves revelatory awareness as well as the products of the story, the metaphor, and the music.

Healing is the realization, knowledge, and appreciation of the inherent wholeness in life that elucidates prospects of clarified understanding and opportunities for action. The unitary scientist/practitioner seeks knowing the pattern to know wholeness. The appreciation context orients the practitioner/scientist to perceiving, being aware of, and being sensitive to the unique manifestations of wholeness available in human encounters. It challenges him or her to express the full force and delicate distinctions of unitary pattern and its wholeness in representing the human experience. It requires a sympathetic recognition of the excellence of wholeness an experienced in gratefulness, enjoyment, and understanding. The essential features of the process of pattern appreciation are a synoptic stance toward pattern information, a participatory engagement with people in exploration of wholeness, and a transformative process that illuminates the possibilities in wholeness—the embodiment of healing.

References

1. Reinharz S. *Feminist Methods in Social Research.* New York: Oxford University Press; 1992.

2. Engebretson J. Comparison of nurses and alternative healers. *Image J Nurs Schol.* 1996;28(2):95–100.

3. Kritek PB. Healing: A central nursing construct—reflections on meaning. In: Kritek PB, ed. *Reflections on Healing: A Central Nursing Construct.* New York: National League for Nursing; 1997.

4. Rogers ME. Nursing science and the space age. *Nurs Sci Q.* 1992;5:27–33.

5. Newman MA. Experiencing the whole. *ANS.* 1997;20(1):34–39.

6. Cowling WR. Unitary case inquiry. *Nurs Sci Q.* 1998;11:139–141.

7. Cowling WR. Unitary pattern appreciation: The unitary science/practice of reaching for essence. In: Madrid M, ed. *Patterns of Rogerian Knowing.* New York: National League for Nursing; 1997.

8. Cowling WR. Unitary practice: Revisionary assumptions. In: Parker MS, ed. *Nursing Theories in Practice*, Vol. 2. New York: National League for Nursing; 1993.

9. Cowling WR. Unitary knowing in nursing practice. *Nurs Sci Q.* 1993;6:201–207.

10. Wheeler CE, Chinn PL. *Peace and Power: A Handbook of Feminist Process.* Buffalo, NY: Margaret-Daughters; 1984.

11. *Oxford English Dictionary* [CD-ROM]. New York: Oxford University Press; 1994.

12. Murphy M. *The Future of the Body: Explorations into the Further Evolution of Human Consciousness.* San Francisco: Tarcher Press; 1992

13. Broad CD. *Religion, Philosophy and Psychical Research.* New York: Harcourt Brace & Company; 1953.

14. Reason P. Three approaches to participative inquiry. In: Denzin NK, Lincoln YS, eds. *Handbook of Qualitative Research.* Thousand Oaks, CA: Sage; 1994.

15. Cooperrider DL, Srivastva S. Appreciative inquiry in organizational life. *Res Organ Change Dev.* 1987;1:129–169.

16. Schaef AW. *Beyond Therapy, Beyond Science.* New York: HarperCollins; 1992.

17. Moss R. *The Second Miracle: Intimacy, Spirituality, and Consciousness.* Berkeley, CA: Celestial Arts Publishing; 1995.

18. Wilber K. The problem of proof. *Revision J Consciousness Change.* 1982;5(1):80–100.

19. Monti EJ, Tingen MS. Multiple paradigms of nursing science. *ANS.* 1999;21(4):64–80.

20. Cash R. Paralyzed. *From Interiors* [CD]. New York: Columbia Records; 1988.

21. Gold J, performed by Griffith N. Southbound train. From *Flyer* [CD]. New York: Elektra Entertainment; 1994.

22. Stewart JC. Calling all angels. From *When I Was a Boy* [CD], performed by Siberry J. Burbank, CA: Reprise Records; 1993.

Chapter 18

Relational Narrative: The Postmodern Turn in Nursing Ethics

Sally Gadow,
RN, PhD

A philosophy of nursing requires an ethical cornerstone. I describe three dialectical layers of an ethical cornerstone: subjective immersion, objective detachment, and relational narrative. Dialectically, the move from immersion to detachment is the turn from communitarian to rational ethics, replacing traditions with universal principles. The move from universalism to engagement is the turn from rational to relational ethics, replacing detached reason with engagement between particular selves. Conceptually, the three layers correspond to premodern, modern, and postmodern ethics. I propose that the layers be viewed not as stages, but as elements that coexist in an ethically vital profession, and I conclude with an illustration of their coexistence in a clinical situation.

A philosophy of nursing requires an ethical cornerstone because a profession is informed by moral ends. Discussions of ethics in nursing usually are framed in the categories of philosophical ethics, such as deontology, virtue, and consequentialism. Although useful for locating nursing ethics within the disciplinary context of philosophy, the categories are not helpful because they manifest no internal relationship to each other, no connection within an encompassing framework. Without a coherent framework, ethics cannot provide the cornerstone for a philosophy of nursing.

In the hope that establishing philosophical connections among different ethical approaches will lead to the construction of an ethical corner-

stone, I offer a method for understanding different ethical views within a dialectical framework. The framework I describe is a triad of ethical layers: subjective immersion (ethical immediacy), objective detachment (ethical universalism), and intersubjective engagement (relational narrative)—corresponding, respectively, to premodern, modern, and postmodern ethics (see **Figure 18-1**). After a brief discussion of dialectic, I describe each of the three layers and conclude with an illustration of their coexistence in a clinical situation.

Dialectic

The method of developing a philosophical dialectic is adapted here from the work of Hegel (1807/1977). A brief elaboration of method is important to the thesis of this discussion, namely, that premodern, modern, and postmod-

Source: Gadow, S. (1999). Relational narrative: The postmodern turn in nursing ethics. *Scholarly Inquiry for Nursing Practice; 13*(1)57–69. Used by permission of Springer Publishing Company, Inc.

Figure 18–1 TRIAD OF ETHICAL LAYERS

bilitation negotiates a new relationship between body and self. While the body remains an other for the self (an otherness the injury produced), harmony between them is cultivated through attentiveness to the injured part. That cultivated unity based on care entails the possibility for climbing stairs as a cooperative, rather than an unconscious, activity of body and self.

A characteristic rhythm is associated with dialectic because of the three phases of simplicity, opposition, and reconciliation. The formulaic description of dialectic as thesis–antithesis–synthesis, however, can be deceptive; it masks the principle of ongoing self-negation at the heart of dialectic. No phase is exclusively thesis, antithesis, or synthesis. Each phase serves as antithesis of the one before, and each synthesis becomes a new thesis as its own unity is further differentiated. The rehabilitated body, for example, can train for a marathon, involving further cycles of immediacy, opposition, and reconciliation.

If an inherent telos is assumed, a dialectic will move inexorably toward culmination. Hegel insisted on a telos, but I do not. Without a telos, the movement of mediation can proceed

ern ethics represent a dialectical relationship among different ethical approaches in which none of the three can stand alone and only their coexistence constitutes a sound basis for practice.

The nature of dialectic can be expressed as mediation. Mediation is the negation of simplicity, resulting in increasing complexity as each new level of differentiation is in turn negated, producing further distinctions. At the same time, the opposition among distinctions is itself mediated. Negativity, in other words, becomes increasingly positive as the original opposition is qualified by a new relationship in which once antithetical elements are no longer mutually exclusive but become mutually enhancing.

A clinical example of dialectic is the experience of injury and rehabilitation (Bloom, 1992; Gadow, 1982).Before injury, the body is experienced as a taken-for-granted immediacy that accomplishes the aims of a person, such as climbing stairs, without reflection or even awareness. An injury negates that immediacy in two ways: the body opposes the aims of the self by its inability to climb, and the inability is itself the antithesis of the lost immediacy. Rehaindefinitely. Without closure, a dialectic of ethical levels such as I propose can give rise to further cycles of differentiation. Ethics, in other words, need not culminate in the postmodern. Indeed, the most interesting question evoked by a dialectic of premodern–modern–postmodern ethics may be, "What now?" Given the nihilism sometimes associated (mistakenly, I believe) with postmodern ethics, treating it as the thesis for a new set of negations might be a fruitful sequel to the discussion that follows.

Premodern Immersion: Ethical Immediacy

In a dialectical framework the first level is immediacy. In ethical terms, immediacy is an unreflective and uncritical certainty about the good. A certainty powerful enough to resist reflection originates outside an individual in order to avoid being undermined by particularity. Certainty about the good, if it is to be more than personal conviction, must derive from a source that transcends the individual, such as religion, family, customs, or the ethos of a profession.

Ethical immediacy is an experience of certainty that needs and allows no explication; it is nondiscursive. That, in fact, is its power. A discursive description of a morally good nurse can be argued and revised, requires consideration, and has to be consciously accepted in order to have power. In contrast, a nondiscursive portrayal—an image rendered in film, a virtue modeled by a mentor—bypasses deliberation to gain acceptance. With a cultural, professional, or religious basis for certainty, a nurse intuits the good directly, without recourse to reflection. That immediacy is the phenomenon I call immersion: a nurse is immersed in a tradition that provides an ethical appraisal of the situation, as well as immersed in the situation itself. Depending on the tradition, that appraisal may dictate, for example, that nurse-assisted suicide is wrong (or

that it is right). Whatever the tradition, immersion offers a degree of certainty unavailable to the other ethical layers because it is nonreflective. It needs no defense.

The strength of immersion as an ethical approach is the solidarity it achieves. Nurses and patients sharing an unquestioned view of the good are united in their attempt to realize that good. Differences in interpretation may arise between individuals, but the foundational unity that grounds their values prevents differences from becoming divisive. Similarly, within an individual, ethical immediacy prevents fragmentation of the self that can result from self-questioning and critique. Immediacy serves to maintain the self—and the group—as a coherent, harmonious whole. Immersion and immediacy, in other words, describe community. "In community persons cease to be other, opaque, not understood, and instead become mutually sympathetic, understanding one another . . . fused" (Young, 1990, p. 231).

Immediacy, like a spell, would be broken by the detachment needed to explain or defend it. Defense is unnecessary in a community characterized by a common tradition, but few nurses practice in such a community. One of the hallmarks of contemporary nursing is the decline of moral immediacy (Benjamin & Curtis, 1992). In place of actual groups united by a single worldview, there are diffuse disciplines (Foucault, 1975/1979) and discourses (Bordo, 1993). They invite a form of immersion, but they unite individuals through abstract ideology rather than community identity (Gouldner, 1978).

Community-based certainty is not obsolete, however. Its contemporary form is communitarian ethics. Communitarians regard individuals as situated within a natural community such as the family, neighborhood, or nation, a community of origin that anchors personal identity and guarantees moral certainty (MacIntyre, 1981). For communitarians, immersion is the ideal form of moral knowledge and the only basis for ethical certainty.

Because the likelihood of a shared community is low for contemporary nurses, ethical immediacy will be challenged in most settings. Merely identifying an ethical issue (should we allow this person to die?) undermines immediacy because ethical issues do not arise in a premodern approach. Once a question is posed, there are two choices. One is to reinforce certainty using force, such as shame or exclusion, against the questioner, thereby ending inquiry and reinstating immediacy. The other option is to answer the challenge by articulating the basis for certainty. That response, however, entails translating subjective certainty into objective forms (language and reasons) that another could understand, and, in so doing, immediacy is shattered. When a person surfaces from ethical immersion to defend a view of the good, certainty is compromised and immediacy is lost.

Modern Detachment: Ethical Universalism

Dialectically, the move away from immediacy produces its opposite, rational objectivity. Historically, the rational turn is symbolized by the Enlightenment celebration of reason as liberator from the Dark Ages of superstition, parochialism, and feudalism (Poole, 1991). In health care, too, an ethics based on rational principles has been heralded as a moral enlightenment following an era of professional feudalism known as paternalism (Beauchamp & Childress, 1994).

Because immersion in unquestioned certainty is an extreme form of ethical knowing, its antithesis too is uncompromising. Rationality counters subjectivity with principles that are categorical and unconditional. Detachment provides the distance needed for objectivity, for viewing from a vantage point outside, instead of inside, a situation. Freed from the limiting perspective of particularity, reason equals universality. The modern turn in ethics aims at overcoming the relativity of competing parochial certainties by producing one incontestable system of universal principles.

The strength of ethical universalism is epitomized by the principle of respecting individuals equally. Respect for individuals is based on the rational autonomy that each person possesses, the ability to transcend personal feelings in making universalistic choices. Formulated another way, ethical choices respect others as ends in themselves, affirming them as rationally autonomous and capable of transcendence; individuals are equivalent units of universality (Friedman, 1993). The principle is blind to actual identities of both the agent and the other, not unlike the double-blind design that assures objectivity in science. In nursing, the principle restrains us from discriminating against patients; prevents us from coercing, oppressing, or lying to them and prevents our treating them as mere objects, material, or means to others' ends. In short, it commits us to a contract of reciprocity in which we respect the value that they and we share as universal, free persons.

Despite the appeal of rational principles, especially in health care, they provide less certainty than they promise. Three limitations of rational ethics can be identified. First, interpretations of a principle can conflict in clinical situations. A requirement to protect life can be interpreted as maintaining physiologic functioning or as alleviating suffering. One way to reconcile the conflict involves redefining terms so that life means quality of life, but for some nurses, a life is more than its quality, whereas for others, suffering enhances the quality of a life. For still others, a nurse's view of life is irrelevant because only the patient's view matters. Application of a principle, in other words, compromises its universality because interpretation is required, and interpretations differ according to the perspectives of the people involved.

A second limitation is the contradiction that universalism, alleged alternative to force, governs by force when it insists on the suppression of particularity, stripping from persons and situations their lived reality. Universal principles provide ethical knowledge in a situation only if all cases are alike but actual issues and the people involved are not identical. The only way a principle could provide solutions would be by force, that is, by requiring a nurse to suppress particular knowledge about a situation and blindly apply the principle; but that reduces a professional from an ethical agent to an automaton.

A feminist critique of universalism identifies a third limitation of rational ethics. That critique exposes the cultural hegemony of reason, specifically the oppressive authority of those whose status affords them the luxury of transcendence as long as others remain bound by conditions of hunger, exhaustion, or pain (Benhabib, 1992). Ethical universalism is founded on a dualist metaphysics in which reason is the essence of humanness, and other aspects (especially emotions and the body) are inessential, unruly, and, ideally, transcended. Because universalism values persons as transcendent, it devalues those experiences, already marginalized by dualism, that are not fully controllable, such as illness and suffering. The moral high ground of rationality becomes synonymous with privilege and power instead of the equality it promised.

The question raised by a critique of rationalism is whether nondualist respect is possible, valuing persons as irreducibly ambiguous: particular and universal, embodied and intellectual, emotional and rational. Dialectically, nondualist respect represents an ethical level beyond both immersion and detachment as sources of certainty, a third level characterized by uncertainty and engagement.

Postmodern Engagement: Relational Narrative

The move beyond rational objectivity in ethics can be considered an existential or postmodern turn. In existentialist ethics, the uniqueness of individuals is their essential feature. A self has a particular perspective as a situated subject. Transcendence is only the ability to imagine and appreciate different perspectives, not to assume a universal view from nowhere. The situated self encompasses not only rationality but also emotion, imagination, memory, language, the body, and even other selves. Individuals are intrinsically relational; existential subjectivity is intersubjectivity.

Respect for persons as existential selves involves more than detached regard for abstract autonomy; it entails attentive discernment and valuing of an individual as unique. Dillon (1992) describes this discernment as care respect because its valuing of particularity parallels that of care ethics. The valuing of persons requires perception of each one's uniqueness, and perception involves engagement. In contrast to rational ethics, which demands detachment in order not to perceive people concretely or respond to them personally, care respect conveys "cherishing, treasuring, profoundness of feeling" (p. 120).

The engagement of care respect is the opposite of ethical objectivity; it is personal responsiveness to the particular other, a relation between individuals that is grounded in the ambiguity of their being at once encumbered and free, situated and transcendent. Engagement cannot be regulated by principles; they would remove the relation from its grounding in actual persons and orient it toward external authority. Codes have no authority to command engagement. The only form that moral authority takes is authorization, the call from the other commanding concern simply by being the other. "The moral call is thoroughly personal . . . the command is not universalizable" (Bauman, 1993, p. 51).

The move from rational principles to existential engagement is a postmodern turn. Postmodern ethics can be characterized as embracing contingency, refusing certainties, and resisting the modern drive for unity, order, and foundations (Bauman, 1995; Tester, 1993). Postmodernism expresses its resistance by dismantling the fixed meanings rationalism has constructed. Every form of order becomes a target for deconstruction, from the social, sexual, and political to the epistemological and metaphysical, but none is as inimical to postmodern ethics as the hermeneutic order, the modern hierarchy of meanings. In that hierarchy, rational meanings are authoritatively assigned, fixed rather than fluid, and ranked by their degree of objectivity. A diagnosis of HIV, for example, is assigned its correct meaning by clinical experts, the meaning remains constant among experts, and the assigned meaning ranks higher on the hermeneutic scale than an emotional or imaginative interpretation by a person with the diagnosis. Significantly, experiences that pose the greatest threat to rational control—dying, illness, pain, dementia—become objects of the strictest hermeneutic control, often with disabling consequences. A social construction of aging, for example, as decline and deterioration can be more disabling than physical changes accompanying aging. From a postmodern perspective, the modern oppression through meanings represents hermeneutic terrorism in which experience is held hostage to authority.

Postmodernism destabilizes the hierarchy of meanings by displaying them as contingent, demonstrating that any interpretation of an experience can be revised because other meanings are always available. Moreover, no uninterpreted basis exists from which to decide objectively among meanings, "no neutral ground on which to stand and argue that either torture or kindness is preferable" (Rorty, 1989, p. 173). Our most trusted ethical certainties are our own creation. We may choose kindness rather than torture, but there is no authorization for our choice. Without a higher authority than ourselves, we have no certainty that our meanings are better than those of others. Ethically, we are on our own, without a metaphysical warrant from either religion or reason.

Meanings are contingent because they are human creations, but the most radical contingency is that of meaningfulness itself. The very enterprise of making meaning is conditional, never assured. It depends on our continuing acts of interpretation, always subject to the possibility that we may be overwhelmed into silence and incapable of interpretation. Scarry (1985) describes intense pain as world destroying. Grief, fear, and despair also can unmake the meanings that comprise a person's world, including the central meaning of the person as meaning maker. If disintegration of both world and self are possible, then meaningfulness itself, not just one or another meaning, is radically uncertain.

Radical contingency is not captured by the nihilist certainty that life is meaningless. That certainty in fact reassures us that there is no possibility of meaninglessness. Radical contingency is more serious. It lacks the comfortable universality of nihilism. It is the concrete possibility in each situation that meaning might not be created, a human interpretation might not be voiced in time to keep the world from ending. If I can say, at least, "this pain is meaningless," I am safe from meaninglessness. If I can say nothing because language is powerless or my voice is silenced, then my world ends.

Dismissing end-of-the-world talk is hubris, the modern certainty that there can be no gap in the plenum of meanings, no abyss into which one could fall. Nurses rarely indulge in that hubris. Most have glimpsed the abyss through a patient's eyes. At the edge of the abyss ethical certainties fail, and nothing remains except possible engagement between nurse and patient; but engagement is enough (without it a patient is alone, no matter how many nurses are present). The ethical narrative a nurse and patient compose through their engagement interprets the situation, saving it, for the moment, from meaninglessness.

Narrative meaning is communicative, the saying of something another can understand; it represents a "moral party of two" (Bauman, 1993, p. 82). Beyond that, it requires that at least one of the two is not silenced by their situation, remaining able to imagine and voice an interpretation: one of the two serves as their poet. "In times of strangeness . . . by being strangers together, people and poet reconstitute an internal homeland" (Cixous, 1993, p. 26). That homeland for nurse and patient is the narrative they compose together, the words of their engagement.

Engagement includes the danger that the poet too will fall silent. By joining another in vulnerability, I myself become vulnerable, and the other's pain may silence me. Wordless, I can only turn to the other for meanings, as did the poet Akhmatova (1983), waiting with the other mothers outside Leningrad prisons, writing her poems with their words. In engagement, even authorship is contingent; "If Akhmatova, mother among mothers, writes with the mothers' meager words, then the mothers are also poets among poets" (Cixous, 1993, p. 27). In composing a narrative between nurse and patient, it does not matter who is author, because each is poet; it matters only that there are enough words between them to make a story.

The attempt to compose meanings, given their contingency, is flawed from a modern standpoint. The ethical knowledge created through a relational narrative is particular, contextual, and nongeneralizable; even its authorship is ambiguous when one person speaks with the other's words. An ethical narrative fails all criteria for objective knowledge, and terms like poem or story only further demean it in the rationalist view.

Dialectically, however, rationalism is flawed by its suppression of engagement as avenue to ethical knowledge. From a postmodern standpoint, modern ethics fails to grasp a significant feature of human experience, its narrative nature (Carr, 1986). To claim that "we lead storied lives" (Connelly & Clandinin, 1990, p. 2) is not only to point out that crafting stories is an important human activity but, more fundamentally, to assert that an experience, in order to be my experience, has narrative form; it has to be fitted into the rest of my experience with a connecting meaning, a thread of sense, even if sensible only for me. To make sense of experience is to make the narrative connection, to relate otherwise inchoate events to my story, the life I am living as mine (LeGuin, 1989).

Nursing has (re)discovered narrative as a form of coherence in the absence of encompassing certainties. Through narrative intervention patients can be helped to create emancipatory narratives, that is, to revise disabling into enabling views that allow movement toward a self with possibilities (Sandelowski, 1994). Ethical narratives are emancipatory in their portrayal of a good toward which a person can move. Because individuals are particular, situated, and self-interpreting, the most faithful way to know the good they seek is through their own accounts, their personal ethical narratives. At times of vulnerability, however, personal narratives can fail, just as ethical certainties fail in the face of radical contingency. In those moments, a new narrative is needed, and help may be needed to compose it. Ethical narratives created by patient and nurse from the homeland of their engagement are thus more than individual accounts: they are relational narratives.

Because a relational narrative expresses engagement, it extends beyond the particularity of either person alone but does not extend beyond their relationship; it is more than personal but not universal (Gadow, 1994, 1995). It embodies intersubjectivity, an alternative to both the subjectivity of immersion and the objectivity of detachment. The paradox of a relational narrative is that it narrates uncertainty, but in so doing can offer a safer home, existentially, than would be found in subjective or objective certainty. Either of those would cost the nurse and patient their relationship. Their lived reality together would be displaced. The aim of relational narrative is to provide a place of shared, and therefore safer, contingency. By combining contingencies through engagement, persons are able to coauthor an interpretation that may be more inhabitable than either of their individual narratives as they seek a new form of the good.

A Dialectical Framework in Practice

I have proposed that the philosophical cornerstone of nursing is dialectically layered rather than unitary. The question now emerges: What would the dialectic among different ethical layers look like in practice?

A dialectic can be reduced to ideology by theorizing a telos that draws the movement toward a final level. To avoid that reduction and its coerciveness, I suggest that the three ethical approaches be regarded not as successive stages in the profession's advance, but as possibilities coexisting in an ethically vital practice. Dialectic offers a way of envisioning contradictory approaches as intrinsically related. None of the three is fully intelligible without its connection to the others. Each complements the limitations of the other two. Dialectic as a philosophical framework is more than a heuristic device for conceptualizing nursing. It is a also a framework for the continuing development of the discipline. If otherwise opposing approaches can be appreciated as inseparable, they may then be acknowledged in practice as being mutually enhancing instead of oppositional. Nursing becomes more than a moral high ground from which difference is excluded. It becomes, instead, a region of existence large enough to accommodate, even encourage, diversity among those who live there.

Just as a geographic region cannot be conveyed in its totality by a map, an existential region cannot be captured in a theory, but something of its vitality can be rendered by images. In a beginning attempt to answer the question of how a dialectical framework might look in practice, I offer instead of theory a metaphor and a clinical example that may serve as an impetus to further exploration.

The flourishing of premodern, modern, and postmodern ethics in nursing can be imagined metaphorically as the biodiversity of a coral reef where different life forms integrate and where organisms even after their death provide a structure that supports life. At the level of immediacy, we are immersed in ethical currents that carry us safely through situations where reflection would be impossible. When crosscurrents require us to reflect and to hold a position, an edifice of ethical principles offers a structure for steadying ourselves. Finally, there are situations where no edifice can alleviate our vulnerability, and in those cases we can only turn to each other and together compose a fragile new form of the good.

To illustrate, I consider the reef-like situation described by Schroeder (1998) in which Carole (mother) and Morgan (daughter) found themselves while Morgan spent the first 3 months of life undergoing surgical heart repairs, inept and relentless technical procedures, and near-fatal nursing and medical errors. Schroeder's description does not indict professionals for being unethical, but displays instead the inevitable collisions when a mother's immersion in her daughter's danger meets the detachment of ethical objectivity.

"How can she be in congestive heart failure if I'm rooming-in?"

He looked impatiently at me. "You're a nurse. Call the intensive care nursery if her respirations go over 60."

Instead of calling, Carole brought her baby into bed with her, pulled the blanket over them, and unplugged the phone, mutely sinking into the quicksand of isolation that immersion becomes when no hand is offered.

Hands eventually were offered from each of the three ethical layers. All of them were essential to the survival of both mother and child.

1. From the urgency of another mother's immersion in her own child's situation: "Get her out of here no matter what," she whispered. . . . "Get her out of here if she is getting better at all."

   And from the same mother, the offer of community in an informal group where mothers' stories to each other kept them from drowning in the immediacy of their children's pain.

2. From the honesty of a nurse who countered institutional hierarchy with her own ethical autonomy:

   One day, Lea told me that the physicians at this hospital were unable to do anything further for Morgan. . . . Although she merely confirmed what I had already been thinking, I was unable to summon the strength to act upon my thoughts without her support. I now know that Morgan would have died in that hospital cubicle if Lea had not risked angering the physicians and telling me the truth.

3. From a nurse whose overtures opened the door to a different story, to engagement instead of isolation:

   Carolyn would ignore my hostile looks and sit with me at Morgan's bedside on work breaks. . . . Her words and presence began to fill some of the emptiness inside me. Although I would never admit it to her, I began to look forward to her visits, and eventually we began to communicate on a level very foreign to our previous working relationship

   And from a nurse who transcended moral duties:

Cathy came out of the ICU and said that they were trying to get her off the heart–lung machine now; "I'll be right back to let you know," she said, and walked back into the ICU. I stared at the door, awestruck at her bravery. She'll have to let me know, I marveled, now she can't just stay behind those doors and let someone else tell me the news. I felt ready to handle anything, almost exhilarated that someone would risk so much when it wasn't even required.

The coral reef that I believe Schroeder describes is ethically layered. Modern, premodern, and postmodern elements alternately prevailed. The situation would have been ethically diminished by an absence of any of the elements. Philosophically, the dialectical nature of nursing entails the presence of all of them. Without a telos to drive the dialectic, there is no basis on which to insist that nursing limit itself to one. The postmodern turn only makes explicit an element that has been implicit; it does not establish a superior ground from which to dismiss the others. In the case of Carole and Morgan, no single element was decisive in determining the ethical course to pursue. They did escape, as the first mother urged, but not before a nurse had urged moving to a better hospital where surgery was successful, and not until other nurses had offered engagement as alternative to immersion.

A dialectical ethical narrative such as Schroeder provides is the equivalent of a relational narrative that a nurse and patient together create. Both narratives are layered with voices from immediacy and objectivity in a continuing tension that cannot be resolved in favor of either without destruction of the narrative's relational nature, its contingency and vitality. The postmodern turn is not an advance that dismisses immersion and detachment as ethical approaches. It is instead a turn toward the absurd, as Camus (1955) would call it, the cultivation of a life "without appeal" (p. 39) in which the longing for certainty and the impossibility of certainty are both embraced passionately. From a modern or premodern perspective, that contradiction is absurd in the sense of being hopeless. From the postmodern perspective, an absurd life is filled with "a wild kind of hope" (Schroeder, 1998, p. 20).

The practice of an absurd life, an absurd ethics, is dialectical because it grants at once the validity of subjective and objective ethics. In nursing the story of that practice can only be intersubjective, a relational narrative. The narrative is layered with voices of immersion and detachment like a medieval motet in which several voices simultaneously sing parts of the text that counter and complement one another (Gadow, 1999). Perhaps the fact that a philosophical cornerstone can be compared metaphorically to a phenomenon as ephemeral as a song is one more indication of the postmodern turn in nursing ethics.

References

Akhmatova, A. (1983). *Poems.* New York: Norton.

Bauman, Z. (1993). *Postmodern ethics.* Oxford, UK: Blackwell Publishers.

Bauman, Z. (1995). *Life in fragments: Essays in postmodern morality.* Oxford, UK: Blackwell Publishers.

Beauchamp, T., & Childress, J. (1994). *Principles of biomedical ethics* (4th ed.). Oxford, UK: Oxford University Press.

Benhabib, S. (1992). *Situating the self: Gender, community and postmodernism in contemporary ethics.* London: Routledge.

Benjamin, M., & Curtis, J. (1992). *Ethics in nursing* (3rd ed.). Oxford, UK: Oxford University Press.

Bloom, L. R. (1992). How can we know the dancer from the dance?: Discourses of the self-body. *Human Studies, 15,* 313–334.

Bordo, S. (1993). *Unbearable weight: Feminism, western culture, and the body.* Los Angeles: University of California Press.

Camus, A. (1955). *The myth of Sisyphus and other essays.* New York: Vintage Books.

Carr, D. (1986). *Time, narrative, and history.* Bloomington, IN: Indiana University Press.

Cixous, H. (1993). We who are free, are we free? In B. Johnson (Ed.), *Freedom and interpretation: The Oxford Amnesty Lectures, 1992* (pp. 14–44). New York: HarperCollins.

Connelly, F., & Clandinin, D. (1990). Stories of experience and narrative inquiry. *Educational Researcher, 19*(5), 2–14.

Dillon, R. (1992). Respect and care: Toward moral integration. *Canadian Journal of Philosophy, 22,* 105–131.

Foucault, M. (1979). *Discipline and punish: The birth of the prison* (A. Sheridan, Trans.). New York: Vintage Books. (Original work published 1975)

Friedman, M. (1993). *What are friends for? Feminist perspectives on personal relationships and moral theory.* Ithaca, NY: Cornell University Press.

Gadow, S. (1982). Body and self: A dialectic. In V. Kestenbaum (Ed.), *The humanity of the ill: Phenomenological perspectives* (pp. 86–100). Knoxville, TN: University of Tennessee Press.

Gadow, S. (1994). Whose body? Whose story? The question about narrative in women's health care. *Soundings, 77,* 295–307.

Gadow, S. (1995). Clinical epistemology: A dialectic of nursing assessment. *Canadian Journal of Nursing Research, 27,* 25–34.

Gadow, S. (1999). I felt an island rising: Interpretive inquiry as motet. Manuscript submitted for publication.

Gouldner, A. (1978). *The dialectic of ideology and technology: The origins, grammar, and future of ideology.* Oxford, UK: Oxford University Press.

Hegel, G. W. F. (1977). *The phenomenology of spirit* (A. V. Miller, Trans.). Oxford, UK: Clarendon. (Original work published in 1807)

LeGuin, U. (1989). Some thoughts on narrative. In U. LeGuin (Ed.), *Dancing at the edge of the world: Thoughts on words, women, places* (pp. 37–45). New York: Harper & Row.

MacIntyre, A. (1981). *After virtue.* Notre Dame, IN: University of Notre Dame Press.

Poole, R. (1991). *Morality and modernity.* London: Routledge.

Rorty, R. (1989). *Contingency, irony, and solidarity.* Cambridge, UK: Cambridge University Press.

Sandelowski, M. (1994). We are the stories we tell: Narrative knowing in nursing practice. *Journal of Holistic Nursing, 12,* 23–33.

Scarry, E. (1985). *The body in pain: The making and unmaking of the world.* Oxford, UK: Oxford University Press.

Schroeder, C. (1998). So this is what it's like: Struggling to survive in pediatric intensive care. *Advances in Nursing Science, 20,* 13–22.

Tester, K. (1993). *The life and times of post-modernity.* London: Routledge.

Young, I. (1990). *Justice and the politics of difference.* Princeton, NJ: Princeton University Press.

Part Four

NURSING'S METAPARADIGM: PERSON AND ENVIRONMENT

Fawcett (2000, p. 5) states that the concept of *person* "refers to the individuals, families, communities, and other groups who are participants in nursing." *Environment* "refers to the person's significant others and physical surroundings . . . the setting in which nursing occurs, which ranges from the person's home to clinical agencies to society as a whole. . . . [It] also refers to all the local, regional, national, and worldwide cultural, social, political, and economic conditions that are associated with the person's health" (p. 5). Clearly, both concepts must be interpreted extremely broadly on a discipline-wide basis. In Part IV, two chapters on *environment* and two chapters pertaining to *persons* are included.

In Chapter 19, Butterfield explains why nurses and other health professionals must look beyond individuals' immediate behaviors, when considering health behaviors, to the societal contexts in which these occur. In many cases in which population health is negatively impacted, improvement stems not from actions at the individual level to change behaviors among those affected but rather from social actions aimed at significant changes in socioeconomic structures and processes that may affect thousands or millions. Butterfield's conceptualization of environment captures all of the dimensions that Fawcett outlined.

In Chapter 20, Kleffel further expands the concept of environment by explicating an ecocentric paradigm in contrast to an egocentric paradigm and a homocentric paradigm. The ecocentric approach is "grounded in the cosmos" and represents a view of environment as whole, living, interconnected, and one with humanity. Clearly, environmental perspectives offer many opportunities for both values-based practice with populations and evidence-based care for populations, but in ways that are qualitatively different from practice with individuals.

Representations of the human person as a bio–psycho–social–spiritual organism are replete in the literature of many disciplines and are undoubtedly familiar, in some form, to all graduate students in nursing. In Part IV, I have sought to introduce only novel conceptualizations that expand the received view. In Chapter 21, Boykin and Schoenhofer, whose framework of *nursing as caring* posits enhancing personhood as a goal of nursing, discuss how enhancing personhood can be viewed as an outcome of nursing practice. Personhood is here defined as "a process of living grounded in caring." Although "outcomes" represents a buzzword and a necessity in today's healthcare universe, it has rarely been defined qualitatively. This chapter challenges us to "suppose that nursing is not a quantity but a quality."

Articles about the "graying of America" and related themes frequently report on the prevalence of various chronic diseases, the necessity of more forms of gerontological care, and a myriad of concerns. In Chapter 22, McCormack introduces a conceptual framework for person-centered practice with older people. The central idea of person-centered practice is respect for persons and their right to self-determination, which McCormack links to the concept of autonomy as authentic consciousness, an explicitly value-laden view. Collectively, these articles represent the need for advanced practice nurses to place persons and their experiences at the center of the caring process, while maintaining a broad perspective of their environments, communities, and societies. This all-at-once seemingly contradictory stance is actually core to nursing as a scholarly discipline, and it must be understood for the advanced practice nursing to have a scholarly understanding of the discipline. These four chapters offer ample opportunities for reflection.

Chapter 19

Thinking Upstream: Nurturing a Conceptual Understanding of the Societal Context of Health Behavior

Patricia G. Butterfield, RN, MS

This chapter addresses the issue of overreliance on theories that define nursing in terms of a one-to-one relationship at the expense of theoretical perspectives that emphasize the societal context of health. When individuals are perceived as the focus of nursing action, the nurse is likely to propose intervention strategies aimed at either changing the behaviors of the individual or modifying the individual's perceptions of the world. When nurses understand the social, political, economic influences that shape the health of a society, they are more likely to recognize social action as a nursing role and work on behalf of populations.

Despite acknowledgment that an understanding of population health is essential in professional nursing, descriptions of one-to-one relationships predominate in the literature read by most nurses. Such portrayals often emphasize the evolution of the relationship between nurse and client with minimal attention to forces outside the relationship that have been paramount in shaping the client's health behaviors. Yet for most people, their cultural heritage, social roles, and economic situations have a far more profound influence on health behaviors than do interactions with any health care professional. Examination of nursing problems from a "think small" perspective[1(p. 504)] fosters inadequate consideration of these social, environmental, and political determinants of health. This perspective results not only in a restricted range of intervention possibilities for the nurse, but also

in a distorted impression of clients' behaviors. An understanding of the complex social, political, and economic forces that shape people's lives is necessary for nurses to promote health in individuals and groups. If nurses are not given an opportunity to appreciate the gestalt of populations and societies, they will be unable to develop a basis for analyzing problems.

This chapter addresses the issue of overreliance on theories that define nursing primarily in terms of a one-to-one relationship and the inherent conflict between these theories and the goal of enabling nurses to promote health through population-based interventions.

Nursing's Role in Pushing Upstream

In his description of the frustrations of medical practice, McKinlay[2] uses the image of a swiftly flowing river to represent illness. In this analogy, physicians are so caught up in rescuing victims

Source: Butterfield, PG. Thinking upstream: Nurturing a conceptual understanding of the societal context of health behavior. *Advances in Nursing Science* 1990;12(2): 1–8.

from the river that they have no time to look upstream to see who is pushing their patients into the perilous waters. The author uses this example to demonstrate the ultimate futility of "downstream endeavors,"[2(p. 9)] which are characterized by short-term, individual-based interventions, and he challenges health-care providers to focus more of their energies "upstream, where the real problems lie."[2(p. 9)] Upstream endeavors focus on modifying economic, political, and environmental factors that have been shown to be the precursors of poor health throughout the world. Although the analogy cites medical practice, it also aptly describes the dilemmas of a considerable portion of nursing practice, and although nursing has a rich historical record of providing preventive and population-based care, the current American health system, which emphasizes episodic and individual-based care, has done woefully little to stem the tide of chronic illness, to which 70 percent of the American population succumbs.

What is the cost of a continued emphasis on a microscopic perspective? How does a theoretical focus on the individual preclude understanding of a larger perspective? Dreher[1] maintains that a conservative scope of practice often uses psychologic theories to explain patterns of health and health care. In this mode of practice, low compliance, broken appointments, and reluctance to participate in care are all attributed to motivation or attitude problems on the part of the client. Nurses are charged with the responsibility of altering client attitudes toward health, rather than altering the system itself, "even though such negative attitudes may well be a realistic appraisal of health care."[1(p. 505)] Greater emphasis is paid to the psychologic symptoms of poor health than to socioeconomic causes; "indeed the symptoms are being taken as its causes."[1(p. 505)] The nurse who views the world from such a perspective does not entertain the possibility of working to alter the system itself or empowering clients to do so.

Involvement in social reform is considered to be within the realm of nursing practice.[3] Dreher[1] acknowledges the historical role of public health nurses in facilitating social change and notes that social involvement and activism are expected of nurses in this area of practice. The American Nurses' Association (ANA) Social Policy Statement delineates, among other social concerns, the "provision for the public health through use of preventive and environmental measures and increased assumption of responsibility by individuals, families, and other groups"[3(p. 4)] and addresses nursing's role in response to those concerns. However, in her review of the document, White[4] notes an incongruence between nursing's social concerns, which clearly transcend individual-based practice, and the description of nursing as "a practice in which interpersonal closeness of the professional kind develops and aids the investigation and discussion of problems, as nurse and patient (or family or group) seek jointly to resolve those concerns."[3(p. 19)] White[4] also notes the document's neglect of the population focus and possibilities for modifying the environment. Clearly, nursing has yet to reconcile many of the differences between operationalization of a population-centered practice and policies that define nursing primarily in terms of individual-focused care.

Three theoretic approaches will be contrasted later here to demonstrate how they may lead the nurse to draw different conclusions not only about the reasons for client behavior, but also about the range of interventions available to the nurse.

The Downstream View: The Individual as the Locus of Change

The health belief model evolved from the premise that the world of the perceiver determines what he or she will do. The social psychologists[5,6] who outlined this model were strongly influenced by Lewin and the view that a person's daily activities are guided by processes of attraction to positive valences and avoidance of negative valences. From these inceptions evolved a model that purports to explain why people do or do not engage in a preventive health action in response to a specific disease threat. The model places the burden of action exclusively on the client; only those clients who have distorted or negative perceptions of the specified disease or recommended health action will fail to act. In practice, this model focuses the nurse's energies on interventions designed to modify the client's distorted perceptions. Although the process of promoting behavior change may be masked under the premise of mutually defined goals, passive acceptance of the nurse's advice is the desired outcome of the relationship.

Although the health belief model was not designed to specify intervention strategies, it can lead the nurse to deduce that client problems can be solved merely by altering the client's belief system. The model addresses the concept of "perceived benefits versus perceived barriers/costs associated with taking a health action."[6(p. 563)] Nurses may easily interpret this situation as a need to modify the client's perceptions of benefits and barriers. For example, clients with problems accessing adequate health care might receive counseling aimed at helping them see these barriers in a new light; the model does not include the possibility that the nurse may become involved in activities that promote equal access to all in need.

True to its historical roots, the model offers an explanation of health behaviors that, in many ways, is similar to a mechanical system. From the health belief model, one easily concludes that compliance can be induced by using model variables as catalysts to stimulate action. For example, an intervention study based on health belief model precepts sought to increase follow-up in hypertensive clients by increasing the clients' awareness of their susceptibility to hypertension and of its danger.[7] Clients received education, over the telephone or in the emergency department, that was designed to increase their perception of the benefits of follow-up. According to these authors, the interventions resulted in a dramatic increase in compliance. However, they noted several client groups that failed to respond to the intervention, most notably a small group of clients who had no available child care. Although this study demonstrates the predictive power of health belief model concepts, it also exemplifies the limitations of the model. The health belief model may be effective in promoting behavioral change through the alteration of clients' perspectives, but it does not acknowledge responsibility for the health-care professional to reduce or ameliorate client barriers.

In fact, some of the proponents of the health belief model readily acknowledge the limitations of the model and caution users against generalizing it beyond the domain of the individual psyche. In their review of 10 years of research with the model, Janz and Becker[8] remind researchers that the model can only account for the variance in health behaviors that is explained by the attitudes and beliefs of an individual. Melnyk's[9] recent review of the concept of barriers reinforces the notion that, because the health belief model is based on subjective perceptions, research that adopts this theoretic basis must take care to include the subjects', rather than the researchers', perceptions of barriers. Janz and Becker[8] address the influence of other factors such as habituation and nonhealth reasons on making positive changes in health behavior, and they acknowledge the influence of environmental and economic factors that prohibit individuals from undertaking a more healthy way of life.

The health belief model is but a prototype for the type of theoretic perspective that has dominated nursing education and thus nursing practice. The model's strength—its narrow scope—is also its limitation: One is not drawn outside it to those forces that shape the characteristics that the model describes.

The Upstream View: Society as the Locus of Change

Milio's Framework for Prevention

Milio's framework for prevention[10] provides a thought-provoking complement to the health belief model and a mechanism for directing attention upstream and examining opportunities for nursing intervention at the population level. Milio moves the focus of attention upstream by pointing out that it is the range of available health choices, rather than the choices made at any one time, that is paramount in shaping the overall health status of a society. She maintains that the range of choices widely available to individuals is shaped, to a large degree, by policy decisions in both governmental and private organizations. Rather than concentrate efforts on imparting information to change patterns of individual behavior, she advocates national-level policy making as the most effective means of favorably affecting the health of most Americans.

Milio[10] proposes that health deficits often result from an imbalance between a population's health needs and its health-sustaining resources, with affluent societies afflicted by the diseases associated with excess (obesity, alcoholism) and the poor afflicted by diseases that result from inadequate or unsafe food, shelter, and water. In this context, the poor in affluent societies may experience the least desirable combination of factors. Milio notes that although socioeconomic realities deprive many Americans of a health-sustaining environment, "cigarettes, sucrose, pollutants, and tensions are readily available to the poor."[10(p. 436)]

The range of health-promoting or health-damaging choices available to individuals is affected by their personal resources and their societal resources. Personal resources include one's awareness, knowledge, and beliefs, including those of one's family and friends, as well as money, time, and the urgency of other priorities. Societal resources are strongly influenced by community and national locale and include the availability and cost of health services, environmental protection, safe shelter, and the penalties or rewards given for failure to select the given options.

Milio notes the fallacy of the commonly held assumption in health education that knowing health-generating behaviors implies acting in accordance with that knowledge, and she cites the lifestyles of health professionals in support of her argument. She proposes that "most human beings, professional or nonprofessional, provider or consumer, make the easiest choices available to them most of the time."[10(p. 435)] Therefore, health-promoting choices must be more readily available and less costly than health-damaging options if individuals are to be healthy and a society is to improve its health status.

The opportunities for a society to make healthy choices have been a central theme throughout Milio's work. In a recent book she elaborated on this theme:

> *Personal behavior patterns are not simply "free" choices about "lifestyle," isolated from their personal and economic context. Lifestyles are, rather, patterns of choices made from the alternatives that are available to people according to their socioeconomic circumstances and the ease with which they are able to choose certain ones over others.*[11(p. 76)]

Milio is critical of many traditional approaches to health education that emphasize knowledge acquisition and consequently expect behavior change. In addressing the role of public health in primary care, Milio voices concern that "health damage accumulates in societies too, vitiating their vitality . . . [and charges nurses to redirect energies] so as to foster conditions that help people to retain a self-sustaining physiological and social balance."[12(pp.188,189)]

One cannot help but note the similarities between Milio's health resources and the concepts in the health belief model. The health belief model is more comprehensive than Milio's framework in examining the internal dynamics of health decision making. However, Milio offers a different set of insights into the arena of health behaviors by proposing that many low-income individuals are acting within the constraints of their limited resources. Furthermore, she goes beyond the individual focus and addresses changes in the health of populations as a result of shifts in decision making by significant numbers of people within a population.

Critical Social Theory

Just as Milio uses societal awareness as an aid to understanding health behaviors, critical social theory employs similar means to expose social inequities that prohibit people from reaching their full potential. This theoretic approach is based on the belief that life is structured by social meanings that are determined, rather one-sidedly, through social domination.[13] In contrast to the assumptions of analytic empiricism, critical theory maintains that standards of truth are socially determined and that no form of scientific inquiry is value free.[13,15] Proponents of this theoretic approach posit that social discourse that is not distorted from power imbalances will stimulate the evolution of a more rational society. The interests of truth are served only when people are able to voice their beliefs without fear of authority or retribution.[13]

Allen[14] discusses how nursing practice can be enriched by enabling clients to remove the conscious and unconscious constraints in their everyday lives. He states that women and the economically impoverished are especially vulnerable to being labeled by pseudodiseases that are rooted in social formations, such as hysteria and depression. Health care providers often frame such problems only within the context of the individual or, at best, the family. But critical social theory can enable a nurse to reframe such an interpretation to gain an understanding of the historical play of social forces that have limited the choices truly available to the involved parties. Through exploration of the societal forces, traditions, and roles that have created the meanings of health and illness, clients may be freed of the isolation and alienation that accompany individual problem ownership.

At the collective level, Waitzkin asserts that the current emphasis on lifestyle diverts attention from important sources of illness in the capitalist industrial environment; "it also puts the burden of health squarely on the individual rather than seeking collective solutions to health problems."[16(p. 664)] Salmon[17] supports this position by noting that the basic tenets of Western medicine promote the delineation of individual factors of health and illness, while obscuring the exploration of their social and economic roots. He states that critical social theory "can aid in uncovering larger dimensions impacting health that are usually unseen or misrepresented by ideological biases. Thus, the social reality of health conditions can be both understood and changed."[17(p. 75)]

Because the theory holds that each person is responsible for creating social conditions in which all members of society are able to speak freely, the nurse is challenged, as an individual and as a member of the profession, to expose power imbalances that prohibit people from achieving their full potential. Nurses versed in critical theory are equipped to see beyond the perpetuation of status quo ideas and may be able to generate unique ideas that are unencumbered by previous stereotypes.[14]

Other Examples of Upstream Thinking

Recent nursing literature provides several other examples of upstream thinking. In a thought-provoking commentary on an intervention program for middle-aged women experiencing subclinical depression, Davis[18] (cited in Gordon and Ledray) notes a lack of congruence between the study's portrayal of depression as a problem with societal roots and its instruction in coping strategies as the intervention program. While recognizing the merits of the intervention program, she comments that, "if our principal task as progressive nurses is to develop and utilize interventions that will ameliorate these social problems, then the emphasis in nursing education and practice might well be on those social actions that aim to change basic social factors such as ageism and sexism."[18(p. 277)]

Chopoorian[19] takes a different tack, emphasizing the concept of environment and suggesting that nurses develop a consciousness of the social, political, and economic aspects of environment. She maintains that a static portrayal of the environment precludes nurses from acting as advocates for people who lack adequate housing and health care and live in intolerable circumstances. She charges nurses to move beyond a psychosocial conceptualization of the environment into a sociopolitical–economic conceptualization. Through this reconceptualization, nurses will see that human responses to health and illnesses "are related to the structure of the social world, the economic and political policies that govern that structure, and the human, social relationships that are produced by the structure and the policies."[19(p. 46)]

The Need for Alternative Perspectives

The danger of the conservative perspective lies not within its content, but rather in the omission of other, larger theories that enable nurses to view situations from both a microscopic and a macroscopic perspective. In discussing the dilemmas of "studying health behavior as an individual phenomena [sic], rather than in the context of a broader social change phenomena [sic]," Cummings[20(p. 93)] reminds us that the approaches are complementary, and both are necessary to a comprehensive understanding of health promotion. The strengths and utility of each theoretic approach are most clearly revealed through an understanding of alternative approaches.

Nursing needs conceptual foundations that enable its practitioners to understand health problems manifested at community, national, and international levels as well as those at the individual and family levels. The continued bias in favor of individual-focused theories robs nurses of an understanding of the richness and complexity of forces that shape the behavior of populations. The omission of theories that relate nursing to the social context of behavior may leave nurses with a minimal understanding of their responsibilities to facilitate change at this level and without the tools to promote such change in an effective and systematic manner.

Maglacas[21] provides a global perspective on the health conditions of societies throughout the world and draws attention to the gaps in service access between the rich and the poor. She then charges nurses within each society and culture to act in response to the inequities in health within that society. If nurses are to be able to enact change at the societal level, they need to be provided with theoretic frameworks that are consistent with such ends and with theoretic perspectives in which social, economic, and political forces are given equal weight with the interpersonal aspects of nursing. Through these means, nurses gain insight into the social precursors of poor health and restricted opportunities and learn rationales for engaging in social action. By tipping the scales of nursing back toward consideration of theories that address health from a societal perspective, nurses can receive not only a richness of understanding but also the means by which to enact this kind of change.

References

1. Dreher MC. The conflict of conservatism in public health nursing education. *Nurs Outlook.* 1982;30:504–509.

2. McKinlay JB. A case for refocussing upstream: The political economy of illness. In: Jaco EG, ed. *Patients, Physicians, and Illness*, 3rd ed. New York: Free Press; 1979:9–25.

3. American Nurses' Association. *Nursing: A Social Policy Statement.* Kansas City: American Nurses' Association; 1980.

4. White CM. A critique of the ANA social policy statement. *Nurs Outlook.* 1984;32:328–331.

5. Rosenstock IM. Historical origins of the health belief model. In: Becker MH, ed. *The Health Belief Model and Personal Health Behavior.* Thorofare, NJ: Charles B. Slack; 1974:1–8.

6. Becker MH, Maiman LA. Models of health-related behavior. In: Mechanic D, ed. *Handbook of Health, Health Care, and the Health Professions.* New York: Free Press; 1983:539–568.

7. Jones PK, Jones SL, Katz J. Improving follow-up among hypertensive patients using a health belief model intervention. *Arch Intern Med.* 1987;147:1557–1560.

8. Janz NK, Becker MH. The health belief model: A decade later. *Health Educ Q.* 1984;11:1–47.

9. Melnyk KM. Barriers: A critical review of recent literature. *Nurs Res.* 1988;37:196–201.

10. Milio N. A framework for prevention: Changing health-damaging to health-generating life patterns. *Am J Public Health.* 1976;66:435–439.

11. Milio N. *Promoting Health Through Public Policy.* Philadelphia: F.A. Davis; 1981.

12. Milio N. *Primary Care and the Public's Health.* Lexington, MA: Lexington Books; 1983.

13. Allen D, Diekelmann N, Bennet P. Three paradigms for nursing research. In: Chinn P, ed. *Nursing Research Methodology: Issues & Implementation.* Rockville, MD: Aspen Publishers; 1986:23–28.

14. Allen DG. Nursing research and social control: Alternate models of science that emphasize understanding and emancipation. *Image: The Journal of Nursing Scholarship.* 1985;17:58–64.

15. Allen DG. Critical social theory as a model for analyzing ethical issues in family and community health. *Fam Commun Health.* 1987;10:63–72.

16. Waitzkin H. A Marxist view of health and health care. In: Mechanic D, ed. *Handbook of Health, Health Care, and the Health Professions.* New York: Free Press; 1983:657–682.

17. Salmon JW. Dilemmas in studying social change versus individual change: Considerations from political economy. In: Duffy ME, Pender NJ, eds. *Conceptual Issues in Health Promotion: A Report of Proceedings of a Wingspread Conference.* Indianapolis, IN: Sigma Theta Tau; 1987:70–81.

18. Davis AJ. Cited by Gordon VC, Ledray LE. Growth-support intervention for the treatment of depression in women of middle years. *West J Nurs Res.* 1986;8:263–283.

19. Chopoorian TJ. Reconceptualizing the environment. In: Moccia P, ed. *New Approaches to Theory Development.* New York: National League for Nursing; 1986:39–54. Publication 15-1992.

20. Cummings KM. Dilemmas in studying health as an individual phenomenon. In: Duffy ME, Pender NJ, eds. *Conceptual Issues in Health Promotion: A Report of Proceedings of a Wingspread Conference.* Indianapolis, IN: Sigma Theta Tau; 1987:91–96.

21. Maglacas AM. Health for all: Nursing's role. *Nurs Outlook.* 1988;36:66–71.

Chapter 20

Environmental Paradigms: Moving Toward an Ecocentric Perspective

Dorothy Kleffel,
RN, MPH, DNSc

This article examines a taxonomy of three environmental paradigms. The egocentric paradigm is grounded in the person and is based on the assumption that what is good for the individual is good for society. The homocentric paradigm is grounded in society and reflects the utilitarian ethic of the greatest good for the greatest number of people. The ecocentric paradigm is grounded in the cosmos, and the environment is considered whole, living, and interconnected. Historically, nurses have adhered primarily to the egocentric paradigm and to a lesser extent to the homocentric paradigm. However, because the world has become a global community, contemporary nurse scholars are shifting to the ecocentric paradigm. Keywords: ecocentric, environment, paradigm, philosophy.

The environmental focus of nursing has traditionally been centered on clients' immediate surroundings in the hospital or other institution, home, or community. This circumscribed environmental worldview of nursing is undergoing change as nurses become aware of the adverse effects of environmental disasters and degradation on human health. Regional catastrophic environmental events like the Bhopal chemical leak, the Chernobyl nuclear disaster, and the Exxon Valdez oil spill have had immediate and lasting consequences. Global dimensions of the decline of the planet's environment include worldwide temperature rise, ozone depletion, destruction of the world's forests, human overpopulation, depleted fish popula-

tions, soil erosion, worldwide hunger, homelessness, and massive species extinction.[1,2] These are not isolated environmental problems that can be addressed by individual effort; they require the coordinated effort of people across the entire planet. Nurses are beginning to understand the scope of environmental threats that threaten everything that exists, living and nonliving. Nurses' enhanced consciousness of the environment has caused the profession to question its current assumptions about the environmental domain of nursing knowledge.

Nursing scholars are becoming cognizant that the existing environmental paradigm does not provide the knowledge and theoretical base to account for environmental conditions that compromise health promotion and interfere with optimum health. Nurses in general do not understand the interrelations between social,

Source: Kleffel, D. Environmental paradigms: Moving toward an ecocentric perspective. *Advances in Nursing Science*, 1996;18(4):1–10 political, and economic structures and the origins of health and illnesses.[3] Nursing theory does not adequately describe the concept of the environment. Almost all nursing research conducted in the domain of environment involves only the immediate milieu of the client, family, or nurse.[4] Nursing's care theories do not allow for nonhuman interchange of care or caring because of their anthropocentricity. Anthropocentrism results in the subjugation of nonhuman nature, which jeopardizes the quality of the physical world and causes other forms of oppression and domination.[5]

These critiques of nursing's environmental assumptions indicate that the profession is experiencing an environmental paradigm shift. A *paradigm* is the body of values, commitments, beliefs, and knowledge shared by members of a profession. Research guidelines, questions, and methodology emanate from the paradigm. When new knowledge is discovered that no longer fits the paradigm or when the paradigm no longer provides model problems and solutions, an anomaly exists. When anomalies become so numerous and significant that they can no longer be ignored, investigations are initiated by the profession. Theories are explored and rejected until a new paradigm emerges that leads to a new basis for practice.[6]

Contemporary nursing scholars are exploring a variety of new environmental ideas and theories as the profession changes its environmental worldview. To contribute to this dialogue, I examine a taxonomy of three environmental paradigms—egocentric, homocentric, and ecocentric—that summarize the assumptions of Western culture regarding the natural world since the 17th century.[7,8] I propose the inclusion of the ecocentric environmental perspective into a central position in nursing's body of knowledge. This mainstreaming of a global view would encourage and support nurses to act with others in averting worldwide environmental disaster.

Egocentric Approach

The egocentric approach is grounded at the personal level and assumes that what is best for the individual is best for society. It is concerned with liberty, rights, and independent action of the individual. It is the dominant Western worldview. Its philosophical foundation is individualistic and mechanistic and includes the thought of Plato, mainstream Christianity, Descartes, Hegel, George Berkeley, Hobbes, Locke, Adam Smith, Malthus, and Garrett Hardin.[8] The egocentric approach is a mechanistic paradigm and assumes that matter is composed of atomic parts, the whole is equal to the sum of the parts, causation is a matter of external action on inactive parts, quantitative change is more important than qualitative change, and there is dualistic separation of mind–body and matter–spirit.[7] In the egocentric approach, the individual is the focus of change.

Most practicing nurses adhere to the egocentric worldview. Their approach is individualistic. They regard the environment as the immediate surroundings or circumstances of the individual or as an interactional field that individuals adapt to, adjust to, or control.[3] The environment is defined in relation to the individual person rather than in terms of its own essence and intrinsic value.

Because the egocentric approach has been the dominant perspective in the Western world, many nurse theorists incorporated those ideas into their theories. An example of a nurse theorist who adhered to the egocentric paradigm was Roy.[9] She defined the environment as all internal and external conditions, circumstances, and influences surrounding and affecting the development and behavior of individuals and groups. Stimuli emanate from the environment and are categorized as focal (immediately confronting the person), contextual (all other stimuli present), and residual (beliefs and attitudes that impinge on the situation). The purpose of nursing is to enhance the adaptation of the patient to environmental stimuli. Roy[10] believed that the science of nursing focuses on human life processes as the core knowledge to be developed. Roy's theory is considered egocentric because of its emphasis on individual adaptation to the environment and on human beings to the exclusion of the rest of nature.

Egocentrism has been the guiding ethic of private entrepreneurs and corporations whose goal is maximization of profit from the development of natural resources. The egocentric approach is limited because of its assumption that the individual good is the highest good that will ultimately benefit society as a whole and that humans are fundamentally different from other creatures, which they are to dominate and control.[7]

Homocentric Approach

The homocentric approach is the utilitarian ethic and is grounded at the social level.[7,8] Social justice, rather than individual progress, is the key value. Decisions are made based on the common good, which is the greatest good for the largest number of people. Humans are considered stewards and caretakers of the natural world. The philosophical foundations of homocentrism are both materialism and positivism. Its assumptions are that humans have a cultural heritage in addition to their genetic inheritance that results in their being qualitatively different from animals, that the determinants of human affairs are social rather than individual, and that culture is a cumulative progress that can continue indefinitely. All social problems are viewed as ultimately solvable. Exponents of the homocentric approach include John S. Mill and Jeremy Bentham (utilitarian theorists), Barry Commoner (socialist ecology), Karl Marx and Mao Tse Tung (political theorists), and JØrgen Randers and Donella and Dennis Meadows (limits-to-growth theorists).

The body of knowledge derived from epidemiology serves as an information base for the practice of public health nursing. Public health nurses use epidemiology in diagnosing, planning, treating, and evaluating community health problems. The nurse who interacts with individual clients and families uses the information for assessing, planning, intervening, and evaluating at the community level.[11] Epidemiology is considered homocentric because of its emphasis on the health of populations rather than individuals.

In the homocentric view, the environment is the focus of change rather than the individual. The homocentric approach to the environment is basically anthropocentric in that humans are to manage nature for the benefit of humans. The management of nature for the intrinsic benefit of other species is not considered in this paradigm.[7]

Ecocentric Approach

The ecocentric approach is grounded in the cosmos. The whole environment, including inanimate elements such as rocks and minerals, along with animate animals and plants, is assigned intrinsic value. It is rooted in holistic rather than mechanistic metaphysics. It assumes that everything is connected to everything else, that the whole is greater than the sum of its parts, that meaning is dependent on context, that biological and social systems are open, and that humans and nonhumans are one within the same organic system. Exponents of the ecocentric approach include most traditional Eastern systems of thought, traditional Native American philosophies, Thoreau, Gary Snyder, Theodore Rozak, Aldo Leopold, Rachel Carson, Fritjof Capra, deep ecology, the holographic model, and ecofeminism.[7,8]

Within the ecocentric paradigm are four contemporary nursing theorists. Sarter[12] compared the philosophical perspectives of fellow nursing theorists Rogers, Neuman, Watson, and Parse and found common shared holistic themes of process, evolution of consciousness, self-transcendence, open systems, harmony, relativity of space and time, pattern, and holism. *Process* is the evolutionary change of human consciousness; *self-transcendence* is the method of the evolution of human consciousness through higher and higher levels toward unity with the universe. *Open systems* are the dynamic and continuous interactions between the person and the world and are essential for the evolution of human consciousness. *Harmony* is considered to exist both within the person and between the person and the environment. Space and time are considered nonlinear, relative, and fluid, with the past and future merging into the present. *Pattern* is information that represents the whole. Pattern recognition is nursing action that looks for patterns representing the whole rather than parts of the whole. Sarter noted that each of these theorists has been influenced, either directly or indirectly, by Eastern philosophies. She believed that the foundation of a commonly held nursing worldview has been laid.

Watson[13] has continued to develop her ecocentric perspectives, moving toward a unitary–transformative viewpoint. This model has eliminated the subject–object and mind–body duality. It acknowledges unity and integrality between humans and the environment; thus conceptualized, human beings and their worlds are not separated.

Other modern nursing scholars also adhere to the ecocentric paradigm. Schuster[14] advocated for a conscious choice of earth dwelling through self-identification and interconnectedness with all beings, which lead one naturally to care for the world in day-to-day living. It is a way of being in the world that allows for all of creation, not just humans, to emerge.

Kleffel,[15] during a qualitative research study, identified [17] distinguished scholars whose work has addressed broad environmental dimensions related to nursing. All except two explicitly reflected the ecocentric paradigm and perceived

the environment to be alive, whole, interconnected, and interacting. These scholars add strength to the idea of the united nursing worldview described by Sarter.[12]

The ecocentric approach has some philosophical difficulties. The central problem is finding a philosophically adequate justification for the intrinsic value of nonhuman nature. In mainstream Western thought, only humans have intrinsic worth, although the rest of nature has instrumental value as a resource for humans. It is not considered wrong to kill the last of a species or use the last mineral if human survival is at stake.[7]

Ecocentrism in the World's Traditions

The egocentric paradigm has been the dominant worldview of most practicing nurses working in hospitals and other health institutions and is ascribed to by the greatest number of nurses in the profession. The homocentric perspective has influenced far fewer nurses, traditionally those practicing in the field of public health nursing, although there are signs of a shifting of the profession toward the homocentric approach in the form of aggregate and population-based nursing.[16] The ecocentric view is only beginning to inform the profession and has not yet achieved significant prominence in nursing scholarship or practice.

Embracing an ecocentric viewpoint has exhilarating potential for transforming nursing scholarship and practice beyond its traditional boundaries. We are now living in a global culture that is united by economic interdependence, international air transportation, and worldwide communications networks. Contemporary environmental degradation and disasters that adversely affect humans have moved into the global arena. Actions stem from worldviews, and the worldview of nursing has been mostly egocentric. Moving to the ecocentric paradigm will encourage nurses to address worldwide environmental problems that affect the health of everything that exists.

Solving global environmental problems will entail international efforts from a variety of disciplines and from many cultures. Such an approach will entail collaborative problem solving by people with differing traditions and cultural backgrounds. To work together, a common global environmental worldview that can incorporate these diverse perspectives is needed. The ecocentric paradigm, which is compatible with elements of Native American traditional ideas, Eastern philosophies, and contemporary Western thought, holds great promise for a unified worldview to which all humans can subscribe.

Native American Tradition

There are difficulties in universalizing the Native American belief system because it comprises so many different cultures. However, some generalizations can be made.[17] The Native American attitude was to regard all entities in the environment as having consciousness, reason, and volition as intense and complete as humans. These entities included the earth itself, the sky, the winds, rocks, streams, trees, insects, birds, and animals. This pervasive spirit in everything was considered a part of the Great Spirit, which fostered the perception of humans and nature as being unified and akin. The Native American's social circle or community included all nonhuman natural entities as well as other humans.

The consequences of the Native American inspired worldview of nature produced a harmony between them and their environment that restrained their killing of animals and gathering of plants to what was necessary for survival. Although there were occasional examples of destruction of nature during periods of enormous cultural stress, the overall and usual effort was conservation of resources. The Native American cultural traditions were not altruistic; they considered it in their own self-interest to defer to nature, which they believed would withhold its sustenance or actively retaliate if provoked.[17]

Eastern Systems of Thought

Similar themes of a unified, living, conscious, and interacting world are found in almost all Eastern systems of thought. With the exception of Islam, these systems are antihierarchal and anthropocentric. Although Islam maintains that humans are dominant over nature, a view similar to the Judeo–Christian tradition, it instructs its adherents to prevent environmental deterioration because the world is God's creation.[18] Other Eastern philosophies emphasize harmony and balance. All aspects of the environment interact, with the parts being within the whole and the whole being within the parts. Humans are a part of the whole and admonished to live in equilibrium with all other parts of the planet.[19]

Some examples of Eastern thought include the law of Karma of the Advita Vedanta, which binds humans together in continuity with the natural world.[20] The wu wei of Taoism is an awareness that allows one to maximize creative possibilities of oneself as a dimension of the environment.[21] The Chi of Chinese thought is a vital force that is the basic structure of the cosmos and exists in all things. Nature is the result of fusion and merging of vital forces to form the "great harmony."[22]

A popular image for portraying the manner in which things exist is described from the Hua-yen school of Buddhism.[23] From the great god Indra there hangs a marvelous net that stretches out infinitely in all directions. There is a jewel in each eye of the net. Because the net is infinite in dimension, the jewels are infinite in number. When one jewel is selected and carefully looked at, all of the other jewels in the net are reflected. In addition, each of the jewels reflected is also reflecting all of the other jewels, so that an infinite reflecting process occurs.

This image symbolizes the cosmos, in which there is an infinitely repeated interrelationship among all of the members of the cosmos. Thus, the part and the whole are one and the same, for what we identify as a part is merely an abstraction from a unitary whole. There is no part-and-whole duality as in Western thought. This totalistic world is a living body in which each cell derives its life from the other cells and in return gives life to the others.

Western Approaches

The ecocentric environmental themes found in Eastern and traditional Native American worldviews originated in ancient times. Several modern Western ecocentric environmental approaches reflect these ideas. The science of ecology, along with relativity and quantum theory, is creating a postmodern scientific worldview. This emerging worldview is in congruence with the traditional and indigenous environmental paradigms of preindustrial cultures.[24] Naess criticized traditional ecology (an egocentric approach), which he dubbed "shallow ecology,"[25(p. 95)] as being concerned only with pollution control and resource conservation in the interests of people in developed countries. He argued that there are deeper concerns (hence the phrase "deep ecology," also called "radical environmentalism") that touch on the principles of diversity, complexity, autonomy, decentralization, symbiosis, egalitarianism, and classlessness. Deep ecology derives its essence from some Eastern and Native American ideas as well as from feminism, John Muir, and other naturalist literature.[26]

The modern Gaia hypothesis is reminiscent of the ancient living organic theory. This view of the environment was proposed by Lovelock,[27,28] an atmospheric chemist. Lovelock saw the evolution of the species of living organisms as being so closely coupled with the evolution of their physical and chemical environment that together they constitute a single and indivisible evolutionary process. No clear distinction is made between living and nonliving material. The planet's organisms act together as a unity to regulate the global environment by adjusting the rates at which gases are produced and removed from the atmosphere. Lovelock warned that the earth's ability to self-regulate is affected by natural or human activity, which could force the climate into a new and different stable state that would result in the elimination of all living organisms.

The idea of the planet's stable state in the modern Gaia hypothesis reflects the idea of harmony in ancient Taoist thought. In both notions, the balance of the environment of the planet must be maintained, or ecological disaster will result.

Bohm,[29] a physicist and one of the early pioneers of the holographic model, believed that the universe is organized along holographic principles. Everything in the universe is part of a continuum, a seamless extension of everything else. There are no separate parts, just as a geyser in a fountain is not separated from the water from which it flows. However, the universe is not an undifferentiated mass. Things can have their own unique qualities and still be part of an undivided whole. Similarly, consciousness is present in all matter in various degrees. The universe cannot be divided into living and nonliving things. All things are interconnected; like a hologram, every portion of the universe contains the whole.

There are similarities of imagery between the holographic model and Indra's net. The giant hologram and Indra's net symbolize the cosmos. All parts of the hologram are interconnected; each jewel in Indra's net is connected with every other jewel. The parts of the hologram and each jewel of Indra's net reflect the whole. The whole of the hologram and the whole of Indra's net reflect each part or jewel. Bohm believed that fragmentation is the cause of most present-day problems. Applied to the environment, one portion of the planet cannot be harmed without resulting damage to the entire planet.

Another modern Western ecocentric view is ecofeminism. Ecofeminism is a theory that women and the environment are interconnected as both share and have been subjected to the same patriarchal domination.[30] A failure to understand these connections will result in the continued exploitation of both women and environment at the theory, policy, and practice levels. Ecofeminists recognize the interconnectedness of women and the environment and recognize the necessity of uniting feminism and ecology. However, feminist theory is not environmentally sensitive. Deep ecology and the Gaia hypothesis share themes of unity and wholeness to which ecofeminists can subscribe; however, both are oriented toward a patriarchal culture. Ecofeminists hold the view that the connections between the twin dominations of women and nature require a feminist theory and practice informed by an ecological perspective and an environmentalism informed by a feminist perspective.[31]

Ecofeminism is against domination of all kinds, including ageism, sexism, and the exploitation of nature. It is contextual and relational and includes consideration of nonhuman relationships with each other, humans, and the community. Ecofeminism identifies human nature within the historical context. It is antireductionist and pluralistic, centralizing on diversity of humans and nonhumans, yet affirming that humans are a part of the ecological community. Ecofeminism provides a central place for values that are typically underrepresented or ignored in our society such as care, love, friendship, and appropriate trust. Ecofeminism views theory building, objectivity, and knowledge as historically and contextually situated and as changing over time.[31,32]

Implementing the Ecocentric Paradigm

Understanding that the environment is alive, whole, interconnected, and interacting and that humans are one with the environment will encourage nurses to practice in an environmentally sensitive manner in whatever setting they work. Nurses working in local settings will understand the relationships between organizational resource use and the worldwide environment. Using the adage "think globally, act locally," they will act within their sphere by doing such things as calling for institutional audits of their work environment, taking client environmental histories, counseling clients regarding the effects of ozone depletion on the incidence of skin cancers and cataracts, reducing the use of toxic materials, purchasing recycled materials and supplies, using products with environmentally friendly packaging, saving water, managing waste safely, using both sides of the paper when copying reports and forms, using reusable products, reducing the use of disposable items, buying rechargeable batteries,[33] and questioning animal experimentation.[34]

Moving to the ecocentric paradigm will mean extending the concept of the nursing client to include the planetary environment. Some nurses will choose to work in the global environmental arena and address international environmental causes of illnesses. For instance, the alarming increase of breast cancer worldwide is an area where nurses could make a difference. In the United States, the risk of breast cancer has increased from 1 in 20 in 1960 to 1 in 8 today. Other industrial countries have similar rates. The incidence in developing countries is also rising, but at a slower rate. Risk factors and lifestyle account for only 20% to 30% of breast cancer cases. Some experts believe that pollutants and chemicals that duplicate or interfere with the effects of estrogen are a possible cause. They point to the fact that in Israel, breast cancer mortality in premenopausal women declined by 30 percent following regulations to reduce levels of DDT and carcinogenic pesticides in dietary fat.[35] Other experts believe that low-level radiation and synthetic chemicals such as chlorines are responsible for the increase in breast cancer in women.[36]

Mainstream medicine and science have ignored the possible environmental causes of breast cancer, focusing on the identification of women with risk factors, early case finding through breast self-examination, routine mammograms, and changing lifestyles (smoking cessation, exercise, and lowering dietary fat intake). In contrast, groups like the Women's Environment and Development Organization and Greenpeace are advocating for public attention to the possible links between the environment and breast cancer.[37] Nurses have followed medicine's lead by emphasizing compliance with breast self-examination, counseling women with risk factors associated with breast cancer, and providing education regarding healthy lifestyles. However, they have not directed their attention toward the relationships between breast cancer and the environment, which are being ignored by most research organizations. Using a global, multidisciplinary perspective, nurses could network with other researchers throughout the world to coordinate investigative efforts to identify environmental causes of breast cancer.

Emerging strains of recurring infectious diseases is another area where nurses could make a difference. AIDS, Lyme disease, the Hanta virus, the deadly Ebola virus, the recurrence of plague in India, and the increases in cholera, tuberculosis, and malaria worldwide are examples of conditions related to environmental alterations, climate changes, rapid international travel, and other human activity.[38] Although these diseases are causing illnesses and the deaths of millions of people, nurses generally do not regard scholarship or action in this arena as part of their domain. It is predicted that the epidemics will get worse as the displacement of wild populations and their habitats caused by development activities continue. International multidisciplinary efforts are required to keep ecosystems intact, minimize habitat alterations, require planners to prepare for unanticipated conse-

quences of development, and establish a reliable global surveillance system. Acting internationally in concert with other nurses, other disciplines, and other organizations, nurses could, if they had a global vision, bring their unique skills and perspectives to addressing this type of global environmental phenomenon.

Moving toward an ecocentric perspective will give nurses a common worldview, already held by a great proportion of the world's peoples, of oneness with a living planet, harmony, balance, interconnectedness, and transcendence. It will empower nurses to move beyond their present domain boundaries to align their efforts with other disciplines and organizations worldwide to address the devastating environmental problems affecting the earth and threatening all of existence.

References

1. Brown LR, Flavin, French H. *State of the World 1995: A Worldwatch Institute Report on Progress Toward a Sustainable Society*. New York: Norton; 1995.

2. Brown LR, Nicholas L, Kane H. *Vital Signs 1995: The Trends That Are Shaping Our Future*. New York: Norton; 1995.

3. Chopoorian TJ. Reconceptualizing the environment. In: Moccia P, ed. *New Approaches to Theory Development*. New York: National League for Nursing; 1986.

4. Kleffel D. Rethinking the environment as a domain of nursing knowledge. *ANS*. 1991;14(1):40–51.

5. Schuster EA. Earth caring. *ANS*. 1990;13(1):25–30.

6. Kuhn TS. *The Structure of Scientific Revolutions*. Chicago: University of Chicago; 1970.

7. Merchant C. Environmental ethics and political conflict: A view from California. *Environ Ethics*. 1990;12(1):45–68.

8. Miller AS. *Gaia Connections: An Introduction to Ecology, Ecoethics, and Economics*. Savage, MD: Rowman & Littlefield; 1991.

9. Roy C. Roy's adaptation model. In: Parse R, ed. *Nursing Science: Major Paradigms, Theories, and Critiques*. Philadelphia: W.B. Saunders; 1987.

10. Roy C. An explication of the philosophical assumptions of the Roy Adaptation Model. *Nurs Sci Q*. 1988;1(1):26–34.

11. Shortridge L, Valanis B. The epidemiological model applied in community health nursing. In: Stanhope M, Lancaster J., eds. *Community Health Nursing: Process and Practice for Promoting Health*, 3rd ed. Chicago: Mosby/YearBook; 1992.

12. Sarter B. Philosophical sources of nursing theory. *Nurs Sci Q*. 1988;1(2):52–59.

13. Watson J. Nursing's caring–healing paradigm as exemplar for alternative medicine? *Altern Therapies*. 1995;1(3):64–69.

14. Schuster EA. Earth dwelling. *Holistic Nurs Pract*. 1992;6(4):1–9.

15. Kleffel D. *The Environment: Alive, Whole, Interacting, and Interconnected*. San Diego: University of California, San Diego; 1994. Dissertation.

16. Moccia P. *A Vision for Nursing Education*. New York: National League for Nursing; 1993.

17. Callicott JB. Traditional American Indian and Western European attitudes toward nature: An overview. *Environ Ethics*. 1982;4(4):293–318.

18. Zaidi IH. On the ethics of man's interaction with the environment: An Islamic approach. *Environ Ethics*. 1981;2(1):35–47.

19. Callicott JB. Toward a global environmental ethic. In: Tucker ME, Grim JA, eds. *Worldviews and Ecology: Religion, Philosophy, and the Environment*. Maryknoll, NY: Orbis Books; 1994.

20. Deutsch E. A metaphysical grounding for natural reverence: East-West. *Environ Ethics*. 1986;8(4): 283–299.

21. Ames RT. Taoism and the nature of nature. *Environ Ethics*. 1986;8(4):317–350.

22. Wei-Ming T. The continuity of being: Chinese visions of nature. In Callicott JB, Ames RT, eds. *Nature in Asian Traditions of Thought: Essays in Environmental Philosophy*. New York: State University of New York Press; 1989.

23. Cook FH. The jewel net of Indra. In: Callicott JB, Ames RT, eds. *Nature in Asian Traditions of Thought: Essays in Environmental Philosophy*. New York: State University of New York Press; 1989.

24. Callicott JB. *Earth's Insights: A Survey of Ecological Ethics from the Mediterranean Basin to the Australian Outback*. Los Angeles: University of California Press; 1994.

25. Naess A. The shallow and the deep, long-range ecology movement: A summary. *Inquiry*. 1973;16:95–100.

26. Devall B, Sessions G. *Deep Ecology*. Salt Lake, UT: Perigrine Smith; 1985.

27. Lovelock J. *Gaia: A New Look at Life on Earth*. New York: Oxford University Press; 1979.

28. Lovelock J. *The Ages of Gaia: A Biography of Our Living Earth*. New York: Norton; 1988.

29. Bohm D. *Wholeness and the Implicate Order*. London, UK: Routledge & Kegan Paul; 1980.

30. Cheney J. Ecofeminism and deep ecology. *Environ Ethics*. 1987;9(2):115–144.

31. Warren KJ. Feminism and ecology: Making connections. *Environ Ethics*. 1987;9(1):3–20.

32. Warren KJ, Cheney J. Ecological feminism and ecosystem ecology. *Hypatia*. 1991;6(1):179–197.

33. Shaner H. Environmentally responsible clinical practice. In: Schuster EA, Brown CL, eds. *Exploring Our Environmental Connections*. New York: National League for Nursing Press; 1994.

34. Todd B. An ecofeminist look at animal research. In: Schuster EA, Brown CL, eds. *Exploring Our Environmental Connections*. New York: National League for Nursing Press; 1994.

35. Platt A. Breast and prostate cancer rising. In: *Vital Signs 1995: The Trends That Are Shaping Our Future*. New York: Norton; 1995.

36. Women's Environment and Development Organization. Does the breast cancer epidemic have environmental links? *News & Views*. 1992;6(1):1,9.

37. Women's Environment and Development Organization. Women's coalitions battle breast cancer and other environmental health problems. *News & Views*. 1995;8(1–2):2.

38. Platt A. The resurgence of infectious diseases. *World Watch: Working for a Sustainable Future*. 1995;8(4): 26–32.

Chapter 21

Reframing Outcomes: Enhancing Personhood

Anne Boykin, PhD
Savina Schoenhofer, PhD

The concept of "enhancing personhood" is a key aspect of the theory of nursing as caring. It is tenuously, though importantly, related to the currently popular notion of outcomes of care. While the standard connotation of outcomes as discrete economic results or end products of nursing care is incongruent with nursing as caring, the ethical professional practice of nursing requires attention to value. This article presents a theoretically congruent reconceptualization of valuing of advanced practice nursing. It offers a model for reframing the concept of outcomes within the theoretical context of enhancing personhood. Keywords: caring, education, graduate, intentionality, nursing, outcomes, personhood, values.

Suppose that time is not a quantity, but a quality, like the luminescence of the night above the trees just when a rising moon has touched the tree line . . . in a world where time is a quality, events are recorded by the color of the sky . . . events glide through the space of the imagination, materialized by a look, a desire. (Lightman, 1993, p. 123)

A dilemma exists in advanced nursing practice today in that advanced practice nurses, having acquired an unprecedented base of knowledge on which to draw, are challenged to articulate the way in which this knowledge influences the relationship of care from a nursing perspective. The viability of advanced practice nursing is at stake as nursing professionals struggle to make a recognizably unique contribution and avoid being subsumed in the anonymity of generic primary care providers and midlevel practitioners. Nurse practitioners, clinical nurse specialists, and others in advanced practice nursing roles face the important challenge of advancing the discipline of nursing while simultaneously communicating with the larger world of health care. A crucial aspect of this challenge involves effective languaging of nursing outcomes of care.

While nurses claim to "know" the value added to the health care situations in which they participate, that knowing remains largely tacit. Evidence supporting this conclusion is readily apparent in nursing literature describing various

Source: Boykin, A., and Schoenhoefer, S., *Advanced Practice Nursing Quarterly*, 1997, 3(1), 60–65. Reprinted with permission from © 1997 Aspen Publishers, Inc.

classification efforts over several decades. Nursing Minimum Data Set (NMDS) (Werley & Lang, 1988), the North American Nursing Diagnosis Association (1994), Rush Medicus (Haussman & Hegyvary, 1976), and the Royal College of Nursing's dynamic standard setting system (McFarlane, 1970) are all examples of frameworks used directly or indirectly to generate statements of nursing outcomes. These and similar frameworks effectively address nursing outcomes related to medical diagnosis and treatment activities, thus serving the generic primary care provider and mid-level practitioner well. However, they fail to communicate the richness of experience gained within the context of nursing situations, falling short of specifying the "value added" of the nursing contribution to care.

Why do these existing frameworks tend to disguise rather than disclose the meaningful experiences our patients gain in their relationships with us? Two interrelated explanations are proposed: intention and language. Compliance with the health care industry standard for provider reimbursement is an underlying intention of these frameworks. Thus, the systems use language that closely mirrors outcomes of medical care. To the extent that nursing care creates a different, unique realm of experience, and thus a different and unique value, this generic approach to outcomes has impoverished our ability to advance nursing practice.

What is the nature of the unique nursing contribution to health care situations? This question may be answered from a variety of perspectives in the formal literature of nursing. For example, within the framework of Orem's (1985) self-care deficit theory, the answer is assistance with self-care. From another perspective, nursing's contribution is termed promotion of adaptation (Roy, 1984), and from yet another, it is the provision of culturally congruent care (Leininger, 1988). Although language from these and other organized views of nursing is included along with more medically oriented

diagnoses and standards, statements specifying outcomes of nursing depict the contribution of our practice in rather mechanical, simplistic, and superficial language that fails to satisfy our largely unspoken understanding of the true value of nursing in the lives of those we nurse.

Assumptions underlying one's practice of nursing reflect values and beliefs. They color the lens for being in relationship and direct what one sees. Therefore, it would seem that assumptions ought to influence significantly the experience of being cared for by a nurse. If the approach to practice is grounded in the importance of normative science, with medical diagnosis as guide to prediction of successful care, the outcomes of care will likely depict cause-and-effect relationships, depersonalization, detachment, and objectification of person. Watson (1995) calls us to reflect on this perspective with the following questions, "Does modern science establish the norms and standards of reality for us? Has science determined the norms and standard of the human experience?" (p. 65). Nursing practice grounded in the importance of person-as-person, of person-as-caring, and of person-as-whole-in-the-moment would likely result in outcomes of care—or experiences of having been cared for—that are within the context of person. What is experienced as the result of care would reflect characteristics of personhood: unity—creative evolving of a unifying, consistent, whole awareness; wholeness—creative unfolding of a recognizable self; and intention—blending desire and purpose. This picture of personhood, a core value in the experience of nursing, cannot be adequately described in normative science terms such as objectivity, prediction, measurement, and control. Rather, it requires a language and structure more akin to poetry. Meaningful explication of the values that emerge within the context of a nursing situation will be more subjective than objective, descriptive than predictive, concerned more with illumination than measurement, and intention more than control.

Nursing as Caring

Nursing as caring offers a perspective in which both intention and language center around caring. While not all nurses accept Leininger's (1988) assertion that caring is the central and dominant construct of caring, it is widely acknowledged by nurses and those we nurse that caring is an important aspect of nursing. Formal knowledge of caring as an important aspect of nursing, initiated by Leininger (1978), Watson (1985), Gaut (1983), and others, is currently incorporated into a broad range of nursing theory development (Orem, 1985; Rogers, 1986; Roy, 1988).

The theory of nursing as caring (Boykin & Schoenhofer, 1993) is grounded in several fundamental assumptions: that to be human is to be caring (Roach, 1987), that personhood is a process of living grounded in caring, and that the capacity for personhood can be nurtured in relationship with caring others. Another important underlying assumption is that persons are whole in the moment, growing from moment to moment. From this grounding, nursing as caring posits that the unique focus of nursing is nurturing persons from the understanding that they are living caring in the moment and growing in caring from moment to moment. The nurturance that is nursing involves acknowledging, affirming and celebrating persons as caring, and supporting them in their unique ways of growing in caring.

From the lens of nursing as caring, the living of values of practice and the knowing of nursing occurs within the context of the nursing situation. The nursing situation is a "hard lived experience in which the caring between the nurse and the one nursed enhances personhood" (Boykin & Schoenhofer, 1993, p. 33). The nurse and one nursed bring to this experience the fullness of their being—their wholeness. The intention of the nurse is to know and to nurture the person in his or her wholeness and to know the one nursed

as a person living and caring uniquely in the moment. In the mutuality of the nursing relationship, the nurse too risks allowing self to be known as caring person.

Relationships

Relationships grounded in caring express the value of the importance of person-as-person. Imbedded in this relationship is the intention of wanting to know other, as well as a willingness to be open and receptive to other. Such relationships require the personal investment of both the nurse and the nursed. The nurse's deliberate presence creates an experience for one being cared for in which wholeness is felt. Such presence involves a way of listening and communicating through which one gives of self. It is through this connectedness, inspired by presence, that the nurse hears calls for nursing and responds with unique expressions of caring.

Reflective Practice

The knowing of person is accomplished by being open to knowing and participating in personal stories. Reflective practice (Schon, 1982) is integral to this process. As the nursing situation unfolds, the nurse, drawing on a vast and expanding knowledge base, is sensitive to gathering every cue, every sign, and every hunch, and reflects on the meaning of these in each particular situation. Upon reflection, the nurse communicates emerging understanding of the situation with the one nursed and together they engage in a dialogue to share understanding, meaning, knowing, and planning in the situation. These reflections and dialogues shape the moment and influence the nurturing response of the nurse. As Taylor (1992) states, the "shared sense of humanity helps a nurse stand back quietly, to move in to help where it is appropriate, to speak plainly and sensitively, to provide comfort at subtle levels and to be oneself in spite of professional knowledge and skills" (p. 42).

Through such presence the nurse expresses humility and active patience, allowing the person the freedom to be himself or herself and to share his or her story as it is lived (Boykin & Schoenhofer, 1991).

Intention

Intention is a key aspect of nursing from the perspective of nursing as caring. Practice grounded in this perspective is not concerned with diagnosis of a problem to be addressed through nursing, but rather with participating in a mutual relationship in which the nurse seeks to know the nursed in his or her unique, unfolding expressions of caring. The nurse enters the relationship with the intention of knowing the other as caring person, creating appropriate ways of knowing and of offering nurturance that are in tune with the uniqueness of the person and the situation. The intention to know and to nurture harmoniously opens a context in which caring is allowed to surface and flourish freely and creatively.

Outcomes

The quality of the nursing relationship as described leads to possibilities that are fully nonprobabilistic and unpredictable though recognizable and patterned. The idea of outcomes of nursing care, then, must be viewed in a different way. The concept of outcomes, as it is widely employed, is static, limited to what can be "predicted" and traceable back to those predictions and the circumstances that are guided by predictions. As acknowledged earlier, this sense of outcome is workable when reflection on the nursing situation is held to a superficial understanding of the situation. However, this approach to outcome specification fails to illuminate the significance of the nursing relationship in the lives of these nursed, and thus it sells short the contribution of nursing to the larger arena of health care.

Transformation

Transformation to a richer understanding of nursing contribution requires courage—courage for nurses to reflect upon and note the meaning of their care, courage to go beyond what is currently accepted in delimiting and languaging the value experienced by persons who participate in nursing situations. Courageous discovery and explication of the full value of nursing are responsibilities of those who would wish to call their efforts advanced practice nursing. Intention, knowledge, and skill are required for the fulfillment of these responsibilities.

Knowledge

Intention is the exercise of a commitment to bring the full power of nursing to those persons seeking nursing involvement in their life situations. The basic, enduring values of nursing—respect, caring, openness, intimacy, hope—provide the content of intention. Knowledge is in the moment, ever transforming and being transformed. It encompasses who we are, what we understand, and the challenges encountered for growth in understanding. Knowledge, or more accurately, knowing, is the convergence of many pathways—personal, empirical, ethical, aesthetic (Carper, 1978), unknowing (Munhall, 1993), and spiritual knowing. Knowing is enriched in dialogue, reflection-in-practice, and reflection on-practice, and it is characterized by humility. Skill is developed as nurses live their intention to explicate the value added through their practice knowledgeably, persistently, and in community with other nurses, those nursed, colleagues in other health care practices, and those in related economic and political arenas.

Nursing Situation

The following advanced practice nursing situation was shared by a nurse whose practice is guided by the theory of nursing as caring. It will be used to provide examples of nursing outcomes framed within that theoretical perspective.

Nurses associated with a community health service for migrant worker families in south Florida went weekly to a nearby labor camp where health information and support were offered as an extension of the primary care services for the migrant community. On this particular night, the plan, by request, was to teach infant cardiopulmonary resuscitation (CPR). Upon arriving at the designated place, three men were encountered who had just finished their evening meal after having spent the day in the fields. These men were among those who had left their families in Mexico, Guatemala, and Salvador in May and would not return until the coming April. It was now early February.

After some general conversation, the nurses worked one on one with the men, teaching and demonstrating the techniques of infant CPR. When it came time for the return demonstration, one man told a nurse why he was interested in learning. He had left two small children and a pregnant wife in Salvador, and his third child was born several weeks after he had left. He was eager to learn all he could that would be helpful to his family.

As he accepted the demonstrator doll, the nurse noticed that he cradled it in his arms and gazed into its upturned face. He was very careful and tender as he proceeded through the return demonstration. Relinquishing fears related to the possible language and cultural barriers, the nurse invited him to share his thoughts and feelings about his family, the child he had never seen, and the present experience of holding the doll in his arms. His eyes glistened with tears as he talked and rocked the child—for it was obvious that it was no longer a doll but his own newborn infant he was encountering for the first time. As the sharing continued, the other men gathered around and talked of their own experience of leaving home and family, of their long-

ing and their determined willingness to suffer separation to provide for their families.

What were the outcomes of this situation of nursing? What was the value added to human health and quality of life? The narrative of this nursing situation and the subsequent outcome statements reflect an explicit theory of nursing, nursing as caring, and provide an example of the value of this perspective in recognizing and languaging the richness of nursing. Included in the outcome statements drawn from this nursing situation are three sets of outcomes: one for the nursed, one for the nurse, and one for the health care agency. They are as follows:

1. Nursed
   - affirmation of self as loving father
     - affirmation of self as caring through unique expressions of hope and courage
   - acquisition of knowledge of a lifesaving technique that could be used as an expression of self as one competent in a specific way of caring
   - strengthening of a human bond with coworkers through personal openness
2. Experience of building a trusting relationship with health care providers
3. Nurse
   - confirmation that through intentionality, life stories unfold
   - confirmation that risk-taking on another's behalf facilitated beneficial self-knowing and interpersonal connection
   - sense of personal connectedness in a bicultural situation
4. Health care agency bond established between agency representative and potential consumers
   - demonstration of agency services as valuable and culturally competent
   - health teaching that is culturally congruent decreases the future likelihood of need for acute care services

It should be noted that these exemplar outcomes emerged through observation, reflection, and dialogue with other nurses. A research method is presently being developed in which the nurse, the nursed, and the nurse researcher engage in dialogue to uncover the meaning of the lived experience of nursing. This approach will allow direct input on the value of the nursing experience to the nursed. A similar approach is planned to obtain information about the value of nursing from the health care agency.

Knowledge and Skills

The knowledge and skills needed for advanced practice nursing are many and complex. The nurse uses multiple ways of knowing to create the artistry of nursing. The expert advanced practice nurse understands that knowledge and skills are global and that unless they are distilled in the context of a particular nursing situation they are meaningless. For example, technological expertise has meaning for nursing only in the context of a particular nursing situation. Advanced practice nurses are uniquely positioned to articulate the reality that the essence of nursing lives in the context of an intentional, mutual, caring relationship, a relationship in which the nurse draws forth a breadth and depth of knowledge for the purpose of knowing person(s) and of nurturing them as they live caring.

The resultant value of our service to society would be made manifest not only by the nurse but also by those nursed, from whom we truly know the value of our care. Rather than being detached from meaning to those nursed, outcomes reframed in the perspective of nursing as caring focus on understanding the value of care

to particular individuals, families, and groups. Rather than outcomes extracted from a reducible view of person and causal in nature, outcomes reframed focus on the value of person as whole and caring.

Of all the sample outcomes listed from this nursing situation, the typical framework would have produced only one, acquisition of competence in infant CPR. The value of this outcome is not to be diminished. However, the value accruing from the experience of this nursing situation as expressed in the outcome statements is only truly appreciated when framed within the intention and language of the nursing theoretical perspective of nursing as caring.

This exemplar expresses a new vision of the purpose and structure of nursing outcomes. In addition to the responsibility of seeking appropriate reimbursement for advanced practice nursing, a more comprehensive sense of quality and accountability should concern us. The outcome statements offered can lead the way to the required demonstration of economic value, that is, a cost-benefit accounting of care. However, without an appropriate perspective, coupled with suitable language, the frustration that nurses experience in their attempts to explicate the real value of our nursing will persist—nursing's contribution to care will continue to be depreciated. To paraphrase Lightman (1993), suppose that nursing is not a quantity but a quality, suppose that nursing events that are recorded by the color of the sky, that glide through the space of the imagination, materialized by a look or a desire, could be described in all their richness, clearly seen and understood. This exemplar opens the door to the possibility.

References

Boykin, A., & Schoenhofer, S. (1991). Story as link between nursing practice, ontology, epistemology. *Image: The Journal of Nursing Scholarship, 23,* 245–248.

Boykin, A., & Schoenhofer, S. (1993). *Nursing as caring.* New York: National League for Nursing.

Carper, B. (1978). Fundamental patterns of knowing in nursing. *Advances in Nursing Science, 1,* 13–23.

Gaut, D. (1983). Development of a theoretically adequate description of caring. *Western Journal of Nursing Research, 5,* 312–324.

Haussman, R., & Hegyvary, S. (1976). The relationship of nursing process and patient outcomes. *Journal of Nursing Administration, 90*(10), 18–21.

Leininger, M. (1978). *Transcultural nursing concepts, theories and practice.* New York: John Wiley & Sons.

Leininger, M. (1988). Leininger's theory of nursing: Cultural care diversity and universality. *Nursing Science Quarterly, 1,* 152–160.

Lightman, A. (1993). *Einstein's dreams.* New York: Pantheon Books.

McFarlane, J. (1970). Study of nursing care: The first two years of a research project. *International Nursing Review, 117*(2), 101–109.

Munhall, P. L. (1993). "Unknowing": Toward another pattern of knowing in nursing. *Nursing Outlook, 41,* 125–128.

North American Nursing Diagnosis Association. (1994). *Nursing diagnosis: Definition and classification 1995–1996.* Philadelphia: NANDA.

Orem, D. (1985). *Nursing: Concepts of practice* (4th ed.), New York: McGraw-Hill.

Roach, S. (1987). *The human act of caring.* Ottawa, Canada: Canadian Hospital Association.

Rogers, M. (1986). Science of unitary human beings. In V. Malinski (Ed.), *Explorations of Martha Rogers' science of unitary human beings.* Norwalk, CT: Appleton-Century-Crofts.

Roy, C. (1984). *Introduction to nursing: An adaptation model.* Englewood Cliffs, NJ: Prentice Hall.

Roy, C. (1988). An explication of the philosophical assumptions of the Roy adaptation model. *Nursing Science Quarterly, 1,* 26–34.

Schon, D. (1982). The reflective practitioner. *How professionals think in action.* New York: Basic Books.

Taylor, B. (1992). A comforting nurse–patient encounter. *Advances in Nursing Science, 15*(1), 33–43.

Watson, J. (1985). *Nursing: Human science and human care. A theory of nursing.* Norwalk, CT: Appleton-Century-Crofts.

Watson, J. (1995). Nursing's caring-healing paradigm as exemplar for alternative medicine? *Alternative Therapies, 1*(3), 64–69.

Werley, H., & Lang, N. (Eds.). (1988). *Identification of the nursing minimum data set.* New York: Springer.

Chapter 22

A Conceptual Framework for Person-Centered Practice with Older People

Brendan McCormack, DPHIL(Oxon), BScNsg(Hons), PGCEA, RGN, RMN

This paper presents a conceptual framework for person-centered practice with older people. The research from which the framework was developed was guided by hermeneutic philosophy and integrated processes of conversation analysis and reflective conversation in data collection and analysis. The research findings suggested that nurses need to be able to particularize the person that the patient is, the relationship that exists between them and the patient, and the understandings and expectations implicit in the relationship. From these findings, a conceptual framework for person-centered practice was developed. In the framework, person centeredness is premised on the concept of authentic consciousness and is operationalized through five imperfect duties. The factors that enable person centeredness to operate in practice are identified as the patient's values, the nurse's values, and the context of the care environment. Considerations for implementing the model in practice are highlighted. Keywords: caring, nurse–patient relationship, older people, person-centered, values.

Introduction

This paper explores the issue of person-centered practice with older people. The paper presents a conceptual framework for person-centered practice that has been developed from a larger research study exploring the meaning of autonomy for older people in hospital settings. The framework emphasizes partnership, which works between nurses and older people based on a

Source: McCormak B. A conceptual framework for person-centred practice with older people. *International Journal of Nursing Practice.* 2003;9:202–209. Copyright © 2003 EBSCO Publishing. Reprinted with permission of Blackwell Publishing, Ltd.

"negotiated relationship." The paper presents an overview of the research from which the conceptual framework has been derived, a description of the components of the framework, and an example of the model in use. The conceptual framework presented in this paper makes a significant contribution to the growing body of knowledge that challenges the dominant emphasis on dependency in gerontology.[1–4]

Person Centeredness

In the United Kingdom, the idea of person-centered practice is now embedded in the language of multidisciplinary practice with older people (see, for example, The National Service Framework for Older People[5]). Respect for persons is central to the notion of person-centeredness and is rooted in a Kantian ideal of mutual respect and sympathetic benevolence.[6] Therefore, the rights of individuals as persons is the driving force behind person-centered health care.[4,7] It represents an attitude of respect for ordinary individuals to make rational decisions and determine their own ends. The idea of respecting the patient's right to self-determination has resulted in a shift in thinking about the role of the patient in health care decision making. Hope and Fulford suggest that this philosophical shift requires health professionals to think beyond concepts of cure based on scientific facts and technical competence, to the adoption of a more holistic approach that also incorporates values.[8] Being person centered requires the formation of a therapeutic narrative between professional and patient that is built on mutual trust, understanding, and a sharing of collective knowledge.

Autonomy and Person-Centeredness: A Hermeneutic Study

The original research, from which this paper is derived, explored the meaning of autonomy for older people in hospital settings.[9] The overall research approach was guided by the hermeneutic philosophy of Gadamer.[10] Hermeneutic research does not attempt to interpret the data from an objective position, but instead creates a dialogue where the researcher and research participants' perceptions interact. The hermeneutic process is a dialogical process between the interpreter's understanding and the object being studied. Research participants' active involvement in this interpretative process is important so that a "meeting of understanding" can be achieved between perspectives of the research participants and the interpreter in order to create new understandings.

A convenience sample of four hospital nurses recorded discussions and conversations between themselves and patients, and with doctors and other members of the health care team, for at least three shifts per week over a 1-year period. In addition, interactions between a recognized expert gerontologic nurse (identified by using criteria derived from the work of Benner,[11] Jasper,[12] and Greenwood and King[13]) and patients in a community hospital setting were also recorded as a means of "testing out" initial themes generated from the data collected by the hospital nurses. Fourteen case studies of nurse–patient interactions were achieved. The local research ethics committee (LREC), in the health district where the research was being conducted, approved the research protocol and management plans. Patients with dementia or confusion (scoring 5 or less on a Mini-Mental Health Assessment[14]) were excluded from the study at the request of the LREC.

The data were transcribed, coded, and described using techniques of conversational analysis.[15] Conversation analysis was used as a structured approach to describing the data and deriving interpretive themes, that is, as a tool for the selection and description of the data sets. By using an established framework derived from conversation analysis, decisions about data choices for analysis would in the first instance be informed through the structure of the framework, rather than the researcher's own subjective choices as a "data interpreter." Conversation analysis identifies a limited set of conversational rules within which discourse is constructed and within which participants perform particular acts within the constraints of this rule system. Discourse is action in its own right and not a route to understanding action. Ordinary conversation is viewed as the predominant medium of action in the social world. Follow-up "reflective conversations"[16] with the nurses clarified and developed the researcher's initial descriptions of the data. Rigor in data analysis was maintained through an iterative process between researcher and research participants. Initial themes from the descriptions were developed through focus group discussions with a group of expert nurses and a group of patients. Nurses and patients identified themes from the descriptions prior to further thematic analysis by the researcher. Finally, participating nurses, the group of expert nurses and the patient group agreed on the final themes that were developed.

The research findings, which have been reported in detail elsewhere,[17] included the key issues of the effects of institutional discourse, the dynamics of power and control, patients' access to knowledge, the impact of professional authority, the constraining nature of institutions and the effect of family and careers on decision making. All of these factors were seen to act as constraints on the ability of older people to exercise autonomy. Through the interpretive process with participants, 23 "principles for action" to address these constraints were identified (Appendix 1) and further analysis of these resulted in the development of the conceptual framework for person-centered practice.

Person-Centeredness as Authentic Consciousness

The research findings suggest that nurses need to be able to particularize the person that the patient is, the relationship that exists between them and the patient, and the understandings and expectations implicit in the relationship. It is proposed that this can be achieved through an understanding of the person's authentic values.

Authenticity refers to a way of reaching decisions which are truly one's own: decisions that express all that one believes important about oneself and the world, the entire complexity of one's values.[18]

Authentic consciousness is a consideration of the person's life as a whole in order to help sustain meaning in life. Authentic consciousness is not a hierarchical ordering of possible desires, but a clarification of values to maximize potential for growth and development. Existing evidence highlights the dominance of routine and ritualized practices with older people that do not take account of individual beliefs and values.[17,19–21] When working with beliefs and values, the role of the nurse is to maximize opportunities for growth through authentic decision making, that is, decisions that are true to the person's life as a whole. It is not enough to just take note of another's beliefs, values, views and experiences. They must be integrated into the biography of that individual.

Being conscious of another's beliefs and values does not tell the nurse what to do; rather, it orientates the nurse to a particular way of being. As Gadow argues, the recognition of beliefs and values allows the patient and the nurse to have the kind of caring relationship that they want to have, appropriate to the context of care.[18] This helps the nurse place actions in context, or as MacIntyre suggests, "The act of utterance becomes intelligible by finding its place in a narrative."[22] In the context of this research, what this means is that desires, wishes, and needs of an older person can best be understood by having a picture of the person's life as a whole. Therefore, being person-centered relies on getting closer to the older person and goes beyond traditional notions of respecting individuality and individualized care, such as choices about food and drink, hygiene, waking, and sleeping. In this framework, getting closer to the patient is achieved through consideration of the patient's authenticity, the adoption of "imperfect duties" and the consideration of contextual factors (**Figure 22–1**).

Imperfect Duties

The term *imperfect duties* is derived from Kant, who made a distinction between perfect and imperfect duties.[23] Perfect duties are strict and enforceable. In contrast, imperfect duties are

Figure 22-1 A CONCEPTUAL FRAMEWORK OF PERSON-CENTEREDNESS AS AUTHETIC CONSCIOUSNESS

"wide, broad and limited"—"they leave us a play-room for free choice in following the law,"[23] as there is no means of offering an exhaustive and a priori account of how the duties are to be fulfilled. Such duties as compassion, concern, benevolence, respect, and care would all be imperfect duties as, for example, one cannot force someone to be caring. Kant views such duties as imperfect because, in ethical decision making, one might have to decide between competing duties and account must be taken of the context in which decisions are made. This approach acknowledges the need for guiding principles that are interpreted in the context of the particular relationship. It highlights the important place of emotions in decision making by highlighting the importance of emotional factors being made explicit and acknowledged as influences on the process and outcome of decision making. Issues such as how much the nurse "likes" the patient, the individual nurse's personal experiences, and the behavior of the patient are seen as significant.

Returning to the study previously described[9] from the data analysis, five imperfect duties are considered to be important to the operationalization of autonomy as authentic consciousness:

1. Informed flexibility the facilitation of decision making through information sharing and the integration of new information into established perspectives and care practices.

2. Mutuality: the recognition of the others' values as being of equal importance in decision making.

3. Transparency: making explicit the intentions and motivations for action and the boundaries within which care decisions are set.

4. Negotiation: patient participation through a culture of care that values the views of the patient as a legitimate basis for decision making while recognizing that being the final arbiter of decisions is of secondary importance.

5. Sympathetic presence: an engagement that recognizes the uniqueness and value of the individual by appropriately responding to cues that maximize coping resources through the recognition of important agendas in daily life.

The Nurse as a Facilitator of Authentic Consciousness

The imperfect duties act as guiding universal principles that are interpreted in the context of the particular care situation. Adopting a person-centered approach to practice requires nurses to recognize freedom of self-determination for patients as a fundamental and valuable human right, based on an interdependent and interconnected relationship with each other.[18] Person-centered practice holds central the knowledge and experience that each person brings to the care situation and which is necessary for decisions that will best serve the patient's well-being. Examples of this in the United Kingdom include developments in the assessment of care needs of older people,[5] models for involving older people with dementia in decision making,[4] and person-centered practices in acute care nursing.[19] At the heart of this style of nursing is the therapeutic nurse–patient relationship that requires continuity of care and the acceptance of responsibility for the outcomes of care. Acknowledging and valuing each patient's biography and their individual perception and experience of their health care experience is fundamental to this way of nursing. Its aim is to transform the patient's experience of illness and is considered to be a therapy in its own right.[8] The role of the person-centered nurse is to be there, offering personal support and practical expertise, while enabling the patient to follow the path of their own choosing and in their own way.

However, total connectedness with a patient can lead to "ethical blindness,"[24] and in order to balance the intensity of an individual relationship with a reflective approach to decision making, the nurse needs to move between three "stances" when working with patients.[25] These stances represent different levels of engagement (connectedness) between the nurse and patient.

When engagement is present, the patient and nurse are connected in the relationship. The nurse and patient are extensions of each other and a care partnership exists. Boykin and Schoenhofer describe this as "the dance of caring persons."[26] Caring exists because the nurse and patient hold a deep respect for each other. However, a dilemma could arise in the care relationship that affects the way the nurse and patient are able to work together, such as a difficult decision and ethical dilemma or a disagreement. As a result, partial disengagement occurs while the nurse and

patient take stock of the situation and formulate the problem. Such disengagement then requires a period of contemplation, and for a period of time, complete disengagement occurs. In this stance, the nurse and patient contemplate the available options from their individual perspectives. They reassess the values that underpin the relationship and decision making. Mechanisms such as supported reflective practice,[27,28] clinical supervision,[29] and case reviews[30] all help to achieve this goal. Although the nurse continues to work with the patient in seeking the most satisfactory resolution, the connectedness in the relationship is broken until such time as a resolution can be found. A skilled nurse can adopt these different stances at different times with the patient. Indeed, they were evident in the practice of the expert nurse and the clinical nurse specialist in the research underpinning this framework.[9] In contemplating options and choices, there are three important factors for the creation of an environment that facilitates person centeredness. These are the patient's values, the nurse's values and expertise, and the context of care.

The Patient's Values

Respect for values is central to person-centered practice.[4,7,9] It is important to develop a clear picture of what patients value about their life and how they make sense of what is happening. This provides a standard against which the nurse can compare current decisions and behaviors of the patient with those values and preferences made in life in general. Approaches to patient assessment that include a biographical account, using narrative and story, are one method of establishing a baseline value history. Assisting the individual to find meaning in care might help them to tolerate the incongruity of their illness and plan for a future.[31]

The complexity of many health care decisions coupled with the stresses and fears of illness, with its related anxiety, dependence and regressive tendencies, means that a patient's ordinary decision making abilities are often significantly diminished. Buchanan and Brock argue that if patients hold the ultimate responsibility for their health care decision, then their treatment choices might fail to serve their well-being, as conceived by them.[32] Thus, they argue that the same value of patient well-being that requires patients' participation in their own health care decisions might sometimes also require persons to be protected from the harmful consequences to them of their own choices.

When considered in practice, the risk to autonomous decision making by patients from paternalistic health care workers is significant. Agich asserts that the means of preventing such action is by having a clear picture of what the patient, and others important to them, really value about their life and how they make sense of the things happening to them.[33] In the exercise of their decision-making capacity, patients bring an individual approach to their concept of their own well-being. Health means different things to different people[34] and is accorded various degrees of importance by individuals. Therefore, there is no one single intervention that is best for everyone. While certain procedures might be more appropriate than others in particular cases, it is the individuality of the particular case that determines the most appropriate approach. For this reason, health care decision making ought to adopt a negotiated approach between practitioner and patient.[9]

The Nurse's Values and Expertise

Although the language of partnership is commonplace and nurses are encouraged to soften their professional presentation to the patient, it remains unusual for nurses to present their own views as a component of the array of information that patients are given to assist their decisions.

Although the patient's values should be predominant,[18] the nurse's values also contribute to the process. However, these are seldom open and transparent. Indeed, it could be argued that if a mutual relationship exists between the nurse and patient, then it is especially important that the nurse's values are expressed, particularly when they conflict with the patient's values. If the nurse is truly working in partnership with the patient then there is no reason why the expression of such values should be coercive. Instead, the disclosure of the nurse's values might help the patient to understand particular negotiation positions taken by the nurse and it might offer the patient an alternative view when considering their options. However, it has been argued that despite an intention to consider patient and nursing values, the context of the care environment has a significant impact on the operationalization of person-centered practices.[35,36]

The Context of Care

The context in which care is provided has the greatest potential to enhance or limit the facilitation of person-centered practice. When facilitating person-centeredness, nurses find they not only balance competing care values but often find it necessary to consider organizational values too. Nurses are not free to fulfill a moral obligation to the patient without considering organizational and professional implications,[37] and indeed, they might find themselves having to accept a forced choice on occasion.[38] In contemporary health care, the fundamental moral predicament of nurses is that while they are expected to engage in autonomous decision making, they are often deprived of the freedom to exercise moral authority.[39] While the freedom of the nurse is a significant issue in the facilitation of person-centeredness, other characteristics of context have been found to be of equal significance,[1] such as systems of decision making, staff relationships, organizational systems, power differentials, and the potential of organization to tolerate innovate practices and risk taking. These findings have been supported in a recent analysis of the concept of context.[35]

A Composite Example

In order to illustrate the framework in use, the following example is offered. The example is derived from data extracts from the research underpinning this conceptual framework.[9] These extracts have been taken from the data of one nurse who participated in the study (Pam) and her work with one patient (Ray).

Pam is a lead nurse in a local community hospital that specializes in the rehabilitation of older people following acute illness. The unit utilizes the Burford Nursing Development Unit (BNDU) model of nursing.[40] Ray, a patient transferred from the regional general hospital, was admitted for rehabilitation following a fractured shaft of his left femur. Ray is a gypsy and values his freedom and independence. Staff in the regional hospital reported that he was "difficult," "uncooperative," and "refused to do what he was told!" When admitted, Pam used the key questions from the BNDU model: "who is this person?" and "what information do I need to know to be able to nurse him effectively?" to focus the construction of his biography, assess his care needs, and agree on a care plan. By using these questions, Ray shared his core values of personal freedom, intolerance of authority, and everyone being equal, while Pam shared her core nursing values of self-determination, honesty, and negotiation. Together, they agreed on a plan of care that encompassed these values. Pam and Ray drew up a contract of how they would work together and this was written into the care plan. The contract included the importance of them being honest with each other, that all decisions would be negotiated between them, that all pre-scribed interventions would be fully explained and that his lifestyle would be respected. His care plan included details of when and how he would have physiotherapy, psychosocial activities to assist his transition back to the community, and a program of self-administration of medicines. Although disagreements and challenges arose between Ray and Pam, renegotiations of his care plan occurred on a regular basis and resolutions were found. In addition, Ray attended regular case reviews with the multidisciplinary team and thus felt fully involved in treatment decisions.

This example demonstrates the centrality of values to the relationship between the nurse and patient. Ray felt part of decisions and Pam ensured that she respected his values in the way she worked with him. Pam worked with him using skills of negotiation, openness, honesty, and consultation to ensure that their agreed contract was fulfilled. The imperfect duties of informed flexibility, mutuality, transparency, negotiation and sympathetic presence are evident. The community hospital in which this case example was situated has invested much time in creating a context to support person centeredness.

Conclusions

This paper presents a framework for person-centered practice that holds as central the concept of autonomy as authentic consciousness. By viewing person centeredness in this way, an understanding of caring relationships is achieved that is not based on one person being the final arbiter of decisions but that is, instead, set within a framework of negotiation based on an individual's values base. The nurse as a facilitator of an individual's authentic consciousness engages in a process of dynamic caring that maintains autonomy at a time when for many older people, their sense of independence is under greatest threat.

References

1. Phillipson C, Biggs S. Modernity and identity. Theories and perspectives in the study of older adults. *Journal of Aging and Identity* 1998;3:11–23.

2. Kitwood T. *Dementia Reconsidered: The Person Comes First.* Milton Keynes: Open University Press, 1997.

3. Nolan M, Davies S, Grant G. *Working with Older People and their Families: Key Issues in Policy and Practice.* Buckingham: Open University Press, 2001.

4. Dewing J. From ritual to relationship: A person-centered approach to consent in qualitative research with older people who have a dementia. *Dementia* 2002;1:157–171.

5. Department of Health. *The National Services Framework for Older People.* London: HMSO, 2001.

6. Richards DAJ. Rights and Autonomy. *Ethics* 1981;92:3–20.

7. Williams B, Grant G. Defining "people-centeredness": Making the implicit explicit. *Health Social Care in the Community* 1998;6:84–94.

8. Hope T, Fulford KW. The Oxford Practice Skills Project: Teaching ethics, law and communication skills to clinical medical students. *Journal of Medical Ethics* 1994;20:229–234.

9. McCormack B. *Negotiating Partnerships with Older People: A Person-Centered Approach.* Aldershot: Ashgate Press, 2001.

10. Gadamer HG. *Truth and Method.* London: Sheed & Ward, 1993.

11. Benner P. *From Novice to Expert: Excellence and Power in Clinical Nursing Practice.* CA: Addison-Wesley, 1984.

12. Jasper MA. Expert: A discussion of the implications of the concept as used in nursing. *Journal of Advanced Nursing* 1994;20:769–776.

13. Greenwood J, King M. Some surprising similarities in the clinical reasoning of "expert" and "novice" orthopaedic nurses: report of a study using verbal protocols and protocol analyses. *Journal of Advanced Nursing* 1995;22:907–913.

14. Dick JPR, Guiloff RJ, Stewart A, Blackstock J. Mini-mental state examination in neurological patients. *Journal of Neurology, Neurosurgery and Psychiatry* 1984;47:496–498.

15. Drew P, Heritage J. *Talk at Work: Interaction in Institutional Settings.* Cambridge: Cambridge University Press, 1992.

16. Bergum V. Being a phenomenological researcher. In: Morse J (ed.). *Qualitative Nursing Research: A Contemporary Dialogue.* London: Sage Publications, 1991; 55–71.

17. McCormack B. Autonomy and the relationship between nurses and older people. *Aging Society* 2001; 21.

18. Gadow S. Existential advocacy. Philosophical foundations of nursing. In: Spicker SF, Gadow S (eds.). *Nursing: Images and ideals—Opening Dialogue with the Humanities.* New York: Springer, 1980; 85.

19. Department of Health. *Caring for Older People: A Nursing Priority.* Report of the Standing Nursing and Midwifery Advisory Committee. London: Department of Health, 2001. No. 23668.

20. Davies S, Laker S, Ellis L. Promoting autonomy and independence for older people within nursing practice: a literature review. *Journal of Advanced Nursing* 1997;26:408–417.

21. Davies S, Nolan M, Brown J, Wilson F. *Dignity on the Ward: Promoting Excellence in Care.* London: Help the Aged, 1999.

22. MacIntyre A. *After Virtue: a Study in Moral Theory.* London: Duckworth, 1992.

23. Sullivan RJ. *Immanuel Kant's Moral Theory.* Cambridge: Cambridge University Press, 1990.

24. Benner P, Wrubel J. *The Primacy of Caring: Stress and Coping in Health and Illness.* Wokingham, UK: Addison-Wesley, 1989.

25. Heidegger M. *Being and Time.* Oxford: Basil Blackwell, 1990.

26. Boykin A, Schoenhofer S. *Nursing as Caring: A Model for Transforming Practice.* New York: National League for Nursing Press, 1993.

27. Johns CC. *Becoming an Effective Practitioner through Guided Reflection.* Unpublished PhD Thesis. Open University, Milton Keynes, 1997.

28. Johns C. Caring through a reflective lens: giving meaning to being a reflective practitioner. *Nursing Inquiry* 1998;5:18–24.

29. Bishop V. *Clinical Supervision in Practice: Some Questions, Answers and Guidelines.* Basingstoke: Macmillan, 1998.

30. Robbins DA. *Ethical and Legal Issues in Home Health and Long Term Care: Challenges and Solutions.* MD: Aspen Publishers, 1996.

31. Meyers DT. *Self, Society and Personal Choice.* New York: Columbia University Press, 1989.

32. Buchanan AE, Brock DW. *Deciding for Others: the Ethics of Surrogate Decision Making.* Cambridge: Cambridge University Press, 1989.

33. Agich GJ. *Autonomy and Long-Term Care.* Oxford: Oxford University Press, 1993.

34. Seedhouse D. *Health: The Foundations of Achievement.* Chichester: John Wiley & Sons, 1986.

35. McCormack B, Kitson A, Harvey G, et al. Getting evidence into practice: the meaning of 'context'. *Journal of Advanced Nursing* 2002;38:94–104.

36. Rycroft-Malone J, Harvey G, Kitson A, et al. Getting evidence into practice: Ingredients for change. *Nursing Standard* 2002;29:38–43.

37. Johns C. Unraveling the dilemmas within everyday nursing practice. *Nursing Ethics: An International Journal for Health Care Professionals* 1999;6:287–298.

38. Yarling RR, McEelmurry BJ. The moral foundation of nursing. In: Pence T, Cantrell J (eds.). *Ethics in Nursing: an Anthology.* New York: National League for Nursing, 1990; 335–342.

39. Holm S. *Problems in Clinical Practice: The Ethical Reasoning of Health Care Professionals.* Manchester: Manchester University Press, 1997.

40. Johns CC. *The Burford NDU Model: Caring in Practice.* Oxford: Blackwell Science, 1994.

Appendix 1

Principles for Action

1. Make explicit the care agenda.
2. Recognize that the questioning style adopted affects the ability of the older patient to contribute to the setting of the care agenda and their contribution to a conversation.
3. Be aware that actions to achieve one outcome might have an effect on a previously unrecognized need.
4. Have a repertoire of interactional approaches that will enable patient decision making and participation in the planning of care plans.
5. Pose specific and clearly formulated questions that have a clear aim.
6. Respect individuals' important routines in daily life and negotiate new components of the care agenda each day.
7. Be aware that older patients depend on professionals to minimize or prevent constraints on their autonomy.
8. Listen to patients and allow them to tell their story as a legitimate part of assessment processes.
9. Wherever possible, encourage patients to identify solutions for existing problems and care needs, set within negotiated parameters of risk taking.
10. Get to know patients and establish a negotiated level of engagement before decisions about degrees of risk taking are made.
11. For informed decision making to be facilitated in a patient-centered way, refrain from imbuing decision-making processes with one's own values.
12. Suspend the use of prior knowledge about a patient and their social context until they have been enabled to tell their story.
13. Recognize that the uniqueness of patients' experiences versus nurses' familiarity with organizational routines limits a patient-centered approach to decision making.
14. Accord the patient's perceptions of their care situation equal status as those of health care professionals.
15. Patients' subjective views of their lives should be respected in decision making.
16. To facilitate patient participation, understand and be confident with the boundaries of one's decision-making potential.
17. Adopt a patient-centered approach to risk assessment and risk taking.
18. Be explicit about the intent and motivation for action and the parameters within which decisions are set.
19. Maximize patients' independence through the balancing of patient narrative with established care policies and procedures.
20. Make decision within a framework of negotiation with clearly established care goals that are regularly reinforced and reviewed.
21. Make time to help patients to integrate new care decisions and options into their already established care program.
22. Acknowledge and facilitate patients' emotional responses as an important part of facilitating patient participation.
23. Create opportunities for reciprocity in relationships with patients.
24. Do not allow age-related perceptions of an individual's ability to limit patient participation.

25. Help patients to see beyond their own limited expectations of their involvement in care and their deference to others.
26. Continuously reinforce the value of patients' decisions.
27. Facilitate patients' emotional coping ability in order to enhance their independence.
28. Recognize that while patients want to be consulted about care decisions they do not always want to be the final arbiter of decisions.
29. Recognize that older people should have their beliefs and values considered in the making of decisions but patients being the final arbiter of decisions is not of prime importance.

Part Five

CONTEMPORARY PERSPECTIVES OF NURSING

In Part Five, three chapters are presented that offer innovative ways of addressing the complexity of advanced nursing practice in the contemporary healthcare environment. These three chapters represent three divergent ways of organizing constructs of science, values, and evidence.

My assumption in putting together this part is that readers are passingly familiar with the dominant views of science in Western societies today, by which I mean quantitative, objectivistic, normative science, in which studies and experiments are designed to predict and control the phenomena of concern. Western medicine is certainly dominated by such a view, and Western nursing is certainly dominated by Western medicine. The science that guides practice from this perspective is oriented toward preserving, promoting, and restoring *norms* of structure, function, and behavior in biological, psychological, and sociological realms. The perspectives offered in this chapter differ from this view to various extents.

In Chapter 23, Letourneau and Allen present postpositivistic critical multiplism as the successor to logical positivism in science and a philosophy of science that advocates methodologic pluralism. Letourneau and Allen occupy that space in the mainstream of contemporary science that explicitly values the contributions of alternative views while continuing to adhere for the most part to traditional Western scientific assumptions.

In Chapter 24, Raymond explores the realms of esthetic and personal knowing in Paterson and Zderad's humanistic nursing using an easy-to-follow case example.

In Chapter 25, Mitchell and Cody attempt to specify the meaning of the claim that nursing is and must be a "human science." A human science, after Dilthey, they say, is one that is concerned with humanly lived experiences, meanings, patterns, beliefs, values, representations, and intentions. Its methods are qualitative, and its goal is *understanding* of what it means to be human. Mitchell and Cody examine a range of contemporary nursing frameworks, which are described in some detail, for their adherence to basic assumptions and values of human science. A value for nursing as a human science will shape the practice of the nurse who holds this value.

Careful study of Part Five will lead readers to an understanding of how the orientation of the nurse toward the science and the art of nursing strongly influences his or her practice. The issues are extremely deep and the questions largely a matter for reflection and dialogue, but these explorations are necessary for the advanced practice nurse to understand herself or himself as a nurse in the context of the range of the sciences of our time. All orientations entail taking a stand. The question is this: *What stance toward science and art in nursing best represents what I want to achieve in nursing and the guidance that I need to do it?*

Chapter 23

Post-Positivistic Critical Multiplism: A Beginning Dialogue

Nicole Letourneau, PhD, MN, BN, RN,

Marion Allen, PhD, MScN(Ed), MN, BN, RN

Following the recognition that logical positivism was no longer tenable in modern science, post-positivism and its research methodology, critical multiplism, emerged and offered a new way of thinking about science. Although not a panacea, critical multiplism, in which methodologic pluralism is advocated, offers a way around the debate of which conception of science is appropriate for nursing and, as such, poses advantages for nursing scientific knowledge development. Keywords: critical multiplism, nursing knowledge, nursing science, philosophy of science, post positivism.

Introduction

For three decades, nurse scholars have debated the merits and limitations of various conceptions or views of science for the development of nursing's scientific knowledge. As a result, arguments for competing views of nursing science abound in the nursing literature. Some nurse scholars call for the accommodation of competing views (Silva & Rothbart, 1984; Cull-Wilby & Pepin, 1987; Dzurec, 1989; Fawcett, 1993), whereas others deem these varying views as incommensurable and therefore reject the suggestion of accommodation (Munhall, 1982; Moccia, 1988; Watson, 1988). This debate may cease if post-positivism's attendant methodology of critical multiplism is taken seriously as an approach for the development of scientific nursing knowledge.

The purposes of this paper are to outline the issues surrounding the use of post-positivistic critical multiplism and to argue that post-positivistic critical multiplism is a unifying research methodology that allows for rival theories and methods to be integrated. A beginning dialogue on the potential advantages of critical multiplism for the development of scientific nursing knowledge is presented. Prior to this discussion, a brief overview of post-positivism and critical multiplism is provided so that there is a shared understanding of these perspectives.

Background

Post-Positivism

Following the recognition that the basic foundations of logical positivism were no longer

Source: Letourneau, N., and Allen, M. *Journal of Advanced Nursing*, 1999, 30(3), 623–630. Reprinted with permission © Copyright 1999 Blackwell Science, Ltd.

tenable in modern science (Hempel, 1966; Popper, 1968; Kuhn, 1970; Lakatos, 1970; Laudan, 1977) a new philosophy of science, that of post-positivism, emerged. Post-positivism has been defined as the search for "warranted assertability" as opposed to "truth," traditionally represented by universal laws or absolutes (Lather, 1990; Phillips, 1990a). As such, post-positivism is regarded by many as "eliminating the intractable problem . . . of a forced choice between value-laden/qualitative and value-free/quantitative research methods" (Howe, 1985, p. 10; see also Smith, 1983; Phillips, 1990b; Lather, 1992; Wildemuth, 1993). Instead, post-positivists advocate critical multiplism, which retains many of the methodological achievements of the past while responding to the criticisms of logical positivism (Houts et al., 1986; Guba, 1990).

Post-positivists are critical realists, meaning that although a real world driven by natural causes exists, it is impossible for humans to truly perceive it with their imperfect sensory and intellectual capabilities (Cook & Campbell, 1979; Guba, 1990). Thus, claims about reality must be subjected to the widest possible critical examination (e.g. by scholars) "to facilitate apprehending reality as closely as possible" (Guba & Lincoln, 1994, p. 110). Reality, seen as "out there," can, then be more or less objectified for study (Guba, 1990; Phillips, 1990b). Although this notion of objectivity remains a regulatory ideal that underpins all inquiry, the importance of values and subjectivity in science is recognized (Phillips, 1990a).

Post-positivists view truth as ultimately unknowable because it cannot be claimed that there is any absolutely authoritative foundation on which to base scientific knowledge (Phillips, 1987; Greene, 1990). As a result, knowledge claims are modest and viewed as warranted assertions in that they represent established regularities or probabilities about human phenomena rather than universal laws that govern behavior (Greene, 1990; Phillips, 1990a).

Scientific knowledge claims gain warrant when they are supported by objective evidence and when their argument is credible, coherent, and consensual (Greene, 1990). Warrants provide good evidence for the existence and nature of phenomena (Schumacher & Gortner, 1992; Forbes et al., 1999). If a knowledge claim is deemed to both correspond with what is known of reality (in the sense of approximation) and to be a good basis for action, it gains warrant. Most importantly, post-positivistic knowledge claims are deemed worthy (or warranted) when they have survived the critical tradition of evaluation and challenge (Popper, 1968; Cook, 1985; Greene, 1990; Phillips, 1990a).

Finally, post-positivists equate scientific knowledge with theory, and theory is construed as a model or a "huge fishnet" of complex, mutually interacting relationships among constructs or variables (Cook, 1985; Greene, 1990; Phillips, 1990a). Relationships are assumed to be complex, multiplistic, and interactive (Greene, 1990).

Critical Multiplism

As the methodology of post-positivism (Guba, 1990), critical multiplism is a form of methodological pluralism that gives way to both qualitative and quantitative methods. *Critical* refers to the rational, empirical and consequently inherently social efforts to identify the assumptions and biases present in the options of methods and theories chosen to investigate a phenomenon (Shadish, 1993). Implicit in this notion of critical is the recognition that there is no one correct or perfect scientific method, as all methods have limitations (Wildemuth, 1993). Similarly, theories derived from these methods also have inherent limitations. Post-positivists, thus advocate the putting together of "packages of imperfect methods and theories in a manner that minimizes constant biases" (Shadish, 1993, p. 18). By bias is meant an error "of omission or commission that leaves us with knowledge that is in some plausible respect wrong or misleading or without certain kinds of knowledge that are plausibly needed" (Shadish, 1993, p. 44).

Multiplism refers to the fact that research questions can usually be approached from several perspectives, and frequently "no single way is known to be uniformly best" (Shadish, 1993, p. 18). Thus, multiple perspectives are used to define the research goals, to choose the research questions, methods and analyses, and to interpret the results (Coward, 1990). Methods, that is both qualitative and quantitative approaches, are selected based on the research question addressed and knowledge claims gain warrant by establishing correspondences across many different perspectives and ways of formulating a research question (Cook, 1985).

An assumption underlying this methodological pluralism is that researchers possess knowledge of the strengths and weaknesses of different approaches to research questions. Justifiable options are selected that complement limitations observed in the research conducted thus far (Cook, 1985), thus ensuring that research questions are examined thoroughly from a wide variety of perspectives. Critical multiplism also suggests that research questions, research designs, data manipulations and substantive interpretations should be openly scrutinized from a wide variety of theoretical perspectives, including overtly antagonistic ones (Houts et al., 1986).

Critical multiplism is described by Cook (1985) and Houts et al. (1986) as approach with several strategies or options. These include:

- the use of multiple stakeholders to formulate research questions
- the design of multitargeted research that seeks to probe many different types of issues within a single study
- multiple operationalism
- multimethod research
- the construction of complex multivariate causal models instead of simple univariate ones
- the competitive testing of multiple rival hypotheses rather than single ones

- research programs based on multiple interconnected studies
- the synthesis of multiple studies conducted in different contexts with different measures
- the desirability of multiple analysts examining important data sets
- the use of multiple theoretical and value frameworks to interpret research questions and findings

Shadish (1993) further described the guidelines for conducting critical multiplist research. These include identifying the tasks to be done, the different options for doing each task, and the strengths, biases and assumptions associated with each option. When it is not clear which of several options for doing a task is least biased, more than one option is selected to reflect different biases, to avoid constant biases, and to overlook only the least plausible biases. It is also essential to note convergences or the coming together of results over options with different biases to explain differences of results yielded by options with different biases, and finally to publicly defend any decisions to leave a task homogeneous.

Shadish (1993) noted, however, that individual scientists frequently have difficulty perceiving their own biases and may not be aware of knowledge developed in different disciplines. Consequently, he suggested additional social guidelines aimed at remedying the social and psychological "limitations" of the individual investigator. These include identifying several sources (people, theories, research) whose biases are likely to differ and enlisting the aid of those sources in completing and criticizing the results of the technical component.

Another central feature of critical multiplism is consciousness raising, in that it promises to increase the degree to which research issues are scrutinized for importance and utility (Cook, 1985; Houts et al., 1986). This is a response to the critique that "little attention has been paid to broader questions about the origins and utility of the issues we [researchers] probe" (Houts et al.,

1986, p. 62). The critical multiplist approach, by encouraging multiple stakeholders to provide critique and direction to the development of research questions, increases the likelihood that the subsequent research findings will prove useful (Coward, 1990).

It ought to be noted that this consciousness raising does not imply that all research questions must be designed to solve extant problems, just that more emphasis ought to be placed on extant problems than has been historically. In other words, critical multiplism does not advocate that *all* research questions must necessarily be designed to answer questions with immediate usefulness. Indeed, conscientious critical multiplists, in the spirit of critique and scrutiny, would argue that some research questions ought to be of an anticipatory nature; while the knowledge so developed may not find an immediate use, it is conceivable that it will be useful at some future point.

Issues Surrounding Critical Multiplism

Several issues are raised by post-positivistic critical multiplism. Critical multiplism has been described as merely another form of triangulation, as promoting relativism (which denies objective knowledge of realities independent of the knower) and accommodating incommensurability (an inability of theories from different paradigms to be measured against each other point by point), and as being too costly. In addition, critical multiplism advances a unique view of values and objectivity in science.

Critical Multiplism and Triangulation

Critical multiplism has been called a method of "elaborated triangulation" (Guba, 1990) and, as such, is purported to add nothing new to contemporary research methodology. Post-

positivists counter that triangulation is part of, but not equal to, the critical multiplist approach (Coward, 1990). Triangulation has been defined as the combination of two or more theories, data sources, methods or investigators in the study of a single phenomenon (Kimchi et al., 1991). The goal of triangulation is to circumvent the personal biases of investigators and overcome the deficiencies intrinsic to a single-investigator, single-theory or single-method study to promote greater confidence in the observed findings (Denzin, 1970; Kimchi et al., 1991).

Critical multiplism is also concerned with reducing bias, in the recognition that no one approach or measure is perfect or without bias. As a result, both triangulation and critical multiplism seek to eliminate inherent bias in the research methods chosen. However, critical multiplism goes further in that it encourages the exhaustive study of phenomena from as many different perspectives as possible, given the recognition that theory is a huge fishnet of complex, mutually interacting relationships among constructs or variables. Further, triangulation frequently is presented as being conducted by a lone researcher or a group of researchers working in tandem to study a phenomenon (Kimchi et al., 1991). In contrast, critical multiplism does not require that researchers work in tandem, rather they may be working in vastly different regions of the globe, working in isolation, yet studying similar phenomena in different ways.

It is the essential critique and scrutiny of the multiple ways of studying the phenomena that distinguishes critical multiplism from triangulation. Critical multiplism is an encouragement to all researchers to be open to all of the possible ways of examining phenomena in an effort to arrive at warranted knowledge claims. This openness is part of the reason for critical multiplists' desire to involve multiple stakeholders, beyond mere investigators, in the process of research.

Relativism and Incommensurability

In spite, or perhaps because, of the many ways in which post-positivistic knowledge claims can gain warrant, post-positivistic critical multiplism has been criticized for the potential to degenerate into relativism whereby all options for the interpretation of results are considered equally valid or useful (Houts et al., 1986; Lutz, 1988; Smith, 1990). Although this could pose a problem to the results of research from merely triangulated methods rooted in diverse paradigms, critical multiplistic methods, rooted in the post-positivistic paradigm, avoid this problem.

Phillips (1987) states that post-positivistic critical multiplism avoids relativism through the regulatory ideal of objectivity. By objectivity is meant openness to public scrutiny. Thus the results of investigations are "forced to face the demands of reason and evidence" (Phillips, 1990b, p. 30). Through this public challenge, analysis, critique and debate, assurance is given (though not absolute) that the views put forth do not reflect the bias, misinterpretation or "whim" of any particular group (Popper, 1976; Phillips, 1990a). Similarly, methods are also empirically and logically examined and, for the research question asked, some methods may be deemed better than others, albeit imperfection themselves (Phillips, 1987).

As researchers enter into this critical tradition (Phillips, 1992) of discussion and critique of issues, methods or knowledge claims, objectivity is gained, thereby avoiding relativism, where any knowledge claim is accepted. It remains that while objectivity increases the ability to judge the worth of knowledge claims or to judge arguments put forth to support a position as better or worse, objectivity in no way ensures that knowledge claims are warranted (Phillips, 1990a). Frequently, until evidence mounts to indicate that one knowledge claim is more worthy than others presented, judgment may be suspended. Individuals may make their own judgments, but more evidence is required before the critical consensus of rational opinion decides whether or not a scientific knowledge claim is acceptable.

Comparison of theories and the use of multiple approaches within a program of research have also raised the issue of incommensurability and thus incomparability. The question is posed as to how theories developed within specific paradigms or methods based on apparently different philosophical assumptions can be compared? It is claimed that there is incommensurability between competing paradigms in that there is disagreement about the research problems/issues that a paradigm is to resolve, that terms and concepts and experiments fall into new relationships one with the other, and, as Kuhn (1970, p. 150) notes, "proponents of competing paradigms practice their trades in different worlds."

Bernstein (1983) offers a solution in that while there may be incommensurability of problems and standards there is not incommensurability of meanings. Indeed, there is always some overlap between competing paradigms and, if there was not, debate and argumentation could not take place. It may be that rival paradigm theories are incompatible in that they are in conflict, incommensurable in that they cannot be measured against each other point by point, but they are comparable in that they can be compared with each other in multiple ways. This comparison does not require the assumption that there is or must be a common, fixed grid by which we measure progress (Bernstein, 1983). As Bernstein notes, the belief that there must be determinate, unambiguous criteria to which one can appeal that will help one decide what is a better or worse substantive argument, is tied to Cartesianism.

It is the Cartesian anxiety that post-positivistic critical multiplism helps dispel. There is recognition that there is no absolute authoritative foundation on which to base scientific knowledge, but there are better or worse arguments in support of a theory or hypothesis. Through the critical tradition of evaluation and challenge one can adequately "test" the collective strength of the multiple argumentation that occurs within critical multiplism.

Heterogeneity and Bias: At What Cost?

Critical multiplism is not without its weaknesses. Two major ones are the difficulty in ensuring that bias is ruled out, and the second concerns the absence of "an algorithm" or step by step procedure (Houts et al., 1986, p. 63) for according what needs to be made multiple or heterogenous.

A basic premise of critical multiplism is that bias is decreased through the promotion of heterogeneity or diversity in all research endeavors (Houts et al., 1986). The greater the heterogeneity of situations across which a relationship is demonstrated, the greater the likelihood that threats to validity or rigor can be ruled out. In other words, external validity is enhanced when results are demonstrably stable across populations, settings and times, thereby increasing the likelihood that knowledge claims are warranted (Cook, 1985).

Heterogeneity does not, however, necessarily rule out the potential for having bias (Cook, 1985; Houts et al., 1986). There can still be difficulty in identifying sources of homogeneity that might lead to a consistent or constant direction or source of bias. Constant sources and constant directions of bias can still result when many sources of potential bias have been made heterogeneous in a study or across a set of studies. A constant source of bias results when no one involved in the research can conceive of the bias being a bias (Coward, 1990). A constant direction of bias can result when a bias is operating in the same direction across all of the methods employed (Houts et al., 1986).

In addition, Cook (1985) warns that satisfaction with using the critical multiplist approach may lull researchers out of the critical frame of mind necessary to rule out sources of bias. Researchers may be less likely to inquire whether other sources of bias-inducing homogeneity are still operating to produce repeated convergence on the wrong answer.

The likelihood of avoiding bias depends on identifying all the plausible sources of such bias. This requires examination of the numerous published lists of threats to validity, a well-documented audit trail, as well as public commentary or critique. Commentators must be induced to be as critical as possible in conceptualizing alternative interpretations to those already posited. Indeed, Cook (1985) contends that consensus about alternatives to a relationship can count more in science than consensus about a relationship.

Interdisciplinary consultation also assists in ruling out sources of bias and alternative interpretations. Disbrow (1983) notes that elimination or decrease of bias can accompany the broadening of research perspectives that accompanies interdisciplinary research. Such fruitful interdisciplinary research occurs when researchers recognize the strengths and perspectives that different disciplines bring to bear on a research problem (Kirchoff & Haase, 1995).

One sensitivity to the necessity of avoiding a bias is raised, the problem confronting researchers is what to make heterogeneous. A study that is truly critical-multiplistic requires the capacity to not only answer multiple research questions but also to uncover novel questions and issues (Houts et al., 1986). It requires multiple constructs, multiple measures of each construct, multiple populations of persons, settings and times, multiple mechanisms for triangulating on inferences about cause, multiple data analyses for every important substantive issue, and finally commentary by many people who have unique values and method preferences that relate to research questions and procedures (Cook, 1985; Houts et al., 1986). All of these require substantial expenditure of resources, funds, time and energy.

One approach is the use of meta-analysis in quantitative research and meta-synthesis in qualitative work. Meta-analysis, the analyses of a large collection of results from individual studies, represents a rigorous attempt "to make sense of the often confusing and conflicting findings resulting from studies of the same variable across different contexts, subjects, and numerous other factors" (Waltz & Bausell, 1981, p. 330). Meta-synthesis, the comparative textual analysis of qualitative studies, leads to a synthesis of the commonalities among individual representations of a phenomenon (Jensen & Allen, 1996). By using these techniques, researchers incorporate and build on the work of others as well as achieve the goal of heterogeneity.

Cook (1985) adds that the costs of critical multiplism are partly related to what is being made heterogeneous. For example, frequently it costs considerably more to add sites to a single study design than to operationalize constructs in multiple ways or to collect data at different or heterogeneous times. Collaboration among researchers and those from other disciplines may be a partial solution to the costs of promoting heterogeneity in as many ways as possible. Such research can conserve time and energy as well as provide increased access to the research sites and subjects necessary to promote heterogeneity (Disbrow, 1983; Kirchoff & Haase, 1995). As a result, the multiplicity and thus expense of critical multiplism is shared among many, often disparate, researchers and does not fall on the shoulders of a lone researcher.

Some have suggested that guidelines are needed to help individual researchers decide what to make heterogeneous, because resource and logistical limitations prevent everything from being made heterogeneous (Houts et al., 1986). Indeed, there are no "cookbook" techniques that specify which options should be made heterogeneous, or even how to accomplish such heterogeneity (Houts et al., 1986; Cook, 1985; Coward, 1990). Although one might prefer specific guidelines, as Houts et al. (1986, p. 68) pointed out "specification in cookbook form smacks of a dogmatism like that inherent in [logical positivist] slogans for practice (e.g. all science requires hypothesis testing)."

Values and Objectivity

Critical multiplists recognize that all research is social and necessarily value laden. Value dependence is welcomed by critical multiplists who recognize that individual passion and intellectual commitments provide both the impetus for inquiry and the protection of knowledge claims from premature abandonment (Cook, 1985). Although the notion of objectivity remains a regulative ideal that underpins all inquiry (Phillips, 1990a), it is recognized that any given concept is more or less objective and more or less subjective. This recognition allows researchers from a wide variety of perspectives to enter "into a mutual and fruitful discussion, criticism, and evaluation," the hallmarks of critical multiplism (Phillips, 1990b, p. 27). Indeed, objectivity may be regarded as the social result of scientists' mutual criticism (Phillips, 1990a).

The importance of subjectivity is recognized in post-positivistic critical multiplism. Instead of treating people as on par with inanimate objects, people are studied within their contexts (Phillips, 1992). Further, it is recognized that many subjective views (criticism is an example) combine to form more objective views. In one sense, the sources of bias are partially neutralized as subjective views combine to form more objective views. In the qualitative interview, subjective experience is valued and contributes to the identification of phenomena at the more abstract and thus less objective level. However, by virtue of being studied and identified, the phenomena have become objectified to a degree.

Some phenomena are not amenable to further objectification due to a high degree of complexity or context dependence that precludes the identification and testing of theoretical relationships to further refine the nature of the phenomena. Trading precision for richness may be appropriate in many situations, such as in the study of individuals' high personal, lived experiences of health-related phenomena. Other phenomena, such as biophysical or psychosocial parameters of health, may be highly amenable to further study and more precise refinement. Regardless, the objectivity obtained through the study of phenomena enables the findings from qualitative and quantitative research to be critiqued in the form of evaluation and challenge by other scientists.

To summarize, post-positivistic critical multiplism should not be seen as a panacea, it does have some weaknesses (Guba, 1990). These weaknesses, however, can be minimized by the constant search for alternative explanations. In addition, post-positivists decry research characterized by excessive context-stripping controls and call for this to be replaced by inquiry carried out in more natural settings. The necessity for the use of qualitative methods of inquiry to provide the richness essential to knowledge development is recognized. Similarly, critical multiplists are concerned with the applicability of theory to local contexts and therefore ground theory in local circumstances, as opposed to more general circumstances. In short, post-positivistic critical multiplism achieves balance by embracing both qualitative and quantitative methods.

Advantages of Critical Multiplism for Nursing

The benefits of pluralism, implicit in critical multiplism, have long been advocated for nursing. Pluralism has been construed as a solution to the qualitative-quantitative methods debate, as a way to address concerns about premature closure on research problems, and as a way to explore the many dimensions of the phenomena of concern to nursing (Cull-Wilby & Pepin, 1987; Gortner & Schultz, 1988; Schultz & Meleis, 1988; Riegel et al., 1992; Gortner, 1993; Kim, 1993). Kim (1993, p. 1632) suggests that "pluralism in nursing provides on the one hand, a rich array of scientific knowledge about human phenomena and ways of dealing with nursing problems, while on the other a set of theoretical choices available for knowledge use in practice." Further, pluralism, in the form of critical multiplism, recognizes the legitimacy of multiple ways of coming to know and accepts the complexity and holistic quality of nursing human beings (Gortner & Schultz, 1988; Schultz & Meleis, 1988). As a result, through achieving balance, the critical multiplist approach enables nursing science to better reflect the holistic nature of nursing practice through the development of nursing theory from a rich variety of perspectives. This variety of perspectives also allows for the identification of patterns and for the knowledge thus developed to be more useful in practice.

Pattern Identification

Critical multiplism has the potential to enhance theory and practice by improving the likelihood that patterns or convergences are identified through the process of having questions studied from several perspectives (Cook, 1985). This identification of patterns can occur when not only multiple approaches are utilized but also when sharing occurs among researchers from a wide variety of methodological backgrounds. This process has the potential to promote the rapidity of nursing theory and knowledge development with the gains subsequently felt in nursing practice.

Similarly, critical multiplism will also ensure that lack of convergence is valued, as it helps guard against premature closure on issues of theoretical or practical concern where investigators might otherwise have been prone to over-generalize or limit their inquiry. Further, a lack of convergence might foster communication among researchers. For example, researchers may receive helpful critique about potential sources of bias and lack of heterogeneity in their research. Conversely, other researchers may be encouraged to further their research with other approaches, thus increasing heterogeneity. As well, critical multiplists' encouragement of interdisciplinary research and collaboration allows broader understanding of phenomenon of mutual interest, thereby contributing to knowledge development in each discipline.

Usefulness of Knowledge

Ensuring that knowledge is useful has been heralded as a potential solution to the perceived gap between nursing theory and nursing practice because problems considered important to the development of knowledge for nursing practice are addressed (Hodgman, 1979; Silva & Rothbart, 1984; Kim, 1993; Rolfe, 1993). Within critical multiplism the need for critique of knowledge claims necessitates that knowledge be disseminated widely and to as many stakeholders as possible (Coward, 1990). Similarly, the "consciousness raising" implicit in critical multiplism also ensures that stakeholders such as nurse clinicians and patients find an integrated place in nursing research by providing critique and direction to the nursing research questions posed and by finding that the resultant knowledge is useful to them. The nurse clinician is in a prime position both to assess the degree to which nursing care problems have been addressed by nurse researchers and to be informed about the results of such research, thereby ensuring that links between theory and practice settings are maintained. Patients, as stakeholders, ought to ensure that the results of research are adequately judged for the improvement of their care. Further, the requisite dissemination will ensure that the public is informed of developing nursing knowledge and that links

are maintained between members of the stake-holding public and nurse researchers. Involving multiple stakeholders thereby increases the likelihood that the research findings will be helpful to those most in need of the research knowledge. Further, stakeholders can help prevent premature closure on research problems that are considered important, thus increasing the likelihood that the knowledge claims are both warranted and found to be useful (Engstrom, 1984; Silva & Rothbart, 1984).

Collaboration

Recognizing the importance of both values and objectivity in research, critical multiplism has the ability to accommodate all forms of nursing inquiry and encourages dialogue and collaboration among nurse researchers from varying perspectives. Dialogue and collaboration will improve the likelihood that nursing theories and knowledge claims are thoroughly examined before they are refuted or accepted for the benefit of nursing practice. Described as an excellent way to test theory and to ensure that theory and practice links are maintained (Engstrom, 1984; Silva & Rothbart, 1984; Stevenson & Woods, 1985; Denyes et al., 1989), collaborative research between nurse researchers and nurse clinicians exemplifies the critical multiplist approach. As Stevenson and Woods (1985) suggest, nurse researchers from various perspectives should collaborate to conduct multi-method and triangulation research for the benefit of nursing knowledge development and the improvement of nursing practice.

Recapitulation

Post-positivistic critical multiplism holds considerable potential for scientific nursing knowledge development and nursing practice. Critical multiplism advocates methodological pluralism that gives way to both qualitative and quantitative methods. As a result, nurse researchers can approach the study of health and holistic human beings from a wide variety of perspectives. This results in research that more accurately reflects the nature of holistic nursing practice. Heterogeneity in the research process induces collaboration among nurse researchers and between disciplines in the interest of reducing bias, promoting the best use of resources, promoting the identification of patterns and convergences, and increasing the likelihood that assertions are warranted. Research questions asked from the perspective of post-positivistic critical multiplism are likely to have more utility for nursing practice, given that stakeholder input has considerable influence over what is considered important for nurses to study. Critical multiplism also has the potential to solve more scientific nursing problems and improve nursing practice.

Critical multiplism offers a new way of thinking about science because it is built upon the constant search for alternative explanations, upon humility in acknowledging our biases, and upon the belief that uncertainty and knowledge (Houts et al., 1986). As such, it has much potential to improve the state of scientific nursing knowledge development and nursing practice.

References

Bernstein, R. J. (1983). *Beyond Objectivism and Relativism: Science, Hermeneutics, and Praxis*. University of Pennsylvania Press, Philadelphia.

Cook, T. (1985). Postpositivist critical multiplism. In *Social Science and Social Policy* (Shotland, R., & Mark, M., eds.). Sage, Beverly Hills, California, pp. 25–62.

Cook, T., & Campbell, D. (1979). *Quasi-Experimentation: Design and Analysis Issues for Field Settings*. Houghton Mifflin, Boston.

Coward, D. (1990). Critical multiplism: A research strategy for nursing science. *Image, 22*, 163–167.

Cull-Wilby, B., & Pepin, J. (1987). Towards a coexistence of paradigms in nursing knowledge development. *Journal of Advanced Nursing, 12*, 515–521.

Denyes, M., O'Connor, N., Oakley, D., & Ferguson, S. (1989). Integrating nursing theory, practice and research through collaborative research. *Journal of Advanced Nursing, 14*(2), 141–145.

Denzin, N. (1970). *The Research Act: A Theoretical Introduction to Sociological Methods*. Aldine, Chicago.

Disbrow, M. (1983). Conducting interdisciplinary research: Gratifications and frustrations. In *The Nursing Profession: A Time to Speak* (Chaska, N., ed.). McGraw-Hill, Toronto, pp. 225–236.

Dzurec, L. C. (1989). The necessity for and evolution of multiple paradigms for nursing research: A post-structuralist perspective. *Advances in Nursing Science, 11*, 69–77.

Engstrom, J. (1984). University, agency, and collaborative models for nursing research: An overview. *Image: The Journal of Nursing Scholarship, 16*(3), 76–80.

Fawcett, J. (1993). From a plethora of paradigms to parsimony in world views. *Nursing Science Quarterly, 6*, 56–58.

Forbes, D., King, K., Kushner, K., et al. (1999). Warrantable evidence in nursing science. *Journal of Advanced Nursing, 29*(2), 373–379.

Gortner, S. (1993). Nursing's syntax revisited: A critique of philosophies said to influence nursing theories. *International Journal of Nursing Studies, 30*(6), 477–488.

Gortner, S., & Schultz, P. (1988). Approaches to nursing science methods. *Image: Journal of Nursing Scholarship, 20*(1), 22–24.

Greene, J. (1990). Three views on the nature and role of knowledge in social science. *The Paradigm Dialogue* (Guba, E., ed.). Sage, Newbury Park, California, pp. 227–245.

Guba, E. (1990). The alternative paradigm dialog. In *The Paradigm Dialog* (Guba, E., ed.). Sage, Newbury Park, California, pp. 17–27.

Guba, G., & Lincoln, E. (1994). Competing paradigms in qualitative research. In *Handbook of Qualitative Research* (Denzin, N. K., & Lincoln, Y. S., eds.). Sage, Thousand Oaks, California, pp. 105–117.

Hempel, C. (1966). *Philosophy of Natural Science*. Prentice Hall, Englewood Cliffs, New Jersey.

Hodgman, E. (1979). Closing the gap between research and practice: Changing the answers to the "who," and "where" and the "how" of nursing research. *International Journal of Nursing Studies, 16*(1), 105–110.

Houts, A., Cook, T., & Shadish, W. (1986). The person-situation debate: A critical multiplist perspective. *Journal of Personality, 54*(1), 52–105.

Howe, K. (1985). Two dogmas of educational research. *Educational Researcher, 14*(8), 10–18.

Jensen, L., & Allen, M. (1996). Meta-synthesis of qualitative findings. *Qualitative Health Research, 6*, 553–560.

Kim, H. (1993). Putting theory into practice: problems and prospects. *Journal of Advanced Nursing, 18*(10), 1632–1639.

Kimchi, J., Polivika, B., & Stevenson, J. (1991). Triangulation: Operational definitions. *Nursing Research, 40,* 364–366.

Kirchoff, K., & Haase, J. (1995). The way of the future: interdisciplinary research *Reflections, 4,* 15.

Kuhn, T. (1970). *The Structure of Scientific Revolutions.* University of Chicago Press, Chicago.

Lakatos, I. (1970). Falsification and the methodology of scientific research programes. In *Criticism and the Growth of Knowledge* (Lakatos, I., & Musgrave, A., eds.). Cambridge University Press, Oxford, pp. 91–196.

Lather, P. (1990). Reinscribing otherwise: The play of values in the practices of the human sciences. In *The Paradigm Dialogue* (Guba, E., eds.). Sage, Newbury Park, California, pp. 315–332.

Lather, P. (1992). Critical frames in educational research: feminist and post-structural perspectives. *Theory Into Practice, 31*(2), 87–99.

Laudan, L. (1977). *Progress and its Problems.* University of California Press, Berkeley.

Lutz, F. (1988). The courage to be creative. Paper presented at the Annual Meeting of the American Educational Research Association, New Orleans. *ERIC Document Reproduction Service ED, 297,* 016.

Moccia, P. (1988). A critique of compromise: beyond the methods debate. *Advances in Nursing Science, 10*(4), 1–9.

Munhall, P. L. (1982). Nursing philosophy and nursing research: in apposition or opposition? *Nursing Research, 31,* 176–177.

Phillips, D. (1987). *Philosophy, Science and Social Inquiry.* Pergamon, Oxford.

Phillips, D. (1990a). Postpositvistic science: myths and realities. In *The Paradigm Dialogue* (Guba, E. ed.). Sage, Newbury Park, California, pp. 31–45.

Phillips, D. (1990b). Subjectivity and objectivity: an objective inquiry. In *Qualitative Inquiry in Education: The Continuing Debate* (Eisner, E., & Peshkin, A., eds.). Teachers College Press, New York, pp. 19–37.

Phillips, D. (1992). *The Social Scientist's Bestiary. A Guide to Fabled Threats to, and Defenses of Naturalistic Social Science.* Pergamon Press, New York.

Popper, K. (1968). *Conjectures and Refutations: The Growth of Scientific Knowledge.* Harper & Row, New York.

Popper, K. (1976). The logic of the social sciences. In *The Positivist Dispute in German Sociology* (Adorno, T., *et al.,* eds.). Harper, New York.

Riegel, B., Omery, A., Calvillo, E., et al. (1992). Moving beyond: A generative philosophy of science. *Image, 24,* 115–120.

Rolfe, G. (1993). Closing the theory-practice gap: A model of nursing praxis. *Journal of Clinical Nursing, 2,* 173–177.

Schultz, P., & Meleis, A. (1988). Nursing epistemology: Traditions, insights, questions. *Image: Journal of Nursing Scholarship, 20,* 217–221.

Schumacher, K., & Gortner, S. (1992). (Mis)conceptions and reconceptions about traditional science. *Advances in Nursing Science, 14*(4), 1–11.

Shadish, W. (1993). Critical multiplism: A research strategy and its attendant tactics. *New Directions for Program Evaluation, 60,* 13–57.

Silva, M., & Rothbart, D. (1984). An analysis of changing trends in philosophies of science on nursing theory development and testing. *Advances in Nursing Science, 6*(2), 1–13.

Smith, J. (1983). Quantitative versus qualitative research: an attempt to clarify the issue. *Educational Researcher, 12*(3), 6013.

Smith, J. (1990). Goodness criteria: Alternative research paradigms and the problem of criteria. In *The Paradigm Dialogue* (Guba, E., ed.). Sage, Newbury Park, California, pp. 167–187.

Stevenson, J., & Woods, N. (1985). *Strategies for the Year 2000: Synthesis and Projections. Setting the Agenda for the Year 2000: Knowledge Development in Nursing.* Proceeds from the American Academy of Nursing Advisory Group on Knowledge Development and Utilization. American Academy of Nursing, Kansas City.

Waltz, C., & Bausell, R. B. (1981). *Nursing Research: Design, Statistics, and Computer Analysis.* F. A. Davis, Philadelphia.

Watson, J. (1988). *Nursing: Human Science and Human Care: A Theory of Nursing.* National League of Nursing, New York.

Wildemuth, B. (1993). Post-positivist research: Two examples of methodological pluralism. *Library Quarterly, 63,* 450–468.

Chapter 24

Esthetic and Personal Knowing Through Humanistic Nursing

Dianne Pelletier
Raymond

Carper (1978) discussed four fundamental patterns of knowing in nursing:

1. empirics, the science of nursing
2. ethics
3. personal knowledge
4. esthetics, the art of nursing

Paterson and Zderad's (1976) humanistic nursing model offers a method for fostering the development of knowledge through personal and esthetic patterns. Empirical science cannot adequately address all phenomena encountered in nursing. Nursing is concerned with such human experiences as suffering, guilt, anger, hopelessness, and fear. The phenomenological approach proposed by Paterson and Zderad (1976) provides the nurse with a method to attend to lived experiences such as these. Phenomenology, however, can neither replace other measures of inquiry in nursing nor account for all its goals (Oiler, 1982). The purpose of this paper is to briefly describe Paterson and Zderad's phenomenological approach, to offer a commentary on McKinnon's 1991 article related to humanistic nursing, to explore a specific nursing situa-

tion utilizing the humanistic nursing paradigm, and to advocate use of the model in qualitative research and theory development.

Humanistic Nursing Model Describes Lived Experiences

The humanistic nursing model (depicted in the figure "Humanistic Nursing Model"), as proposed by Paterson and Zderad (1976), has its own phenomenological method for describing lived experiences. The authors call their approach phenomenological nursology. According to Paterson and Zderad (1976), phenomenological nursology is a medium through which concept and theory development can take place.

Phenomenologic nursology is comprised of five phases. The first four phases involve assessment and the final phase is analogous to the nursing diagnosis. The lived experience as viewed by the patient unfolds through the therapeutic relationship itself. The phases are identified as follows (Paterson & Zderad, 1976):

- Phase I: Preparation of the nurse knower for coming to know (the patient)
- Phase II: Nurse knowing the other (the patient) intuitively

Source: Raymond, D. P. (1995). Esthetic and personal knowing through humanistic nursing. *N & HC: Perspectives on community.* 16(6):332–336. Reprinted with permission from the National League for Nursing.

- Phase III: Nurse knowing the other (the patient) scientifically
- Phase IV: Nurse complementarily synthesizing known others
- Phase V: Succession within the nurse from the many to the paradoxical one (conclusion)

McKinnon (1991) contended that Paterson and Zderad's model offered neither guidelines for administering patient care nor a means of evaluating its effectiveness. Further, the author stated that a main weakness of the model is its failure to hold the nurse accountable for the quality of patient care. One may argue that the nurse who does not also consider the lived experience of the patient in approach to care may not be totally accountable to the patient. Without a consideration of needs as the patient views it, there is a danger of addressing needs only from an outsider's perspective, which may be narrow or inaccurate. Further, one may argue that fostering the kind of relationship necessary for understanding the worldview of the patient may potentially enhance the quality of patient care delivered. The ethical dictum of phenomenology is the imperative to turn to the people who actually live the experience (Swanson-Kauffman & Schonwald, 1988).

It is important to note that the humanistic model is at a descriptive level in theory development (Brouse & Laffrey, 1989). The aim of the model is to describe the human experience as it is lived by the patient. The model does not attempt to predict or to control nursing phenomena. In other words, the model does not claim to provide all of the guidelines necessary in administering nursing care. According to Brouse and Laffrey (1989), "The phenomenological method is complementary to but operates at qualitatively different levels from empirical science" (p. 207). Empirical science provides a view that is logically deduced, while phenomenology emphasizes the view of the subject (the lived experience). One view should not necessarily discount the other, but may be seen as a complement to the other. Thus, the phenomenological approach attempts to address questions that cannot be answered by empirical science.

The following paragraphs illustrate the application of the humanistic nursing model to a clinical situation in order to demonstrate its usefulness in practice. "Elise" was a patient who I encountered while working as a staff nurse on a psychiatric unit.

Figure 24–1   MODEL DEPICTS HUMANISTIC NURSING FRAMEWORK DEVELOPED BY PATERSON AND ZDERAD (1976) AS VIEWED BY AUTHOR.

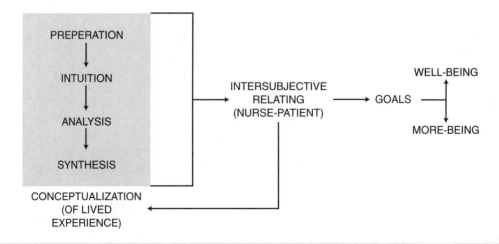

Clinical Situation as Lived by "Elise"

Elise was a 17-year-old woman of Acadian descent living in a rural community. Elise was referred to the psychiatric unit via the helpline by her mother, who had noted progressive withdrawal in Elise and failing grades in school. Elise lived at home with her mother and her brothers. Her father had died five years prior to the admission. She had been very close to her father. Elise's conversations with her mother were obsessed with thoughts of her father's death and God. She was described as reclusive to her room. Upon admission, Elise made it obvious to all staff that she did not want to be there with much crying and expressions of anger. She experienced auditory hallucinations. Her affect was flat with a mask-like expression on her face. She would sit for hours at a time looking straight ahead, immersed in her own world. Elise was tried on antipsychotic medication with little initial response. After one week on the psychiatric unit, she began to verbalize paranoid delusions of staff wishing to "lock" her up forever and the food being "poisoned." She began to gag on her food and medication and reported nausea. Her appearance further deteriorated.

Phase I: Preparation of the Nurse for Coming to Know

Through my years of nursing experience and years of education, as well as life experiences, I have prepared myself for coming to know the human condition. Through these experiences, I have developed the ability to empathize—to experience the feelings of another. The key to practice utilizing phenomenology is to have a nurse who is willing to operate in a methodology that mandates an investment of the personal self

(Swanson-Kauffman & Schonwald, 1988). The outcome depends on the nurse's ability to engage in another's reality in an empathic sense. I had attended a case review where all the disciplines involved in Elise's care discussed her lack of progress. I was assigned to work with Elise. The most recent subjective data from her chart contained statements such as "I want to go home now!" and "I'm not getting better here." The chart noted that she was only sleeping two or three hours per night. I chose a time when Elise was sitting quietly in the solarium to approach her, respecting her need to maintain the distance between us. I approached her openly, leaving all of the accumulated database behind—e.g., DSM-III-R diagnosis and increasing distrustful and aggressive behavior. A nurse that can be open provides a model for the patient (Berger, 1977). By approaching Elise openly, I encouraged her to be open with me. I introduced myself to Elise as her staff person for the day.

Phase II: Nurse Knowing Other Intuitively

After a few superficial exchanges, Elise identified me as an authority figure on the unit and as a person who gave her medication. She proceeded to tell me that she felt that staff was deceiving her. She stated, "They tell me that if I take the medication that I'll get better and then I can go home. I think they tell me that so I'll take it. I don't want to take the medication. It will make me sick." I responded by providing Elise with a brief explanation of her medication and the symptoms that needed to be controlled before discharge was possible.

This was the beginning of an intersubjective relationship with Elise. I intuitively grasped her situation—allowed myself to feel what she must be feeling. Elise was losing her sense of contact with the people and the things in her world. She felt that she was forced into the hospital and forced into strange routines. She was eating unfamiliar food and ingesting medications that she was unaccustomed to taking and had equated to making her feel ill. I allowed myself to experience the situation subjectively through her worldview. Hospitalization was an identifiable source of stress for Elise. I experienced the apprehension that arises from being separated from familiar people, personal possessions, and the safety and security of home.

Phase III: Nurse Knowing Other Scientifically

I reflected on what I knew of Elise intuitively and examined the experience objectively. During our dialogue, I had observed her dilated pupils, her look of bewilderment, her trembling hands, and her guarded, withdrawn manner. I recalled the elevated vital signs and nausea. I analyzed the available data.

Phase IV: Nurse Complementarily Synthesizing Known Others

I compared Elise's experience with that of other patients with similar symptoms and with what I had read in the literature. I recalled what Gibson described as a "need/fear dilemma" (Berger, 1977). Patients who are out of touch with reality need others desperately to strengthen their inadequate egos. Yet they feel threatened by others and find it hard to maintain a clear picture of reality. Thus, they may try to avoid other people to escape their feeling of being engulfed by them, which explains the withdrawal that they manifest (Berger, 1977).

Phase V: Succession Within the Nurse from the Many to the Paradoxical One

In relating to Elise's experience, I concluded that she was experiencing the phenomenon of fear. Once isolated, the nursing diagnosis of fear can be approached via the nursing process. McKinnon (1991) contended that the humanistic nursing process does not include the development of a plan of care or mutual goal setting with patients of any age. Humanistic nursing practice, however, does call for intersubjective relating where the patient expects to be helped and the nurse expects to give help (Paterson & Zderad, 1976). The plan includes the establishment of a therapeutic relationship that forms the basis of all other treatment that follows. The plan of care utilizing the humanistic model may be supplemented by other theories and approaches. Although phenomenological nursology, an empathic approach, continued to be an important therapeutic approach with Elise, an interdisciplinary treatment approach was critical to her care as well, which included the collaborative efforts between nursing, psychiatry, occupational therapy, social worker, and dietician. The treatment approach focused on reassuring her of her safety.

Planning Involves the Patient in Making Responsible Choices

The effectiveness of the phenomenological approach with Elise was validated through her admission of fear and through direct observation of her behavior. She did not react with hostility. She stated her agreement to continue to take the medication. She acknowledged that she was hearing voices and that she wanted them to go away. Through continued intersubjective encounters with Elise, combined with the other treatment modalities, one could notice a gradual improvement in her mental status. She stayed on the unit for a total of two months. As she was able to relax and to see her own progress; the aggressive behavior disappeared. She began to show trust in staff and to actively involve herself in unit activities. Her affect improved markedly. Although the planning, implementation, and evaluation stages of the nursing process are not directly addressed by Paterson and Zderad, these stages may be inferred. The planning involved eliciting the active involvement of the patient in making responsible choices. The therapeutic relationship that was one of collaboration not only was an important intervention, but facilitated the implementation of other treatment modalities. Evaluation occurred through validation with the patient. The goal of well-being was met through Elise's steady improvement in mental status and her participation in health maintenance behaviors. She was discharged from the hospital and returned to live with her family. As long as Elise can be functional and maintained within the community, there can be continual movement toward the goal of more-being or the maximization of her human potential.

Philosophy of Science and Nursing Theory Are in a "State of Transition"

Traditionally, logical empiricism with its quantitative methodologies has dominated theory development and testing (Silva & Rothbart, 1984). However, the philosophy of science and nursing theory are in a "state of transition" (Silva & Rothbart, p. 294). According to Silva and Rothbart (1984), a new philosophy of science known as historicism has emerged. While logical empiricism provides a logical explanation of the nature of scientific knowledge, historicism is a philosophy of science that provides a historical explanation (Silva & Rothbart, 1984). According to Silva and Rothbart, historicists attempt to understand science in terms of research traditions. The authors defined a research tradition as "a broadly based foundation of many theories and [as] an accepted way of viewing fundamental phenomena within a discipline" (p. 295). Further, the authors noted that research traditions are global and changeable within the boundaries of an ontological commitment or nature of being. According to these authors, a methodological commitment that defines the legitimate method of inquiry suitable to a research tradition's ontology is essential. For example, Silva and Rothbart (1984) questioned whether the case study method of inquiry may be better suited to the ontological commitment of holism than a traditional experimental design method of inquiry with its built-in reductionism. Theories based on research traditions view the person as a holistic being as opposed to looking at parts. Thus, according to the authors, the logical empiricists with their deductive approach emphasize science as product, whereas, the historicists place emphasis on science as process.

In addition to the shift in the philosophy of science espoused in the nursing literature, Silva and Rothbart (1984) identified a shift in emphasis from quantitative to qualitative methodologies as another trend. Grounded theory research is an example of a current break from tradition. In grounded theory research, the researcher becomes immersed in the world of the research subject (Bowers, 1988). According to Bowers, the researcher attempts to discover how subjects experience their world. Through bracketing, researchers are able to temporarily relinquish their perspectives and assume the perspective of the research subject (Bowers, 1988). The similarity between grounded theory research and the phenomenological approach proposed by Paterson and Zderad is clearly evident. Moreover, there are other methodologies such as ethnomethodology and ethnography that employ a strategy which allows researchers to apprehend experiences as they are perceived by those who live them (Swanson-Kauffman & Schonwald, 1988).

Further, Silva and Rothbart (1984) suggested that historicism and alternative research methodologies hold promise in helping to bridge the gap to contend with phenomena dealing with humanism and holism. Thus, phenomenological nursology may serve as a valuable tool for qualitative research and for the identification of concepts and further theory development.

Interestingly, Paterson and Zderad published their conceptual framework in 1976, but their model received little attention in the nursing literature (Silva & Rothbart, 1984). Silva and Rothbart (1984) speculated that this may be due to its existential–phenomenological perspective and ontological commitment, which was out of the mainstream of current thinking about philosophy of science at that time. Thus, Paterson and Zderad's humanistic nursing model reflected progressive thinking in keeping with the historicist philosophy.

The humanistic nursing model must not be dismissed due to its unique perspective and nontraditional approach. The model serves as a valuable framework in the development of knowledge through esthetic and personal patterns of knowing. Empathy is an important mode in the esthetic pattern of knowing (Carper, 1978). Further, through the "therapeutic use of self," the nurse develops personal knowledge. Without question, phenomenological nursology is an empathic process that requires the "therapeutic use of self." Moreover, Carper (1978) stated that the more skilled the nurse becomes in empathizing, the more knowledge will be gained in alternative perceptions of reality.

According to Chinn and Kramer (1991), there should be an integration of all patterns of knowing. The authors suggested that there has been little attention given to developing forms of expression for personal and esthetic knowing. Further, they asserted that all patterns of knowing are legitimate sources of knowledge for a collective body of nursing knowledge and for nursing practice.

Humanistic Nursing Complements Other Approaches in Patient Care

There is no one theory that serves as a panacea for all nursing problems. All paradigms have their particular strengths and weaknesses. A model is neither all good nor all bad. The phenomenological approach serves as a form of expression for the development of knowledge acquired through esthetic and personal patterns of knowing. The humanistic nursing approach complements other approaches in patient care. It offers a philosophical framework in the therapeutic nurse-patient relationship. Further, the model provides a methodology for qualitative research and for describing human phenomenon derived directly from the lived experiences of patients, which is important to clinical nursing practice.

References

Berger, M. (1977). *Working with people called patients.* New York: Brunner/Mazel Publishers.

Bowers, B. J. (1988). Grounded theory. In B. S. Sarter (ed.), *Paths to knowledge* (pp. 33–59). New York: National League for Nursing Press.

Brouse, S. H., & Laffrey, S. C. (1989). Paterson and Zderad's humanistic nursing framework. In J. J. Fitzpatrick & A. L. Whall, *Conceptual models of nursing: Analysis and application* (2nd ed.). Norwalk, CT: Appleton and Lange.

Carper, B. A. (1978). Fundamental patterns of knowing in nursing. *Adv Nurs Sci, 1*(1): 13–24.

Chinn, P. L., & Kramer, M. K. (1991). *Nursing's patterns of knowing: Theory and nursing: A systematic approach* (3rd ed.). St. Louis: Mosby-Year Book.

McKinnon, N. C. (1991). Humanistic nursing: It can't stand up to scrutiny. *Nursing and Health Care, 12*(8): 414–416.

Oiler, C. (1982). The phenomenological approach in nursing research. *Nursing Research, 31*(3): 178–181.

Paterson, J., & Zderad, L. (1976). *Humanistic nursing.* New York: John Wiley & Sons.

Silva, M. C., & Rothbart, D. (1984). An analysis of changing trends in philosophies of science on nursing theory development and testing. In L. H. Nicoll (ed.), *Perspectives on nursing theory* (pp. 293–302). Glenview, IL: Scott, Foresman and Company.

Swanson-Kauffman, K., & Schonwald, E. (1988). Phenomenology. In B. S. Sarter (ed.), *Paths to knowledge* (pp. 97–105). New York: National League for Nursing.

Chapter 25

Nursing Knowledge and Human Science: Ontological and Epistemological Considerations

Gail J. Mitchell,
RN, MScN

William K. Cody,
RN, MSN

Increasingly, nursing is being referred to as a human science (Connors, 1988; Gortner &
Schultz, 1988; Meleis, 1990; Munhall, 1989; Parse, 1981, 1987; Watson, 1985). The
meaning of this term as it is used in the literature, however, is not clear. Munhall (1989),
Parse (1981), and Watson (1985) refer to human science as distinct from natural science and
as bearing specific views, concepts, and methods. In contrast to this position, Connors (1988)
and Gortner and Schultz (1988) refer to human science as the fields of biology, psychology,
anthropology, and sociology. Is human science inclusive of any inquiry about human beings, or
is it a distinctive philosophical foundation for science? Is nursing currently a human science or
is this an ideal to be esteemed and aspired to? The purpose of this chapter is to examine the
meaning of human science as originated by Dilthey (1961, 1976, 1977a, 1977b, 1988)
and explicated by Giorgi (1970, 1971, 1985) and to compare selected works from nursing's
extant theoretical base with the explicit attributes that constitute "human" science.

Defining Human Science

The origins of the term *human science* can be traced to the philosopher Wilhelm Dilthey (1833–1911). The German term for human science, *Geisteswissenschaften,* has also been translated as "human studies." Translators frequently note the linguistic challenge involved in capturing the meaning of freshly coined and esoteric German expressions in English. Also noted in

Dilthey's works is his tendency to refer to "psychic" life in a nineteenth-century fashion while writing of the coherent whole of lived experience. Dilthey did, however, describe life as a unity, a living nexus, and he consistently referred to individuals as wholes and to human life as interconnected with others and history. The intent of the authors here is to offer an admittedly hermeneutical interpretation of Dilthey's view, in what is believed to be the unitary perspective of human beings that he intended.

Dilthey in the late 1800s was very concerned about what he called a "crisis in science," a crisis of modern consciousness, thought, and values (Ermath, 1978). The industrial society had already concretized the successes of the natural sciences, and the developing science of *Anthropologie*, with no other model, was rapidly abandoning any interest in human consciousness in favor of a crude "mindless" naturalism (Ermath, 1978). Dilthey (1977a) described what he saw as a sterile empiricism that disconnected life from knowledge. His fears were stoked by the growing trend to regard human behavior and culture as susceptible to the methods of natural science, which, he thought, stripped life of human meaning and purpose (Dilthey, 1977a). He proposed that "the deepest problem of modern thought and culture is to understand life as it is lived by man" (Ermath, 1978, p. 17).

Dilthey (1977a, 1977b, 1988) believed that the development of a human science held the only hope for understanding life as it is humanly lived. He proposed that the human sciences required concepts, methods, and theories that were fundamentally different from those of the natural sciences (Dilthey, 1977a, 1988). Dilthey viewed human beings as the preeminent source of knowledge. His philosophy took as its basis the whole of lived experience, the coherent nexus of life as it is humanly lived (Dilthey, 1977a). He wrote about "living" knowledge and "reflective" life. History and culture were, for Dilthey, manifestations of patterns of human life, pervaded with meaning. The natural sciences, concerned with the elaboration of physical laws from observation and experimentation, were, for Dilthey, very different from the concerns a true human science would focus on meaning, values, and relationships within the coherent texture of humanly lived experience. The subject matter of the human sciences is "the interrelation of life, expression, and understanding" (Dilthey, 1976, p. 175).

Dilthey proposed that the lived experience should be "the basic empirical datum of the human sciences" (Ermath, 1978, p. 97). Further, the researcher, a living being too, is inexorably and unequivocally "in" and "of" what is investigated. There could be no meaningful objective/subjective dichotomy and no analytic reduction beyond experience as humanly lived. Human experience is a coherent whole to which subjectivity is fundamental; objectivity is a human creation. Dilthey maintained that life is a process, a continuous becoming that manifests itself in the dynamic unity of experience (Dilthey, 1976). Human beings were described as individual wholes with intrinsic value (Dilthey, 1977b). Dilthey (1977b) referred to the self as a "life–unity" that is free yet also determined by history. The concept of free will is a fundamental assumption of human science. On free will, Dilthey (1988) wrote, "This is an immediately given actuality. *It cannot be denied.* . . . {O}ne cannot explain the fact of free will, for it is precisely its hallmark that we cannot break it down in a conceptual system" (p. 270).

More recently, the psychologist Giorgi (1970, 1971, 1985) has reasserted the need for an approach to the human sciences fundamentally different from conventional empirical methods. He proposed to study human beings as persons, as experiencing participants. He challenged the prevailing positivistic methods of psychology, contending that human experience must be understood in the way that it reveals itself, and he maintained that the study of lived experience could be done scientifically (Giorgi, 1985).

According to Giorgi, understanding life experiences requires a focus on meaning within the context of the person's experience of the phenomenon. Human beings cannot be known as objects, nor as separate from their lives. Echoing Dilthey, Giorgi maintained that a person is not "a passive receiver of physical energies, but rather his or her behavior reflects intentionality" (Giorgi, 1971, p. 23). Giorgi also addressed the influence of the researcher in conceptualizing research and the impact of the researcher on study findings. For Giorgi, the most important variable in the human sciences is the meaning of the lived experience for the subject. An exposition of the major thinkers and scholars, such as Gadamer (1976), Geertz (1973), Heidegger (1962), Ricoeur (1974), Schutz (1967), and Winch (1958), who have built on the tradition of which Dilthey is the foremost progenitor, is beyond the scope of this article.

The domination of twentieth-century social science by positivistic approaches in stark contrast to human science philosophy has been well documented (Polkinghorne, 1983) and contributes to the contexthual situation in which this article emerges. The philosophical stance of human science outlined here has underpinned or strongly influenced the works of the six seminal scholars mentioned above and many others in the tradition of human science. These scholars have recognized the manifest necessity for the human sciences to explore and understand lived experience, the full complexity of human meanings and values, with no more fundamental reference than the human lives which are the phenomena of concern; indeed, this formidable undertaking is the very mission of human science.

Based on the above explications of human science by Dilthey and Giorgi, specific ontological and epistemological attributes emerge as crucial to this approach for nursing science. Human science, in view of its origins and its philosophical foundations, cannot be viewed as a generic term for any and all disciplines studying human beings. It is proposed here that for a scientific discipline to be considered a "human science" logically it must incorporate the ontology and epistemology of its philosophical underpinnings, as described in **Table 25–1**.

A distinction must be made between a "humanistic" philosophy of science and "human science." According to Webster (1985), "humanism" entails a rejection of supernaturalism and asserts "the essential dignity and worth of man [*sic*] and his capacity to achieve self-realization through the use of reason and scientific method." Humanism thus is seen to acknowledge human

values and potentialities without requiring a critique of "scientific method." Human science, in contrast, unequivocally rejects the methods of natural science (Dilthey, 1976, 1977a, 1988; Giorgi, 1985) and asserts from the outset that lived experience, the world as experienced, meaning, and understanding are all aspects of a unitary process of human life and cannot be adequately described, explained, or analyzed through objectification, measurement, or reduction.

Significance of Human Science for Nursing

If nurses embrace the human science paradigm, activities in theory development, research, and practice will change to reflect the new philosophical perspective. An examination of nursing's philosophical and theoretical body of literature reveals that, in the past decade, such a change has already begun. In order to explore to what extent nurses are incorporating beliefs of the human science paradigm in theory, research, and practice, four nursing frameworks were selected for analysis. These frameworks are Paterson and Zderad's (1988) humanistic nursing, Newman's (1986a, 1990) model of health as expanding consciousness, Watson's (1985) human science and human care, and Parse's (1981, 1987, 1990a) theory of human becoming (formerly man–living–health, 1981). These frameworks were selected because all their authors claim a unitary conceptualization of human beings, thereby evincing some degree of interfacing with the human science perspective. Further, these authors have publicly renounced the natural science approach and have called for new and different methods more congruent with nursing's philosophical foundations.

Critical to the development of nursing theories underpinned by the human sciences would be the acknowledgment of human beings as individual wholes who are situated in the world and who are respected as intentional, free-willed persons.

Table 25-1 ONTOLOGY AND EPISTEMOLOGY OF THE HUMAN SCIENCE PARADIGM

Ontology	Epistemology
Human beings are unitary wholes in continuous interrelationship with their dynamic, temporal, historical, cultural worlds.	Research and practice focus on the coherent experience of the person's meanings, relations, values, patterns, and themes.
Human experience is preeminent and fundamental and reality is the whole complex of what is experienced and elaborated in thinking, feeling, and willing.	Lived experience is the basic empirical datum, as gleaned from the participant's description free of comparison to objective realities or predefined norms.
Human beings are intentional, free-willed beings who actively participate in life continuously.	The person's coparticipation in generating knowledge of lived experience is respected, and no more fundamental reference than what is disclosed by the person is sought.
The researcher is inextricably involved with any phenomenon investigated.	The researcher seeks knowledge and understanding of lived experience and is cognizant of the other's lived reality as a unitary whole.

Source: Synthesized and condensed from Dilthey, 1961, 1976, 1977a, 1977b, 1988; and Giorgi, 1970, 1971, 1985.

Any theoretical principles and concepts used to structure a theory would need to incorporate these beliefs. Also essential would be approaches which view the individual's lived experience as the focus in both practice and research and which honor the person's lived experience as reality. Researchers and practitioners would be regarded as coparticipants with persons in inquiry and practice in a human science paradigm.

Analysis of the Nursing Frameworks

Inquiry into the four frameworks above revealed a definite commitment to the human science paradigm. Parse's theory of human becoming was found not only to be consistent with the human science beliefs but to clarify, expand, and develop this approach. Consequently, an in-depth analysis of Parse's theory will be offered at a later point. Analysis of the works of Newman, Paterson and Zderad, and Watson illuminated consistencies and inconsistencies in relation to

the beliefs of human science. Consistencies and commonalities included affirmation, to varying degrees, of the wholeness of the human being, the significance of subjective experience, and mutual participation in the creation of reality.

The inconsistencies took two main forms. In some instances, the author(s) acknowledged an inability to reconcile traditional objectivist beliefs with beliefs congruent with human science, and consequently they incorporated conflicting beliefs in theoretical conceptualizations. Alternately, the author(s) extended and elaborated on beliefs essential to the human science tradition, leading to significant dissidence with the core philosophy. These two inconsistencies are discussed with specific examples to illustrate logical incongruencies with the human science tradition. The intent here is not to rebuke the nursing theorists for their philosophical obscurities, for obscurity engenders clarification. Rather, the intent is to illuminate the inconsistencies in order to foster clarity and further the development of nursing science.

Incorporating Diverging Beliefs

As previously noted, the nursing frameworks revealed both consistencies and inconsistencies with the foundational beliefs of the human science paradigm. Perhaps reflecting the evolutionary nature of knowledge and theory development, several of the authors incorporated diverging beliefs in their work, leaving the reader unclear as to their philosophical underpinnings. The inconsistencies arise in three main areas: the human being's wholeness, the intentionality and free will of the person, and the nature of reality. Each of these will be explored in relation to the works of Paterson and Zderad (1988), Newman (1986a, 1990), and Watson (1985).

Wholeness of Human Beings

Paterson and Zderad (1988) in their humanistic nursing practice propose that "the nurse sees the patient as a whole, a gestalt" (p. 25). Human beings are described as "in-the-world" and nurses are guided to recognize the complexity and uniqueness of each person's relating and experiencing. Paterson and Zderad note, however, that this view of the person as a whole conflicts with the evaluative stance of the conventional nursing process. They address this conflict by positing that "both subject–subject and subject–object relationships are essential for clinical nursing" (Paterson & Zderad, 1988, p. 27) in which focusing on discrete parts rather than the whole person is sometimes necessary. This attempt to incorporate human science beliefs with biomedical traditions leads to conceptual inconsistencies. It is suggested here that nurses cannot switch their very beliefs according to the nature of the practice situation. What seems to be overlooked by Paterson and Zderad is that nurses can live according to human science beliefs and still perform tasks related to the execution of medical orders. There

need not be the subject–subject, subject–object dilemma as espoused by these authors. Although Paterson and Zderad reflect on the inadequacy of the labeling process for capturing lived experiences, they accept the linear, causal nursing process and the diagnosing of human responses as necessary evils, required for economic reasons. Paterson and Zderad maintain that the natural science tradition is inappropriate for nursing, yet they do not reconcile the inconsistencies between reductionistic and unitary approaches with human beings.

Newman explicitly expresses a belief in the unitary nature of human beings, yet she also discusses the human being as a "system" made up of physiological structures and functions, such as the immune system and the genetic code, reflecting a natural science orientation. The unity of the human "system," for Newman, is predicated on the idea that "mind and matter are made of the same basic stuff" (1986a, p. 37). It is apparently quite appropriate within Newman's model to discuss the physiological, psychological, and emotional processes of the "human system" in conventional terms, so long as one remembers that everything, from the atom to the human being and beyond, is a manifestation of the implicate order, or "absolute consciousness" (pp. 33–37). Similarly, Watson (1985) maintains that the person is conceptualized as an irreducible whole, yet she repeatedly refers to body, mind, spirit and soul, and physical, emotional, and spiritual spheres. Her definitions of health and illness are dependent on the harmony or disharmony within these aspects. Watson also refers to several selves; the "real self," the "inner self," and the "ideal self" are presented as distinct entities. She refers to the "I" and the "Me" of the person and the potential disharmony of these aspects. It is not consistent to maintain that a person is a unitary whole and then to define the person according to these separate parts or spheres. Dilthey (1977a) maintained that "we continually experience a sense of connectedness and totality in ourselves" (p. 53). The authors' struggles to incorporate the concept of the unitary human being into nursing theory and practice parallel a long and complex tradition of discourse in the human sciences.

Intentional Free-Willed Beings

Human science conceptualizes human beings as intentional and inherently free willed; therefore the nurse would seek no more fundamental reference than the lived experience of the person. Paterson and Zderad (1988) address the *nurse's* intention and free will to commit authentically to another. The authors also regard the human being as free willed, yet they suggest, "The nurse is alert to opportunities for the patient to exercise his [*sic*] freedom of choice within the limits of safe and sound practice" (p. 17). The nurse is guided to monitor the patient's choices and to determine if they are responsible ones. To carry out this monitoring, the nurse would have to rely on some schema of normative standards or beliefs in order to judge what is "responsible," which is an inconsistent practice if the nurse wishes to respect the human science belief that the individual is an intentional being possessing free will.

Newman's (1986a) conceptualization of freedom describes an arc-like progression as consciousness expands. Human beings first *lose* freedom as they "come into being," are "bound in time" and "find . . . identity in space," until they reach a stage in which choice is engendered through movement (p. 46). "Restriction of movement forces one into a realm beyond space and time" (p. 62). Thereafter one throws off self-concerns, recognizes one's own "boundaryless-ness" and "timelessness" and *gains* the freedom of returning to "absolute consciousness" (p. 46). It is essentially the movement toward spirituality that imbues the human being with freedom, which is relative to the extent that consciousness is expanded.

The notion that human freedom underpins human science is quite different, in that freedom is never "lost," and there is no requisite for expanding consciousness to "gain" it. Human beings are believed to be free to choose meaning and direction because they make such choices continuously in living everyday life (Dilthey, 1988). "It is true," writes Dilthey (1988), "that the will depends on intellect, but the will can choose or not choose what the intellect understands. . . . In fact the will is free precisely inasmuch as in it the search for a reason ends" (p. 270). Newman's (1986b) proposal for "the diagnosis of pattern" would appear to be hinged on her notion of freedom as relative to expanded consciousness. She states, "The role of the nurse within a paradigm of pattern is to help clients recognize their own patterns," a process in which a "burst of insight" occurs that "opens up" a "pathway of action" (pp. 55–56). From a human science perspective, in contrast, the pathway of action is always open.

Watson (1985) says that human beings are free to self-determine and free to choose. Nurses are guided to hold nonpaternalistic values, which respect human autonomy and freedom. Yet this belief is violated in two ways. First, there are references to the nurse's helping, integrating, and "correcting" the patient's condition to increase harmony and to try to find meaning in the situation. Second, Watson maintains that "*ideally* [italics added], a person should have the opportunity for self-determination of the meaning of a health-illness experience *before professionals make decisions* [italics added] about treatments and interventions" (1985, p. 66). Human science philosophy abdicates the position of science as the arbiter of truth; the human scientist is a seeker of truth, a seeker rather than a dispenser of wisdom. Dilthey maintained that "understanding constitutes the goal of the human studies in the way that explanation defines the natural sciences" (cited in Makkreel, 1977, p. 7). Knowledge is not used or applied to the person, but rather knowledge enhances understanding for participating with the person in the process of becoming. Dilthey (1976) proposed, "In everything there is the same limitation of possibilities and yet freedom to choose between them, and the beautiful feeling of being able to move forward and to realize new potentialities in one's own existence" (p. 245).

The Nature of Reality

In a human science ontology, human beings and their worlds as experienced cannot be separated. Human science does not distinguish between subjective and objective realities because the focus of scientific activities is the humanly lived experience of the world, in which subjectivity is primal. Paterson and Zderad suggest that "nurses are drawn toward two realities—the reality of the objective scientific world and the reality of the subjective–objective world" p. 36). The authors' endorsement of the traditional nursing process automatically places the person in the position of object and the nurse in the role of arbiter of truth. Again, this reflects the conflicting views proposed with respect to the nurse–patient relationship.

Newman's (1986a) view of the nature of reality draws on Bohm's (1980) theory of the implicate order. All humanly experienced phenomena comprising the explicate order are posited as manifestations of an unseen, unknowable implicate order which comprises the unity of all that is. According to this view, patterns of human experience are reflective of this underlying primary reality. Newman writes, "We need to remind ourselves that our manifest reality is a small portion of the total enfoldment of the pattern in time–space" (1986a, p. 15). Her model theoretically eliminates the subject–object duality, according to its ontology. However, Newman's (1986a, 1986b) view is that neither objectivity nor subjectivity has any validity, as the perspective adapted from Bohm says there are no boundaries to (physical) reality. From a human science perspective, this is still essentially an objectivist reality, founded on the basis of the speculations of physical scientists that the nature of reality is a complex, multidimensional whole. The human being in such a model is defined by what physical science says about matter and energy. In contrast, human science directly asserts that human reality as lived is itself a complex multidimensional whole (Dilthey, 1977a).

The preeminence of the human experience is ostensibly highly valued in Watson's theory. She speaks of developing knowledge about the lived world of human experience and contends that the phenomenological research method is most congruent with her theoretical perspective. However, Watson distinguishes the person's experience of the world (phenomenal field) from the world as it actually is. For example, she proposes that nurses "help integrate the person's subjective experience and emotions with the objective external view of the situation" (Watson, 1985, p. 65). Watson also suggests that there can be incongruencies between the person and nature (world). For example, she states, "If a person does not feel congruent with mind, body, and soul . . . or rejects the self . . . or is obsessed with an ideal self, the person will be dissatisfied and maladjusted" (p. 57). These distinctions reveal a belief in an objective reality separate from the person's experience of it. This essentially dichotomous view is inconsistent with human science philosophy, in which being human means participating in the creation of reality. Human consciousness already is the unity of the person's subjective–objective relationship with the world; it is not something to be aspired to (Dilthey, 1977a). The use of the conventional subjective–objective constructs speaks to the exigencies of traditional science but is inconsistent with the understanding of humanly lived reality that underpins human science.

Extending Essential Beliefs

In several instances within the frameworks examined, departures from the human science tradition were noted in areas where some congruence might be expected based on the overall presentation and central concepts. Paterson and Zderad (1988) move from focusing on the human being's lived experience to focusing on nurses' lived experiences and their descriptions of human beings. Both Newman (1986a) and Watson (1985) go well beyond the lived experience as the primal foundation of human knowledge by assigning higher order importance to metaphysical concepts.

It is clear that the basic empirical datum in Paterson and Zderad's humanistic nursing is the nurse's experience, "the between" of existentially experienced nursing situations. The authors address the importance of meanings, patterns, values, and themes, but it is not clear whose experiences are paramount, the nurse's or the patient's. Paterson and Zderad contend that nursing must be described phenomenologically, that nurses' descriptions of nursing situations with patients will build the knowledge and "make explicit a science of nursing" (1988, p. 3). This is a description of the practice of nursing, however, not of a nursing science based on the health experience of human beings. Giorgi (1985) proposed that a discipline is not ready-made in the world and simply viewed and studied. Rather, it is created by a unique knowledge base that is housed within its theories. Thus, to study the nursing act phenomenologically as Paterson and Zderad suggest is to study the particular nurse's view of nursing. It is suggested in this article that nursing science focuses on the concepts of human–environment and health, not the nurse's views of the between. To be consistent with the human science approach nurses must rely on the person's description as it is given, and not on what that experience is assumed to be. Paterson and Zderad's focus on the practitioner's experience reflects a serious departure from beliefs related to the practice of a human science, which investigates lived experiences and life expressions of human beings.

Human consciousness is an important concept in human science; it is the origin of all knowledge about lived experience (Dilthey, 1988). The ontology of Newman's theory is largely metaphysical, in that the key concept of "absolute consciousness" is beyond the realm of lived experience. Newman (1986a) ascribes consciousness to atoms, rocks, plants, animals, and unspecified "astral" and "spiritual" entities (pp. 33–37). In human science philosophy there is no way of knowing a more fundamental ground behind or beyond the lived experience of the person. One wonders why Newman (1986a), whose central thesis is "health as expanding consciousness," has completely ignored continental European philosophy and theory on consciousness throughout her work. Instead, Newman cites works of speculative physics as underpinning her theory, even when addressing human experience. Dilthey (1977a) maintained that "consciousness cannot go behind itself" (p. 75). It is the structure of consciousness that sheds light on the coherent unity of human life.

In human science, humanly lived experiences elaborated in thinking, feeling, and willing are the complex whole of reality. Watson emphasizes the significance of human experience as it is lived. However, her emphasis on the metaphysical, spiritual realm clouds the issue of the primacy of lived experience. Watson (1985) states that "the human soul is more than physical, mental, emotional existence. . . . The soul exists for something larger than physical life" (p. 45). She maintains, "The soul, inner self, spiritual self is tied to a higher degree of consciousness . . . that transcends time and space" (p. 46). This soul, which "may be underdeveloped and in need of reawakening" (p. 45), reflects a reality beyond that which is directly experienced by human beings and is in conflict with the purported human science origins of Watson's theory.

Watson explicitly presents her framework as emerging from the human science paradigm. Paterson and Zderad refer to their work as humanistic, a related term but not synonymous with human science. Although the concepts Newman uses are abundantly addressed in human science, the ontology underpinning her theory is derived instead from speculative physics. The selective extraction of inconsistencies with the human science paradigm in these authors' works is not intended to suggest a failing on their part but is intended to foster greater conceptual clarity and is offered in the spirit of scholarly questioning and debate. The purpose of this analysis was to determine to what extent the values and beliefs of the human science paradigm were currently evident in nursing's extant knowledge base. The authors conclude that the human science tradition is present to varying degrees in nursing science.

Of the four theories explored here, Parse's (1981, 1987, 1990a) theory of human becoming remained consistent with the fundamental ontology and epistemology of the human science tradition. The theory can be seen to have expanded and clarified major ideas of the human science tradition. Parse's (1981) work was the first publication in nursing to specify nursing as a human science in Dilthey's traditional sense. Parse's theory is analyzed here with regard to both its adherence to and expansion of the human science tradition.

Parse's Theory of Human Becoming

Parse's first chapter begins, "To posit the idea of nursing rooted in the human sciences is to make explicit an alternative to the traditional practice of nursing as a medical model grounded in the natural sciences" (1981, p. 3). Parse describes nursing as a human science focusing on the unitary human being's experience of living and creating health, and she cites Dilthey in her explication of the concepts of her theory. She states that the methodologies of human sciences focus on "uncovering the meaning of phenomena as humanly experienced" and "on understanding the connectedness of life itself," (1981, p. 11). Dilthey (1977b) suggested that explicating human interrelatedness connects that which is universally human with that which is individual.

Parse (1981) synthesized concepts from Rogers' (1970) science of unitary human beings and tenets of contemporary existential phenomenology in such a way that the fundamental notion of human science proposed by Dilthey was brought to fruition for nursing science in the theory of human becoming. The tenets of human subjectivity and intentionality, and the concepts of human coexistence, coconstitution, and situated freedom, drawn from existential phenomenology, reflect the development of ideas germinated by Dilthey and others in the philosophy of human science. The synthesis of concepts from Rogers' work with concepts from existential phenomenology to form a unique, coherent theory of nursing underscores the compelling fit between human science philosophy and nursing as a unique and autonomous discipline. Parse (1987) avoided conceptual inconsistencies by inventing nursing practice and research methodologies that flow directly from the ontological and epistemological foundations of her theory. In this way there is no need to reconcile human science beliefs with biomedical traditions. Parse's theory and her practice and research methodologies express and structure the beliefs that underpin human science in a new way specifically for nursing science.

Parse's (1981, 1987, 1990a) theory of human becoming has three central themes: meaning, rhythmicity, and cotranscendence. Her explication of these themes moves her theory beyond human science as described by Dilthey (1961). Parse describes the human being as an open unity who freely chooses meaning in situations, bears responsibility for choices, and co-constitutes with the environment rhythmical patterns of relating in the process of co-transcending with emerging possibilities. Health is described as a "process of becoming, a cocreated process of living value priorities" (1981, p. 31). Health is the day-to-day living of rhythmical patterns reflecting the person's unfolding and co-transcending with the possibles (the moving onward in life in a chosen way) (Parse, 1981).

The goal of practice in Parse's theory is the quality of life from the person's perspective (1987). Nurses in true presence with people live the practice method, which revolves around the all-at-once of illuminating meaning through "explicating," synchronizing rhythms through "dwelling with," and mobilizing transcendence through "moving beyond" (1987, p. 167). Parse's research method is rooted in phenomenology and is structured to be congruent with the assumptions and principles of the human becoming theory. It focuses on uncovering the structures of universal lived experiences in the human–universe–health interrelationship. The goal of the method is to enhance understanding of lived experiences of health.

Critique of the Theory of Human Becoming

Parse presents her theory as emerging from the human science paradigm, and she remains congruent with those philosophical underpinnings throughout her work. The human being is viewed as unitary, mutually interrelating with environment, and there is no reference to human beings other than as living unities. The person's lived experience is clearly regarded as the preeminent ground of human health. The researcher

explores universal lived experiences of health, with the goal of enhancing understanding. This is consistent with Dilthey's concern "to understand life as it is lived by man" (Ermath, 1978, p. 17). Both the research and practice methods focus on the lived experience of human beings. There is no subject–object dichotomy; reality is viewed as cocreated with the universe and others while experienced uniquely by the person. Nursing is seen as a scientific discipline in which the concepts of unitary human beings, mutual unfolding, human coexistence, intentionality, free will, and intersubjective sharing of meaning may at last be fully elaborated and incorporated in praxis. Dilthey consistently maintained that all theory was theory for praxis (Ermath, 1978).

Parse suggests that persons "unfold with contemporaries the ideas of predecessors . . . in a continuity that connects past with future" (1981, p. 26). The "way the person lives in interrelationship with others reflects chosen meanings and reveals cherished values" (1981, p. 48). Individuals freely choose the meaning of situations and freely live personal values by choosing ways of being/becoming from among possibilities. Again, this is consistent with Dilthey's (1961) view of human interconnectedness, yet it goes beyond his view.

Guided by Parse's theory, the nurse in true presence with the person focuses on the individual's own meaning without judging, labeling, or trying to change the person. The nurse goes with the person as he or she explores options, imagines consequences of choices, and plans to live hopes and dreams. In the true presence of the nurse, the individual clarifies the meaning of the situation and new meanings are uncovered; new insights generate new possibles, the understanding of opportunities and limitations in light of what is truly valued. The nurse coparticipates with the person in the process of moving beyond the now moment, guided by the theory to understand that the person chooses his or her own way (Parse, 1987). Parse maintains that individuals know their own way, reflectively and prereflectively. The nurse in true presence bears witness to the person's unfolding and becoming (Parse, 1990b). In creating the theory of human becoming, Parse has uncovered the intrinsic relevance of the human science perspective, which is centrally concerned with what it means to be human for the discipline of nursing.

In Parse's (1987) research methodology, the researcher "lives" dialogical engagements with participants. This is described as "an intersubjective being with, in which the researcher and participant live the I–Thou process as they move through an unstructured discussion about the lived experience" (1987, p. 176). The researcher views the participant as the expert on the lived experience being explored and remains focused on the phenomenon as it is revealed by the person. The researcher participates in generating enhanced understanding of the phenomenon by creatively abstracting the structure of the lived experience in the language of science.

In summary, Parse's theory, intentionally structured as a human science theory of nursing, accurately reflects the ontology and epistemology of human science philosophy. Parse's theory lays a foundation for a nursing science that is grounded in the meaning of lived experiences in the human–universe process. The theory focuses on the lived experience of unitary human beings in continuous interrelationship with their worlds. Reality as perceived by the person is not compared to an "objective" reality but is respected, as is the free will of the person, in choosing ways of becoming. Parse's theory is thus congruent with yet goes beyond the ontology and epistemology of human science as posited in this article and is an emergent, a newly created theory for praxis that uncompromisingly incorporates the beliefs of human science into nursing research and practice.

Conclusion

Nursing science is currently undergoing change as new views emerge that challenge the traditional methods of natural science-based, biomedical nursing. The human science paradigm is one such view. This perspective is surfacing in nursing at a time when nurse scholars are questioning the precepts of the natural science paradigm and, in doing so, are expressing many of the concerns that led Dilthey to propose a different approach to human science over a hundred years ago. It has been suggested in this article that the human science tradition is not merely any study of human beings, but a particular way of studying human life that values the lived experience of unitary persons and seeks to understand life in all its interwoven patterns of meanings and values.

Nurse scientists are defining boundaries and seeking knowledge that is unique to nursing. This knowledge is currently organized in conceptual and theoretical frameworks, some of which reflect the values and beliefs of the human science paradigm. Of the four frameworks explored here, one, Parse's theory of human becoming, was found not only to be congruent with but to go beyond the human science perspective. The other three frameworks, Paterson and Zderad's humanistic nursing, Newman's model of expanding consciousness, and Watson's human science and human care, demonstrated both consistencies and inconsistencies with the philosophy of human science. Continued explication of the assumptions, values, and beliefs that underpin different theoretical approaches is needed so that nurses can understand with depth and clarity the foundations of the unique knowledge base of nursing. Only through contemplative consideration of the philosophical basis of the extant body of theory and through open critique and discourse can nurses choose which paths to follow in the quest for knowledge.

References

Bohm, D. (1980). *Wholeness and the implicate order.* London: Routledge.

Connors, D. (1988). A continuum of researcher–participant relationships: An analysis and critique. *Advances in Nursing Science, 10*(4), 32–42.

Dilthey, W. (1961). *Pattern and meaning in history: Thoughts on history and society* (H. P. Rickman, Ed. and Trans.). New York: Harper & Row.

Dilthey, W. (1976). *Selected writings* (H.P. Rickman, Trans.). Cambridge: Cambridge University Press.

Dilthey, W. (1977a). Ideas concerning a descriptive and analytic psychology. (Original work published 1894). In R. M. Zaner & K. L. Heiges (Trans.), *Descriptive psychology and historical understanding* (pp. 23–120). The Hague, Netherlands: Nijhoff.

Dilthey, W. (1977b). The understanding of other persons and their expressions of life. (Original work published 1927). In R. M. Zaner & K. L. Heiges (Trans.), *Descriptive psychology and historical understanding* (pp. 123–144). The Hague, Netherlands: Nijhoff.

Dilthey, W. (1988). *Introduction to the human sciences* (R. J. Betanzos, Trans.). Detroit: Wayne State University Press. (Original work published 1883)

Ermath, M. (1978). *Wilhelm Dilthey: The critique of historical reason.* Chicago: University of Chicago Press.

Gadamer, H. G. (1976). *Philosophical hermeneutics* (D. E. Linge, Trans.). Berkeley: University of California Press.

Geertz, C. (1973). *The interpretation of cultures.* New York: Basic Books.

Giorgi, A. (1970). *Psychology as a human science.* New York: Harper & Row.

Giorgi, A. (1971). Phenomenology and experimental psychology: II. In A. Giorgi, W. Fischer, & R. von Eckartsberg (Eds.). *Duquesne studies in phenomenological psychology* (vol. 1, pp. 3–29). Pittsburgh, PA: Duquesne University Press.

Giorgi, A. (1985). Sketch of a psychological phenomenological method. In Fischer, & R. von Eckartsberg (Eds.). *Phenomenology and psychological research* (pp. 8–22). Pittsburgh, PA: Duquesne University Press.

Gortner, S. R., & Schultz, P. R. (1988). Approaches to nursing science methods. *Image: Journal of Nursing Scholarship, 20,* 22–24.

Heidegger, M. (1962). *Being and time* (J. Macquarrie & E. Robinson, Trans.). New York: Harper & Row.

Makkreel, R. A. (1977). Introduction. In R. M. Zaner & K. L. Heiges (Trans.), *Descriptive psychology and historical understanding* (pp. 1–20). The Hague, Netherlands: Nijhoff.

Meleis, A. (1990, September). *Directions for nursing theory development.* Paper presented at the National Nursing Theory Conference, Los Angeles, CA.

Munhall, P. (1989). Philosophical ponderings on qualitative research methods in nursing. *Nursing Science Quarterly, 2,* 20–28.

Newman, M. (1986a). *Health as expanding consciousness.* St. Louis: Mosby.

Newman, M. (1986b). Nursing's emerging paradigm: The diagnosis of pattern. In A. M. McLane (Ed.), *Classification of nursing diagnoses: Proceedings of the seventh conference.* St. Louis: Mosby.

Newman, M. (1990). Newman's theory of health as praxis. *Nursing Science Quarterly, 3,* 37–41.

Parse, R. R. (1981). *Man–living–health: A theory of nursing.* New York: Wiley.

Parse, R. R. (1987). *Nursing science: Major paradigms, theories and critiques.* Philadelphia: Saunders.

Parse, R. R. (1990a, September). [Speaker on] *Panel of nursing theorists.* National Nursing Theory Conference, Los Angeles, CA.

Parse, R. R. (1990b). Health: A personal commitment. *Nursing Science Quarterly, 3,* 136–140.

Paterson, J. G., & Zderad, L. T. (1988). *Humanistic nursing.* New York: National League for Nursing.

Polkinghorne, D. (1983). *Methodology for the human sciences: Systems of inquiry.* Albany: State University of New York Press.

Ricoeur, P. (1974). The *conflict of interpretations: Essays in hermeneutics* (W. Domingo et al., Trans.). Evanston, IL: Northwestern University Press.

Rogers, M. E. (1970). *An introduction to the theoretical basis of nursing.* Philadelphia: Davis.

Schutz, A. (1967). *The phenomenology of the social world* (G. Walsh & F. Lehnert, Trans.). Evanston, IL: Northwestern University Press.

Watson, J. (1985). *Nursing: Human science and human care.* Norwalk, CT: Appleton-Century-Crofts.

Webster's ninth new collegiate dictionary. (1985). Springfield, MA: Merriam-Webster.

Winch, P. (1958). *The idea of a social science and its relation to philosophy.* London: Routledge & Kegan Paul.

Part Six

INTERRELATIONSHIPS AMONG NURSING THEORY, RESEARCH, AND PRACTICE

The clarion call for evidence-based practice is but one among many contemporary influences that demand that the advanced practice nurse have a clear and expandable understanding of the interrelationships among nursing theory, research, and practice. In Part Six, these interconnections are explored in six chapters by a large collection of nurse leaders, offering many opportunities for reflection.

As established in Chapter 1 and carried on as a thread throughout this book, a useful distinction can be made between practice and care, although this distinction is rarely observed in the literature. The logic, coherence, and utility of construing *practice as values based and practitioner driven* and *care as evidence based and consumer driven* can certainly be put to the test in this part of the book. The rubric of *values-based practice and evidence-based care* is offered here as a kind of organizing principle. Although the language of the chapters does not match the language of values-based practice and evidence-based care, it may be useful for the reader to evaluate this organizing principle as a means to reach a greater understanding of the issues at stake in identifying guides to practice.

In Chapter 26, five well-known and influential nurse scholars offer a view of nursing theories and evidence that seeks to expand the received view of scientific evidence to admit of philosophical, autobiographical, and aesthetic "evidence." Clearly, the case has been made many times over that the knowledge needed for nursing practice is far greater than scientific knowledge alone. For this author, the question arises as to whether it is necessary or appropriate to expand the notion of evidence from its traditional science base or whether it may be preferable to speak of philosophical, autobiographical, and aesthetic ways of knowing in altogether different ways arising from their different traditions. Does it confuse the issue to introduce notions of multiple kinds of evidence alongside the traditional view of scientific evidence? To those who are familiar with

the processes through which the most objectively rigorous integrative reviews are conducted in order to evaluate evidence and construct standards of care, it is plain that discourses such as this are unlikely to alter the standards by which quantitative research studies are evaluated and counted as solid evidence. Why use the language of evidence for values, beliefs, and lived experiences when these phenomena have their own discursive traditions?

In Chapter 27, the Nursing Philosophy Working Group examines the very notion of evidence in evidence-based practice. Their discussion includes an exploration of the "values inherent in the call for evidence-based practice." They conclude that what is required is a clear understanding of the contributions of different worldviews toward delineating what evidence is or should be.

In Chapter 28, Mitchell offers a critique and alternative view of evidence-based practice. Mitchell asserts that "professional nursing practice requires the risk to embrace the inherent ambiguity of the moment and to be with others with explicit commitment, responsiveness, openness, compassion, and the intent to serve." She goes on to present four principles generated by a long-time patient, which include "I am the only legitimate decision-maker," and "I must have complete information." These assertions resonate harmoniously with the organizing rubric of *values-based practice and evidence-based care* as delineated in this book.

In Chapter 29, Birx explores the process and function of critical thinking in implementing nursing theory-based practice. She devotes considerable attention to the importance of being able to appreciate multiple perspectives and the importance of recognizing the consequences of adopting any one particular perspective.

In Chapter 30, Dunphy and Winland-Brown describe a model developed especially for advanced practice nursing as it exists in North America today. This model necessarily incorporates elements of medical and interdisciplinary healthcare knowledge while attempting to emphasize at the same time the uniqueness that the nursing discipline brings into healthcare.

Finally, in Chapter 31, the late Janet Kenney, sole editor of the first three editions of this book, discusses nursing theory-based advanced practice nursing. Kenney's discussion (left intact for this edition) is broad ranging and thorough, and it offers the reader the opportunity to synthesize all that has come before to construct a personal perspective on the alternative theoretical and philosophical perspectives available in the literature.

Chapter 26

On Nursing Theories and Evidence

Jacqueline Fawcett, PhD, FAAN

Jean Watson, PhD, FAAN

Betty Neuman, PhD, FAAN

Patricia Hinton Walker, PhD, FAAN

Joyce J. Fitzpatrick, PhD, FAAN

Purpose: To expand the understanding of what constitutes evidence for theory-guided, evidence-based nursing practice from a narrow focus on empirics to a more comprehensive focus on diverse patterns of knowing.

Organizing construct: Carper's four fundamental patterns of knowing in nursing— empirical, ethical, personal, and aesthetic—are required for nursing practice. A different mode of inquiry is required to develop knowledge about and evidence for each pattern.

Conclusions: Theory, inquiry, and evidence are inextricably linked. Each pattern of knowing can be considered a type of theory, and the modes of inquiry appropriate to the generation and testing of each type of theory, provide diverse sources of data for evidence-based nursing practice. Different kinds of nursing theories provide different lenses for critiquing and interpreting the different kinds of evidence essential for theory-guided, evidence-based holistic nursing practice. Keywords: nursing theory, patterns of knowing, evidence-based practice.

Evidence-based practice is in the forefront of many contemporary discussions of nursing research and nursing practice. Indeed, the term "seems to be the up-and-coming buzzword for the decade" (Ingersoll, 2000, p. 151). The current call for evidence-based nursing practice has set the debate in a conventional, atheoretical, medically dominated, empirical model of evidence, which threatens the foundation of nursing's disciplinary perspective on theory-guided practice (Walker & Redmond, 1999). More specifically, as Ingersoll (2000) pointed out,

almost all discussions of evidence-based practice are focused on the primacy of the randomized clinical trail as the only legitimate source of evidence. Furthermore, most discussions of evidence-based practice treat evidence as a theoretical entity, which only widens the theory-practice gap (Upton, 1999). Moreover, although multiple patterns of knowing in nursing have been acknowledged at least since the publication of Carper's work in 1978, nurses have ignored this disciplinary perspective and reverted to a medical perspective of evidence when discussing evidence-based nursing practice.

The purpose of this paper is to invite readers to join in a dialogue about what constitutes the evidence for theory-guided, evidence-based nursing

Source: Fawcett, J., Watson, J., Neuman, B., Walker, P.H., Fitzpatrick, J.J.; *Journal of Nursing Scholarship Second Quarter.* 2001; 33:2, 115–119 © 2001 Sigma Theta Tau International. Reprinted with permission by Blackwell Publishing, Ltd.

practice. We are initiating the dialogue by offering a comprehensive description of theoretical evidence that encompasses diverse patterns of knowing in nursing. We advance the argument that each pattern of knowing can be considered a type of theory and that the different forms of inquiry used to develop the diverse kinds of theories yield different kinds of evidence, all of which are needed for evidence-based nursing practice.

On Nursing Theories

Diverse patterns of knowing were identified by Carper (1978), who expanded the historical view of nursing as an art and a science in her classic paper, "Fundamental Patterns of Knowing in Nursing." She identified four ways or patterns of knowing in nursing: empirics, ethics, personal, and aesthetics. Carper's work is significant in that it "not only highlighted the centrality of empirically derived theoretical knowledge, but [also] recognized with equal importance and weight, knowledge gained through clinical practice" (Stein, Corte, Colling, & Whall, 1998, p. 43). Chinn and Kramer (1999) expanded Carper's work by identifying processes associated with each pattern of knowing. Their work has enhanced understanding of each pattern of knowing and has brought Carper's ideas to the attention of a wide audience of nurses.

The pattern of empirical knowing (Table 26–1) encompasses publicly verifiable, factual descriptions, explanations, and predictions based on subjective or objective group data. In other words, empirical knowing is about "averages." This pattern of knowing, which constitutes the science of nursing, is well established in nursing epistemology and methods. Empirical knowing is generated and tested by means of empirical research. The next section of this paper extends the common focus on empirics as the primary focus of evidence, and offers a new lens for considering theory-guided evidence and diverse ways of knowing that can and should be integrated into nurses' evidence-based practice initiatives.

Diverse Patterns of Knowing

In contrast to empirics, the other patterns of knowing are less established, but they are of increasing interest for the discipline of nursing in particular and for science in general. Ethical knowing, personal knowing, and aesthetic knowing are required for moral, humane, and personalized nursing practice (Stein et al., 1998). The pattern of ethical knowing (Table 26-1) encompasses descriptions of moral obligations, moral and nonmoral values, and desired ends. Ethical knowing, which constitutes the ethics of nursing, is generated by means of ethical inquiries that are focused on identification and analysis of the beliefs and values held by individuals and groups and the clarification of those beliefs and values. Ethical knowing is tested by means of ethical inquiries that focus on dialogue about beliefs and values and establishing justification for those beliefs and values.

The pattern of personal knowing refers to the quality and authenticity of the interpersonal process between each nurse and each patient (Table 26-1). This pattern is concerned with the knowing, encountering, and actualizing of the authentic self; it is focused on how nurses come to know how to be authentic in relationships with patients and how nurses come to know how to express their concern and caring for other people. Personal knowing is not "knowing one's self" but rather knowing how to be authentic with others, knowing one's own "personal style" of "being with" another person. Personal knowing is what is meant by "therapeutic nurse-patient relationships." Personal knowing is developed by means of opening and centering the self to thinking about how one is or can be authentic, by listening to responses from others, and by reflecting on those thoughts and responses.

Table 26–1   Patterns of Knowing: Types of Nursing Theories

	Description	Mode of inquiry	Examples of Evidence
Empirics	Publicly verifiable, factual descriptions, explanations, or predictions based on subjective or objective group data; the science of nursing	Empirical research	Scientific data
Ethics	Descriptions of moral obligations, moral and nonmoral values, and desired ends; the ethics of nursing	Identification, analysis, and clarification of beliefs and values; dialogue about and justification of beliefs and values	Standards of practice, codes of ethics, philosophies of nursing
Personal	Expressions of the quality and authenticity of the interpersonal process between each nurse and each patient; the interpersonal relationships of nursing	Opening, centering, thinking, listening, and reflecting	Autobiographical stories
Aesthetics	Expressions of the nurse's perception of what is significant in an individual patient's behavior; the art and act of nursing	Envisioning possibilities, rehearsing nursing art and acts	Aesthetic criticism and works of art

The pattern of aesthetic knowing shows the nurse's perception of what is significant in the individual patient's behavior (Table 26-1). Thus, this pattern is focused on particulars rather than universals. Aesthetic knowing also addresses the "artful" performance of manual and technical skills. Aesthetic knowing is developed by envisioning possibilities and rehearsing the art and acts of nursing, with emphasis on developing appreciation of aesthetic meanings in practice and inspiration for developing the art of nursing.

Carper (1978) and Chinn and Kramer (1999) pointed out that each pattern of knowing is an essential component of the integrated knowledge base for professional practice, and that no one pattern of knowing should be used in isolation from the others. Carper (1978) maintained that "Nursing . . . depends on the scientific knowledge of human behavior in health and in illness, the aesthetic perception of significant experience, a personal understanding of the unique individuality of the self and the capacity to make choices within concrete situations involving particular moral judgments" (p. 22). Elaborating, Chinn and Kramer (1999) pointed out the danger of using any one pattern exclusively. They said

When knowledge within any one pattern is not critically examined and integrated with the whole of knowing, distortion instead of understanding is

produced. Failure to develop knowledge integrated within all of the patterns of knowing leads to uncritical acceptance, narrow interpretation, and partial utilization of knowledge. We call this "the patterns gone wild." When this occurs, the patterns are used in isolation from one another, and the potential for synthesis of the whole is lost. (p. 12)

The current emphasis on empirical knowing as the only basis for evidence-based nursing practice is an outstanding example of a "pattern gone wild."

Patterns of Knowing as Theories

The question arises as to whether the multiple, diverse patterns of knowing can be considered sets of theories. The answer to that question depends, in part, on one's view of a pattern of knowing and a theory. A pattern of knowing can be thought of as a way of seeing a phenomenon. The English word "theory" comes from the Greek word *theoria,* which means "to see," that is, to reveal phenomena previously hidden from our awareness and attention (Watson, 1999). For the purposes of this paper, a theory is defined as a way of seeing though "a set of relatively concrete and specific concepts and the propositions that describe or link those concepts" (Fawcett, 1999, p. 4). Theories constitute much of the knowledge of a discipline. Moreover, theory and phenomena are the lenses through which inquiry is conducted. The results of inquiry constitute the evidence that determines whether the theory is adequate or must be refined.

Collectively, the diverse patterns of knowing constitute the ontological and epistemological foundations of the discipline of nursing. Inasmuch as both patterns of knowing and theories represent knowledge and are generated and tested by means of congruent, yet diverse processes of inquiry (Table 26-1), we maintain that each pattern of knowing may be regarded as a type of theory. These four types of theories are subject to different types of inquiry. Henceforth,

then, we will refer to the patterns of knowing as empirical theories, ethical theories, personal theories, and aesthetic theories. Our decision to regard the patterns of knowing as types of theories is supported by Chinn and Kramer's (1999) reference to ethical theories and Chinn's (2001) articulation of a theory of the art of nursing. Other global perspectives indicate the direction of diverse patterns of knowing as types of theories. For example, Scandinavia nurses view nursing within a caring science model, and they acknowledge personal knowing, personal characteristics, and moral and aesthetic knowing of caring practices as theoretical ways of knowing the elicit diverse forms of evidence (Dahlberg, 1995, Fagerstrom & Bergdom Engberg, 1998; Kyle, 1995; Snyder, Brandt, & Tseng, 2000; von Post & Eriksson, 2000).

Furthermore, we, like some of our international colleagues, maintain that the content of ethical, personal, and aesthetic theories can be formalized as sets of concepts and propositions, just as the content of many empirical theories has been so formalized (Fawcett, 1999; von Post & Eriksson, 2000). Moreover, regarding all four patterns of knowing as types of theories reintroduces the notions of uncertainty and tentativeness that typically are associated with empirical theories (Fagerstrom & Bergdom Engberg, 1998; Morse, 1996; Polit & Hungler, 1995).

The four types of theories constitute much, if not all, of the knowledge needed for nursing practice. A potentially informative analysis, which follows from the conclusion that the patterns of knowing can be regarded as sets of theories, is the examination of extant theories to determine in which pattern of knowing each is located. That analysis is, however, beyond the scope of this paper and will not be pursued here. Rather, we are attempting to make connections between the four types of theories, representing the four patterns of knowing, and what constitutes evidence for nursing practice.

On Evidence

These four types of theories underlie all methodological decisions, and they are the basis for generating multiple forms of evidence. The question of what constitutes evidence depends, in part, on what one regards as the basis of the evidence. We maintain that theory is the reason for and the value of the evidence. In other words, evidence itself refers to evidence about theories. Similarly, theory determines what counts as evidence. Thus, theory and evidence become inextricably linked, just as theory and inquiry are inextricably linked.

Any form of evidence has to be interpreted and critiqued by each person who is considering whether the theory can be applied in a particular practice situation. This view indicates acknowledgment of diverse forms of knowing as inherent in any global or cultural interpretation of knowledge or theory (Zoucha & Reeves, 1999). The four types of theories are diverse ontological and epistemological lenses through which evidence is both interpreted and critiqued. The current emphasis on the technical-rational model of empirical evidence denies or ignores the existence of a theory lens. In contrast, our theory-guided model of evidence requires and acknowledges interpretation and critique of diverse forms of evidence. As shown in Table 26-1, we regard the scientific data produced by empirical research as the evidence for empirical theories. We count as scientific both qualitative and quantitative data and we support the call for palliative outcome analysis (Kyle, 1995; Morse, Penrod, & Hupcey, 2000; Snyder et al., 2000). The evidence for ethical theories is illustrated in formalized statements of nurses' values, such as standards of practice, codes of ethics, and philosophies of nursing. The evidence for personal theories is found in autobiographical stories about the genuine, authentic self. The evidence for aesthetic theories is manifested or expressed as aesthetic criticism of the art and act of nursing and through works of art, such as paintings, drawings, sculpture, poetry, fiction and nonfiction, dance, and others.

Our view of the reason for evidence differs from the prevailing discussion in the literature. In current literature, typically a procedure or intervention is presented in isolation from the theory that undergirds that procedure or intervention, and in isolation from the value of the evidence-hence the term "evidence-based practice." We maintain that the more appropriate term is "theory-guided, evidence-based practice" (Walker & Redmond, 1999). Given the diversity of kinds of theories needed for nursing practice (see Table 26-1), evidence must extend beyond the current emphasis on empirical research and randomized clinical trials, to the kinds of evidence also generated from ethical theories, personal theories, and aesthetic theories.

Our view of the diversity of types of theories and the type of evidence needed for each type of theory addresses, at least in part, current criticisms of the evidence-based practice movement. We agree with Mitchell (1999) that the "proponents of evidence-based practice have . . . grossly oversimplified and misrepresented the process of nursing" (p. 34). Mitchell was particularly concerned that "the notion of evidence-based practice is not only a barren possibility but also that evidence-based practice obstructs nursing process, human care, and professional accountability" (p. 30). We respond to Mitchell's concern by including evidence about personal theories, which include authenticity in nurse–patient interpersonal relationships. Moreover, Mitchell (1999) maintained that "Evidence-based practice does not support the shift to patient-centered care, and it is inconsistent with the values and interests of consumers" (p. 34). Here, we respond to Mitchell's concerns by including evidence about ethical theories, which include the values of nurses. Mitchell (1999) also was concerned that "evidence-based practice, if taken seriously, may restrain some nurses from defining the values and theories that guide the nurse-person process" (p. 31) and relationship. This point relates to our view that the art of nursing is expressed through the nurse–person process and the evidence derived from interpretations of tests of aesthetic theories and ethical theories.

Furthermore, our view of the diversity of types of theories and corresponding types of evidence needed for theory-guided, evidence-based nursing practice elaborates Ingersoll's (2000) definition of evidence-based nursing practice. Her definition is as follows: "Evidence-based nursing practice is the conscientious, explicit, and judicious use of theory-derived, research-based information in making decisions about care delivery to individuals or groups of patients and in consideration of individual needs and preferences" (p. 152). Our view makes explicit the multiple kinds of theories—ethical, personal, aesthetic, and empirical—whereas Ingersoll's reference to theory could easily be construed to mean only empirical theory or, perhaps because of the reference to individual needs and preferences, to include empirical and aesthetic theories.

We maintain the appropriateness of recognizing and appreciating empirical, ethical, personal, and aesthetic theories and the corresponding critique and interpretation of the evidence about each kind of theory. Such critique and interpretation of evidence is crucial for nursing practice because it is embedded in the values and phenomena located within a broad array of nursing theories. Moreover, by recognizing the four types of theories, more nurses and other health professionals may appreciate and use theories. They may agree with us that theories and values are the starting point for the critique and interpretation of any evidence needed to support clinical practices that may enhance the quality of life of the public we serve.

Conclusions

We invite readers to expand the dialogue about theory-guided, evidence-based practice. We urge nurses everywhere to consider the implications and consequences of the current virtually exclusive emphasis on empirical theories and empirical evidence-based nursing practice. We urge our nurse colleagues throughout the world to join us and those who have accurately pointed to the limitations of viewing nursing as a strictly empirical endeavor (Bolton, 2000; Dahlberg, 1995; Fagerstrom & Bergdom Engberg, 1998; Hall, 1997; Zoucha & Reeves, 1999) to consider what might be gained by recognition and development of ethical, personal, and aesthetic theories and by formalization of those kinds of theories. Accordingly, we encourage all nurses to actualize their claim of a holistic approach to practice by adopting a more comprehensive description of evidence-based nursing practice, a descriptive that allows for critique and interpretation of evidence obtained from inquiry guided by ethical, personal, aesthetic, and empirical theories, as well as by any other kinds theories that may emerge from new understandings of nursing as a human science and a professional practice discipline.

References

Bolton, S. C. (2000). Who cares? Offering emotional work as a "gift" in the nursing labor process. *Journal of Advanced Nursing, 32,* 580–586.

Carper, B. A. (1978). Fundamental patterns of knowing in nursing. *Advances in Nursing Science, 1*(1), 13–23.

Chinn, P. L. (2001). Toward a theory of nursing art. In N. L. Chaska (Ed.), *The nursing profession: Tomorrow and beyond* (pp. 287-297). Thousand Oaks, CA: Sage.

Chinn, P. L., & Kramer, M. K. (1999). *Theory and nursing: Integrated knowledge development* (5th ed.). St. Louis: Mosby.

Dahlberg, K. (1995). Qualitative methodology as Caring Science Methodology. *Scandinavian Journal of Caring Science, 9,* 187–191.

Fagerstrom, L., & Bergdom Engberg, L. (1998) Measuring the unmeasurable: A caring perspective on patient classification. *Journal of Nursing Management, 6,* 165–172.

Fawcett, J. (1999). *The relationship of theory and research* (3rd ed.), Philadelphia: F. A. Davis.

Hall, E. O. C. (1997). Four generations of nurse theorists in the U.S.: An overview of their questions and answers. *Vard I Nordeu: Nursing Science and Research In the Nordic Countries, 17*(2), 15–23.

Ingersoll, G. L. (2000). Evidence-based Nursing: What it is and what it isn't. *Nursing Outlook, 48,* 151–152.

Kyle, T. V. (1995). The concept of caring: A review of the literature. *Journal of Advanced Nursing, 21,* 506–514.

Mitchell, G. J. (1999). Evidence-based practice: Critique and alternative view. *Nursing Science Quarterly, 12,* 30–35.

Morse, J. M. (1996). Nursing scholarship: Sense and sensibility. *Nursing Inquiry, 3,* 74–82.

Morse, J. M., Penrod, J., & Hupcey, J. E. (2000). Qualitative outcome analysis: Evaluating nursing interventions for complex clinical phenomena. *Journal of Nursing Scholarship, 32,* 125–130.

Polit, D. F., & Hungler, B. P. (1995). *Nursing research: Principles and methods* (5th ed.). Philadelphia: Lippincott.

Snyder, M., Brandt, C. I., & Tseng, Y. (2000). Measuring intervention outcomes: Impact of nurse characteristics. *International Journal of Human Caring, 5*(3), 36–42.

Stein, K. F., Corte, C., Colling, K. B., & Whall, A. (1998). A theoretical analysis of Carper's ways of knowing using a model of social cognition. *Scholarly Inquiry for Nursing Practice, 12,* 43–60.

Upton, D. J. (1999). How can we achieve evidence-based practice if we have theory-practice gap in nursing today? *Journal of Advanced Nursing, 29,* 549–555.

Von Post, L., & Eriksson, K. (2000). The ideal and practice concepts of "Professional Nursing Care." *International Journal for Human Caring, 5*(3), 14–22.

Walker, P. H., & Redmond, R. (1999). Theory-guided, evidence-based reflective practice. *Nursing Science Quarterly, 12,* 298–303.

Watson, J. (1999). *Postmodern nursing and beyond.* New York: Churchill Livingstone.

Zoucha, R., & Reeves, J. (1999). A view of professional caring as personal for Mexican Americans. *International Journal of Human Caring, 3*(3), 14–20.

Chapter 27

The Notion of Evidence in Evidence-Based Practice by the Nursing Philosophy Working Group

Donna M. Romyn, PhD, RN
Marion N. Allen, PhD, RN
Geertje Boschma, PhD(c), MN, RN
Susan M. Duncan, PhD, RN
Nancy Edgecombe, PhD(c), MN, RN
Lousie A. Jensen, PhD, RN
Janet C. Ross-Kerr, PhD, RN
Patricia Marck, PhD, RN
Mahvash Salsali, PhD
Ann E. Tourangeau, PhD, RN
Fay Warnock, PhD, RN

Questions concerning the nature of evidence in evidence-based practice have kindled debate within nursing and other health care disciplines. Such questions include the ends for which evidence is sought, the form(s) of evidence, and the values underlying evidence-based practice. In this article, some of the issues, contradictions, and tensions implicit in these questions are highlighted. It is imperative for the nursing profession to continue to explore the philosophic perspectives that underscore evidence-based practice and their implications for decision making in nursing practice. Keywords: evidence-based practice; nature of evidence.

Recently, there has been a call for evidence-based practice within nursing and other health disciplines. Some nurses have argued that evidence-based practice is vital to improving clinical practice, providing quality and cost-effective care, optimizing patient outcomes, and enhancing the credibility of nursing. Evidence-based practice is said to integrate the best evidence from research with clinical expertise, patient preferences, and existing resources into clinical decision making about the health care of individuals (DiCenso, Cullum, & Ciliska, 1998; Sackett, Rosenberg, Muir Gray, Haynes, & Richardson, 1996). Although most nurses would agree that nursing practice should be based on the best avail-

able evidence, there is a lack of agreement in the literature as to what the term *evidence* means. Coupled with this is a lack of agreement regarding the ends for which evidence is to be sought and the means by which it is to be acquired. The intent in this article is to explore these issues in light of their implications for evidence-based practice in nursing and to highlight some of the ontologic, epistemologic, and ethical arguments associated with the notion of evidence in evidence-based practice. In so doing, first consider the question, to what end is evidence sought?

To What End Is Evidence Sought?

In 1966, McKay noted that nursing must address two major questions: (1) What is valued

Source: Romyn, D.M., Boschma, G., Edgecombe, N., Ross-Kerr, J.C., Tourangeau, A.E. *Journal of Professional Nursing*, Vol 19, No 4 (July/August), 2003: pp 184–188. Reprinted with permission by Elsevier.

as an end in nursing? (2) What means will most effectively achieve that end? Despite the fact that more than 30 years have passed since McKay posed these questions, they remain equally valid today. The first of these is a question for philosophy and relates to the goods to be sought in nursing. The second is one for science and relates to the way in which those goods are best attained within the profession. Answering the latter demands due and thoughtful consideration of the former. Extant within the nursing literature, however, is substantial disagreement regarding the proper end of nursing. This disagreement stems, at least in part, from differing ontologic perspectives regarding the nature of human beings and the nature of nursing. Flowing logically from these are differing epistemologic beliefs regarding what constitutes knowledge, and hence evidence, in evidence-based nursing practice. In what follows, three different positions and their implications for evidence-based nursing practice are examined briefly.

First consider the view that human beings have common needs with regard to health and that nursing, as a professional discipline, has a social mandate to assist individuals in meeting those needs. Consistent with this is the belief that nursing must seek knowledge of means to attain that end, including the identification of best clinical practices to attain normative health outcomes (Adler, 1989; Kikuchi, 1996). According to this view, evidence from sound empiric research is sought to show the efficacy of clinical practices and to generate nomothetic or law-like explanations that can be generalized in developing prescriptive theories to guide nursing practice (Polifroni & Packard, 1995).

Consider next a second view that posits that human beings are existential beings for whom no common needs or goals exist with respect to health. Consequently, human beings choose their own meanings of health and the means by which they, as individuals, will seek to attain health. Nursing, according to this perspective,

has a mandate to enhance health and quality of life, as defined by the individual. Hence, knowledge is sought neither to promote normative standards of health nor to direct the technical aspects of clinical care, but rather to understand the individual's particular health experience (Cody, 1993; Mitchell, 1999; Parse, 1998). On this basis, Mitchell (1997, 1999) posits that evidence-based practice, which commonly is conceived in the nursing literature as being grounded in the values, assumptions, and findings of empiric science, is inconsistent with and antithetical to the goals and proper accountabilities of nursing. In keeping with this, she further argues that evidence of the benefits of nursing come not from the attainment of normative measures of health but from "client's personal descriptions of how health and quality of life change with nursing care" (1999, p. 33).

Although some nurse scholars, such as Mitchell (1999), Cody (1993), and Parse (1998), maintain that generalizable understanding of individual's lived health experiences should not be sought, Sandelowski (1997) argues that seeking such understanding does not preclude the generation of interpretive or ideographic generalizations that can inform and enlighten nursing practice. She maintains that these kinds of explanations contribute to thoughtful practice by creating more perspectives from which to know and provide information crucial to determining the fit of prescriptive theories in the particular case. Along similar lines, Morse (1999) noted that although the criterion for determining generalizability of qualitative findings, which are oftentimes derived from small, purposefully selected samples, differ from those of quantitative studies characterized by large randomly selected samples, qualitative findings are indeed applicable to similar situations, questions, and problems. To believe otherwise, in her view, is to say qualitative research is "of little use [and] insignificant" (p. 5). Based on similar arguments, some proponents of evidence-based nursing practice have argued that qualitative generalizations be included as an essential component of the evidence constituting evidence-based nursing practice (Estabrooks, 1998).

Yet a third perspective on the question "To what end is evidence sought?" stems from a critical social theory perspective and holds that human beings are oppressed by dominant cultures within society that seek and use empiric science as an instrument of oppression. Proponents of this view argue that critique is essential to understanding (uncovering evidence regarding) how knowledge is constructed and used to perpetuate dominant values and power structures (Habermas, 1971; Kim, 1994; Lutz, Jones, & Kendall, 1997; Morrow, 1985). Such understanding is held to be emancipatory, and as a result, individuals are empowered to use it to change oppressive situations within which they find themselves. Within the context of nursing, critique is deemed essential to both disrupting the status quo and to understanding the value ascribed to different forms of knowledge and specific aspects of nursing practice. According to this perspective, critique and theory are merged in guiding conceptualizations of moral-practical action (Wells, 1995).

The Nature of Evidence

From the preceding, it is evident that there are widely differing perspectives that can and have been taken with respect to the question "To what end is evidence sought?" and to the related question, "What is the nature of evidence?" Following logically from the latter is yet another question: "Are there some kinds of knowledge, and not others, that properly can be termed evidence?" Recently, the Canadian Nurses Association (1998) issued a policy statement on evidence-based decision making and nursing practice. In it, evidence was defined as "information based on historical or scientific evaluation of a practice" and types of evidence were held to include

"experimental, non-experimental, expert opinion, and historical or experiential evidence" (p. 1). These definitions imply that virtually all forms of knowledge ought to be considered evidence for evidence-based decision making provided that they have been subjected to historic or scientific evaluation. In writing this article it became apparent that although our group, the Nursing Philosophy Working Group, agreed that the evidence for evidence-based nursing practice ought to be derived from scientific inquiry, members of the group did not hold to a single, unified view of science. This is not surprising given that defining science is an ongoing subject of debate within nursing. Although discussion of the various views of the nature of science and scientific knowledge is beyond the scope of this article, if it is said that the evidence for evidence-based practice is derived from scientific inquiry, how science is defined within the discipline will have important implications for the kinds of knowledge that will count as evidence and hence be valued in evidence based practice.

Values Inherent in the Call for Evidence-Based Practice

"Values are those assertions or statements that individuals make through their behavior, words, or actions that define what they think is important" (Curtin & Flaherty, 1982, p. 8). Inherent in the call for evidence-based practice are beliefs that deem certain kinds of knowledge as superior to others. For example, the National Forum on Health (1997) purports that evidence should be "relevant, accessible, timely, and of good quality for operational needs" (p. 12). Other values imbedded in this definition of evidence-based practice include those related to quantification, prediction and control, and measurement of outcomes. These values are reflected clearly in the pursuit of nomothetic or law-like generalizations as the basis for decision making in nursing practice. Tensions, however, arise when values such as these are seen as being in conflict with or incongruent with other values, such as those underlying the quest to understand individual lived experiences of health or to eliminate the oppression of others.

Consider, for example, a recent situation involving a 14-year-old Canadian boy undergoing treatment for osteosarcoma. The family was offered, and adamantly refused, the preferred medical option of amputation and continued chemotherapy but chose to undergo nontraditional treatment in a Mexican clinic instead. This case was brought before the Canadian legal system, and questions were raised by the courts about the validity of the treatment chosen and the boy's participation (or lack thereof) in giving informed consent. The court overruled the family's decision based on the belief that is was in the boy's best interest to accept the recommended treatment because scientific evidence suggested that this treatment offered the most favorable outcome (Nichols & Perreaux, 1999; Rogan, 1999).

This situation clearly depicts the tension in values that sometimes is associated with determining what is the best evidence in making health care decisions. Moreover, it aptly shows that the definition of best evidence is value laden and may be subject to personal and/or political agendas. The evidence cited in the court's decision reflects certain values with respect to treatment. It may be argued that values related to seeking a clearer understanding of the complex interplay of family dynamics and beliefs about health, as well as the relations of power that give primacy to certain kinds of knowledge, may have resulted in a more positive outcome for this boy and his family. Considering such knowledge as evidence in decision making serves to uphold core nursing values related to health and well being, individual autonomy, social justice, and professional accountability (Mitchell, 1999). Although

it is apparent that differing values will result in differing views related to nature of evidence and the way in which that evidence is used in particular situations, there is little agreement, both within and between disciplines, as to how (or if) these values ought to be distinguished from evidence or how they ought to be prioritized and subsequently acted on (Muir Gray, 1998). Without doubt, these are issues that require resolution if the notion of evidence-based practice is to be articulated more clearly and understood.

The Implications of Evidence-Based Practice for Nursing

Over 20 years ago, Gortner, Bloch, and Phillips (1976) lamented the lack of evidence derived from research in many areas of nursing practice. They posited that if nurses failed to engage in the philosophic work required to establish our most important ends and, thus, our most necessary questions and modes of inquiry, nursing knowledge would cease to progress. We believe that this charge still is valid. Careful examination of the underlying values and philosophic foundations of evidence-based practice is essential if nursing is to determine how such an agenda ought to unfold to best develop a knowledge base that supports nursing practice in meeting the health care needs of society.

Although many have argued that nursing must seize the opportunity to direct its own agenda with respect to evidence-based practice, a question arises: "Is nursing indeed ready to adopt such an agenda?" Some nurse scholars have suggested that it is premature to adopt such an agenda and that such a move is doomed to failure because nursing does not have what is required to implement that agenda—that is, a body of knowledge that constitutes best available evidence for practice (Mitchell, 1999). Although such a body of knowledge may not yet exist, this does not mean that nursing should not move in this direction. Currently, traditional practices retain a stronghold in nursing and health care. Unless the initiative is taken to develop and search for evidence to uphold or refute these practices, nursing will not be in a position to answer, with confidence, questions about why, or if, these traditional practices ought to be maintained or changed. Exemplifying this is the research conducted by Fahs and Kinney (1991) that called into question, and subsequently discounted, nurses' assumptions and traditional practices related to selecting the abdomen as the preferred site for subcutaneous heparin administration. As Dzurec (1998) noted, "disciplinary consensus, resting on a hierarchy of assumptions, needs to be interrupted from time to time, at least for long enough to support clinicians' consideration of emergent knowledge and theory" (p. 57).

The direction that evidence based nursing practice takes will depend on the kinds of evidence valued by the discipline and the profession of nursing. If it is believed that evidence is required to direct nursing practice, then nursing must continue to develop prescriptive theories that delineate clearly how specific health-related goals are best attained. Empiric evidence from research characterized by scientific rigor is essential to sound decision making in nursing. If this evidence is to be used to direct nursing practice in a contextualized manner, however, it must be interpreted in light of extant theory in its application in practice and should be considered as only one resource to support decision making in practice. Prescriptive theory emanating from well-crafted interventions studies can inform but not replace individual clinical expertise and knowledge of patient preferences. Nor can it be considered in isolation from the human and material resources required for its implementation, regardless of how compelling the scientific evidence may be that underpins it.

Consideration of factors such as these in clinical decision making serves to ensure that if nursing adopts an evidence-based practice agenda, the context of nursing practice and the preferences of individual patients will not be subjugated to generalizability and nursing care will not become routine, dehumanized, or decontextualized, as Mitchell (1999) suggested. We believe that nursing as a professional discipline will best be served by attaining a balanced pursuit and utilization of both prescriptive and interpretive (idiographic) nursing knowledge. Such a balance will serve to ensure that the rigorous conduct of scientific research related to health care outcomes occurs in conjunction with equally rigorous development of qualitative understanding of health experiences and takes into consideration the values and social context, including implicit and explicit relations of power, which undergird nursing practice and the pursuit of nursing knowledge. As Gortner (1993) cautions, no single world view should have primacy in our quest for knowledge to support decision making in nursing practice. What is required instead is a clearer understanding of the substantive contributions different world views lend in delineating the constituent components of evidence in evidence-based nursing practice.

References

Adler, M. J. (1989). Human nature, nurture and culture. *Aspen Institute Quarterly, 1,* 90–110.

Canadian Nurses Association. (1998). *Policy statement: Evidence-based decision-making and nursing practice.* Ottawa, ON: Author.

Cody, W. K. (1993). Norms and nursing science: A question of values. *Nursing Science Quarterly, 6,* 110–112.

Curtin, L., & Flaherty, M. J. (1982). *Nursing ethics: Theories and pragmatics.* Bowie, MD: Robert J. Brady Company.

DiCenso, A., Cullum, N., & Ciliska, D. (1998). Implementing evidence-based nursing: Some misconceptions. *Evidence-Based Nursing, 1,* 38–40.

Dzurec, L. C. (1998). Certainty, leaps of faith, and tradition: Rethinking clinical interventions. *Advances in Nursing Science, 21,* 52–61.

Estabrooks, C. A. (1998). Will evidence-based nursing practice make practice perfect? *Canadian Journal of Nursing Research, 30,* 15–36.

Fahs, P. S. S., & Kinney, M. R. (1991). The abdomen, thigh, and arm as sites for subcutaneous sodium heparin injections. *Nursing Research, 40,* 204–207.

Gortner, S. (1993). Nursing's syntax revisited: A critique of philosophies said to influence nursing theories. *International Journal of Nursing Studies, 30,* 477–488.

Gortner, S., Bloch, D., & Phillips, T. (1976). Contributions of nursing research to patient care. *Journal of Nursing Administration, 6,* 22–28.

Habermas, J. (1971). *Knowledge and human interests.* London, UK: Heinemann.

Kikuchi, J. F. (1996). Multicultural ethics in nursing education: A potential threat to responsible practice. *Journal of Professional Nursing, 12,* 159–165.

Kim, H. S. (1994). Action science as an approach to develop knowledge for nursing practice. *Nursing Science Quarterly, 7,* 134–140.

Lutz, K. F., Jones, K. D., & Kendall, J. (1997). Expanding the praxis debate: Contributions to clinical inquiry. *Advances in Nursing Science, 20,* 23–31.

McKay, R. (1966). *The process of theory development in nursing.* Unpublished Doctoral Dissertation, Columbia University, New York.

Mitchell, G. (1997). Questioning evidence-based practice for nursing. *Nursing Science Quarterly,10,* 154–155.

Mitchell, G. (1999). Evidence-based practice: Critique and alternative view. *Nursing Science Quarterly, 12,* 30–35.

Morrow, R. A. (1985). Critical theory and critical sociology. *Canadian Review of Sociology and Anthropology, 22,* 710–747.

Morse, J. M. (1999). Qualitative generalizability. *Qualitative Health Research, 9,* 5–6.

Muir Gray, J. A. (1998). Evidence based policy making. In A. Haines, & A. Donald (Eds.), *Getting research findings into practice* (pp. 70-77). London, UK: BMJ Publishing.

National Forum on Health. (1997). *Canada health action: Building on the legacy: The final report of the National Forum on Health.* Ottawa, ON: Health Canada Communications.

Nichols, M., & Perreaux, L. (1999). Faith or medicine? A judge orders chemotherapy after a boy says no. *Maclean's, 112,* 78.

Parse, R. R. (1998). *The human becoming school of thought: A perspective for nursing and other health care professionals.* Thousand Oaks, CA: Sage.

Polifroni, E. C., & Packard, S. A. (1995). Explanation in nursing science. *Canadian Journal of Nursing Research, 27,* 35–44.

Rogan, M. (1999, June). Acts of faith. *Saturday Night, 6,* 43–51.

Sackett, D. L., Rosenberg, W. M. C., Muir Gray, J. A., Haynes, R. B., & Richardson, W. S. (1996). Evidence based medicine: What it is and what it isn't. *British Medical Journal, 312,* 71–72.

Sandelowski, M. (1997). "To be of use:" Enhancing the utility of qualitative research. *Nursing Outlook, 45,* 125–132.

Wells, D. L. (1995). The importance of critical thinking to nursing: A description using research concerning discharge decision-making. *Canadian Journal of Nursing Research, 27,* 45–58.

Chapter 28

Evidence-Based Practice: Critique and Alternative View

Gail J. Mitchell, RN, PhD

Recent calls to promote evidence-based practice in nursing raise serious concerns. It has been suggested that evidence should be the primary source of knowledge for nurses. The general literature supporting evidence-based practice indicates that evidence will take nurses away from tradition, intuition, and anecdote to factual, scientific practice. The suggestion is that evidence can provide nurses with directives about how to think and act with patients, families, and groups. However, I contend that the notion of evidence-based practice is not only a barren possibility but also that evidence-based practice obstructs nursing process, human care, and professional accountability.

Prior to presenting arguments against evidence as the guide for nursing practice, let me state up front that evidence, defined here as conclusive statements based on findings from randomized controlled trials, has two areas of relevance. First, evidence may provide direction for development of procedures, techniques, and protocols that nurses and others are asked to perform. Healthcare professionals and nonprofessionals require such knowledge to guide their

performance of tasks, and large systems require protocols to coordinate hospital-based care. Naturally, people who require knowledge and skill in these areas value the most effective techniques for preventing complications or performing tasks such as delivering medication, for instance, but evidence about procedure or service delivery is different from knowledge that informs the nurse–person process. Nurses may use techniques and technologies, but the knowledge base of nursing is not technical.

Second, evidence may provide one more resource for clients and nurses to consider the latest developments in the diagnosis and treatment of illness and disease. This information is available to any person who has access to libraries or to the Internet. Television broadcasts regularly offer the latest developments about links between heart disease and smoking or drug trials and side effects, for example. Health care professionals no longer control access to health-related information, and the general public will have increasing opportunities to consider the latest developments and to weigh their relevance in light of personal life circumstances.

In a general way, evidence may well be useful to people for making decisions about how they wish to approach their care and what options are available. Pharmacological or medical informa-

Source: *Nursing Science Quarterly*, Vol. 12, No. 1, January 1999. 30–35. Reprinted by permission of and copyright © (1999) Sage Publications, Inc.

tion may be a launching pad for discussions with people as they figure things out—but evidence will not build a knowledge base for nursing practice. The usefulness of evidence has been wrongfully cast in the context of legitimizing nursing as a profession instead of describing evidence as one possible resource for supporting clients' processes of decision making.

Rather than legitimizing nursing, evidence-based practice entraps nurses in the role of medical extender or medical technician, but even in these roles, evidence will not provide a foundation for practice. The idea that nurses in practice can access the relevant literature, make the required judgments about credibility of findings, interpret the significance of the findings in light of the guiding theory, and implement changes in practice is inconsistent with current realities. For one thing, nurses are expected to follow procedures written by multidisciplinary groups that are responsible for updating clinical practice in particular medical specialties. In the more technical practice contexts, nurses are rewarded for complying message is that nurses are the experts who intervene (try to manage and control) to create change toward provider-defined goals.

The term evidence-based practice, rather than being restricted to its technical and medical context where it may have some relevance, is being applied to the nurse–person process as the primary mode of knowing for relating with patients and families. Nursing practice happens in the nurse–person process, and to suggest that this process can be directed by evidence is not a supportable position; it is actually inconsistent with professional ethical codes, with current philosophical thought, and with what people say they want from nurses. Once again, it is obvious that nurses require current knowledge and skill for guiding activities involved in the delivery of healthcare, especially in hospitals. However, the nurse–person process is not data based—it is human based and must be guided by values and theoretical principles.

Specific Issues of Concern

Specific issues, then, about evidence and its use for guiding nursing practice are as follows. First, there is no body of evidence that can justify nursing as an applied science; current evidence is contradictory, tentative, unethical, and in some instances absurd. Second, proponents of evidence-based practice do not sufficiently acknowledge that all evidence is value laden and theoretically driven. Third, evidence-based practice is inconsistent with nursing's societal mandate to serve others rather than nurses themselves. Fourth, proponents of evidence-based practice oversimplify and misrepresent the complexities of human relating and the realities of multiple competing values, including those of the client, in the nurse–person process. Each of these points deserves thoughtful and scholarly attention by the nursing community. The following is an attempt to initiate discussion about these four issues.

Where Is the Evidence?

Proponents of evidence-based practice suggest that there is a body of knowledge that, if accessed by nurses, could provide clear direction about how to benefit others. In reality, the evidence does not exist. What do exist are multiple calls for more research and multiple reports that offer generalized statements that in many instances merely confirm the obvious. For instance, research findings about crisis intervention have led to recommendations that nurses should listen to people experiencing crisis, or studies of quality of life have suggested that people with more resources have different health patterns than those who have no resources at all. This confirmation of the obvious is absurd. It should be a fundamental assumption that listening to all clients is essential in nursing practice—listening should be a core value of the nursing discipline. Directives for listening should be explicit in theories and standards that guide nursing practice. As a nurse leader, I prefer directing my time and energy to promoting practices that ensure that all persons experience being listened to by nurses so that the patient's reality provides the foundation for any care offered. If nurses began by listening, they would know how to be helpful and what actions and information might help people in light of their personal health experiences. The unsettling reality is that patients and families consistently report that many nurses, similar to other professionals, do not listen.

Most nursing philosophies specify nursing's commitment to treat all patients as unique human beings who define and live health differently; therefore, should not nurses already know and expect that all people have unique health patterns, not just those reported in research studies? Do we need evidence to know that some percentage of unemployed, single mothers with several children would benefit from more resources in the community? How will the evidence from these sorts of studies help nurses to practice with a particular mother and her children? Will nurses share with the mother that research evidence suggests that if she just had more money or more support she would be better off and her health patterns might improve? Nurses should be offended by the presentation of the obvious; it insults the knowing of both patients and nurses.

I am very concerned that nurses are being portrayed as empty (thoughtless) beings who must be directed when to speak, what to think, and when to listen—based on research evidence. The idea that nurses require evidence to know they should listen or be open to unique patterns of health, for instance, is a dangerous notion—if one can take it seriously at all. It is possible to imagine that evidence-based practice could propel nursing toward a purely technical vocation, which questions the need for professional nurses. Unregulated workers can certainly follow menu-driven directives based on evidence. I concur with White (1997), who suggests that evidence-based practice may represent one more example of how nurses embrace what they think will liberate them when, in reality, the initiative ensures their subservience to other interests and other disciplines.

Professional nursing practice requires the risk to embrace the inherent ambiguity of the moment and to be with others with explicit commitment, responsiveness, openness, compassion, and the intent to serve. Professional practice demands an engagement with the unknown in light of a broad knowledge base and understanding of lived experience and not the enforcement of predefined directives based on generalized and often meaningless statements of evidence. Beneficial outcomes for patients surface in genuine engagements with nurses—as persons (clients) themselves clarify meanings, ask questions, explore concerns, discover strengths, and make plans to change health and quality of life. Patients and families indicate that they want to be treated as human beings, and the essence of this kind of human relationship is unscripted engagement in which nurses live the commitment to be with clients and to listen, respect, provide, and be involved as directed by clients. Knowledge about how to be with others in ways that respect the client's power and direction can only be found in nursing theories, because theories direct the "how" of nursing in light of its human context. Unfortunately, evidence-based practice obscures the critical links among practice, theory, and the client's experience of nursing.

Obscuring the Theory–Practice Link

Contemporary scholars endorse the belief that all thinking is theoretical and value laden, yet many supporters of evidence-based practice fail to acknowledge that nursing practice requires thought and is therefore also guided by theory. All the thinking and acting that happens in nursing moments are already guided by theory. Moments with nurses help or hinder persons as they struggle and plan to change patterns of health. In evolving as a discipline, nursing has relied on theory from other disciplines to guide practice, but it is becoming increasingly obvious that nurses require nursing theories to fulfill their societal mandate to provide a service that enhances health and quality of life. Introducing evidence as the guide for practice obscures the linkages that already exist between practice and theory. This is a critical omission in the literature promoting evidence-based practice because the reality is that, despite evidence, some theories are not appropriate for professional nursing because of what people experience when the theory is used and because the goals of some theories are not consistent with nursing's ethic.

For instance, there may be research evidence to support the use of behavior modification to make patients comply with medical directives, but this evidence does not justify the nurse's choice to reward and punish patients in a paternalistic model of care. In this example, there are clear directives from the theory that shape the nurse–person process and the patient's experience of nursing. Behavior modification, a theory borrowed from psychology, does not uphold nurses' commitment to a dynamic (open and changing), nonjudgmental process that respects human freedom. I have heard nurses describe both the burden of policing patients and the harm to relationships that can accompany behavior modification. Any evidence that is unexamined in light of the guiding theory and uninformed about the client's experience is not consistent with nursing. One need only listen to patients describe what it is like to be on the receiving end of rewards and punishments to know that behavior modification is inconsistent with the mandate of nursing. In my opinion, it

is essential to question who is being served when punitive interventions are used by professionals to bring about desired change.

Self-Serving or Other Serving

I have heard claims that disciplines are merely self-serving. Much of this antidisciplinary sentiment emerged a decade ago in North America when it was discovered that disciplines created large departments and complex care processes that had questionable benefit to the persons being served. Many health disciplines wanted to ensure a holistic approach to care and so their members developed extensive multisystem assessments for problem identification. Meanwhile, patients were being subjected to multiple, redundant questions and interventions that may or may not have been relevant to their immediate concerns and interests. The question of whether disciplines are self-serving is legitimate, and nurses especially must question whose interests they serve in day-to-day practice.

For instance, some nurses perform assessments and use tools that may harm patients or that diminish their quality of living. Nurses may lose sight of the client's experience and focus more on collecting evidence than on satisfying or comforting patients. There are multiple examples of this self-serving phenomenon, but two that are particularly meaningful are linked with nurses doing routine Mini Mental State Examinations (MMSE) and pain scale ratings. The MMSE is a tool for detecting problems with orientation and memory. In some institutions, nurses routinely complete the MMSE daily or weekly to collect evidence of change. Fluctuations in scores, however, are not usually explainable even from a medical perspective, and there is no clear direction about what nurses should do in the nurse–person process in light of any particular score. Furthermore, many patients find the MMSE unsettling at best, and for some, it leads to crying and upset as they try to find the right answer to please the healthcare professional. Nurses must begin to question this routine collection of data that does not inform their practice and that often leads to embarrassment for clients.

Similarly, frustrations have been reported by patients who are asked to rate their pain on a scale of 1 to 10. I recently heard a very compelling story from a patient who was being pressured to rate his pain on a scale of 1 to 10 before staff would respond to his requests for medication. He expressed frustration and anger about being treated as if he were wrong and having to say the right things to get pain medication. The message being given to patients who prefer not to rate their pain on a scale of 1 to 10 is that their language does not count as credible evidence. If a patient prefers to use the word terrible to describe pain, and if the person can only say that the pain is "somewhat" or "mostly better," it should be enough for nurses. From my view, we are already bordering on negligence by forcing patients to comply with our tools so that we can collect numerical evidence instead of attending to patients' concerns and issues with compassion and respect for their choice of words and descriptions. The previous examples about patient dissatisfaction lead one to the following question: Who are nurses serving in their day-to-day practice?

I support the belief that nursing practice should integrate particular values and principles to structure the nurse–person process. The only evidence that can help nurses understand the benefit of nursing will come from clients' personal descriptions of how health and quality of life change with nursing care. The notion of evidence-based practice should be clearly limited to the technical/procedural realm of clinical care so that nurses are not expected to relinquish their responsibility to live certain values and

theoretical principles with all human beings. Nurses must begin to ask clients what difference nurses' attitudes, actions, and expressions make to their experiences of health and quality of life.

There are extensive reports from patients that indicate that they want to be accepted, listened to, involved, respected, and treated as unique human beings (see e.g., Gerteis, Edgman-Levitan, Daley, & Delbancho, 1993; Young-Mason, 1997). One man who spent a great deal of time with healthcare professionals developed his own principles that helped him deal with a medical belief system that consistently ensured staff had power and control (Macurdy, 1997). Macurdy's four principles, which are echoed in many stories from patients, are as follows:

1. As the person with the greatest stake in my healthcare, I make the decisions, and no health professional can overrule my preferences.
2. I am the only legitimate decision maker, and no one else is permitted to speak for me.
3. I must have complete information.
4. Healthcare is a means to a full and meaningful life; it is not an end in itself. I will not allow the medical agenda to rule my life. I choose to lead my life and accept the risks and consequences of a meaningful existence.

The knowledge base for ensuring that all patients have experiences that support their being listened to, involved, respected, and treated like human beings flows from guiding nursing theories rather than evidence. Theories guide how nurses think and act with individual persons and families as clients provide direction by identifying concerns, what is helpful, what information might be useful, what things mean, what is possible, and what choices are most important. The nurse–person process is very complex, and proponents of evidence-based practice have, in my view, grossly oversimplified and misrepresented the process of nursing.

The Misrepresentation of Evidence

To say nursing is evidence based misrepresents what is in reality a complex, intimate, and multidimensional process of interhuman relating. Despite claims that are in contrast (DiCenso et al., 1998), evidence-based practice does indeed promote a routinized process of care that is dehumanizing. Nurses want and need to know how to practice with people in open, nonjudgmental, participative relationships that enhance quality from the client's perspective. If nursing is to remain a human science concerned about quality of life and lived experience, then it is essential that nurses identify the specific values and theories that will guide the nurse–person process toward this goal. Proponents of evidence have not explicitly addressed the influence of values, assumptions, interpretations, intentions, and desired outcomes in practice.

It is also essential that nurse leaders acknowledge that there are higher values in the discipline of nursing (such as respect for self-determination, mutual process, and individual uniqueness). Any evidence or theory selected by nurses should be coherent with such values. The very term evidence flows from certain assumptions that are not consistent with nursing practices that honor situated freedom, human uniqueness, and client as leader. Nursing's responsibility should be first and foremost to develop and sustain knowledge that honors the client's meanings, realities, possibilities, wishes, and choices. The nurse–person process must be informed by values and theories that provide nurses with the knowledge to participate with human beings in changing health and quality of life as directed by people themselves.

Also underestimated by proponents of evidence- based practice are that hospitals, clinics, and other service-oriented centers already embrace some philosophy for practice that influences decisions made by frontline providers.

Nurse leaders are responsible for creating settings that nurture specific values and beliefs about patient care. As a chief nursing officer, I want nurses to practice patient-focused standards that are consistent with the human becoming school of thought (Parse, 1998). The notion that individual nurses could or should practice in ways supported by any evidence is inconsistent with the expectation that nurses should represent specific values and principles when it comes to human care.

Research involving human beings is infinitely complex, open to interpretation, and value laden. If research expands and informs the guiding theory, then findings must be considered in light of the practice prescribed by the theory. The most challenging aspect of nursing is the reasoning and thinking required to be with others in open, participatory, nonjudgmental relationships in which multiple forces and struggles come into play. Therefore, nurses should be given opportunities to look at their practices in light of the values and beliefs of nursing philosophy and theory. Changes in practice happen through personal insights about the linkages among beliefs, values, and actions—not through presentation of data.

The responsibility of all nurses should be to continue to integrate and develop theories that assist practitioners to be helpful and to have meaningful relationships with clients. Evidence in the absence of values and theories about human care and participative relationships is meaningless unless nursing is to be reduced to a purely technical, menu-driven enterprise. It is unfortunate that some nurses have failed to be guided by the concerns and wishes of those served by nursing—patients and families—because there are opportunities for professionals to create practices that enhance quality of life and consumer satisfaction. Some people are coming to hospitals with extensive knowledge and with a greater understanding of their health situations than many professionals. People want dialogue that is relevant to their personal lives. Evidence-based practice does not support the shift to patient-focused care, and it is inconsistent with the values and interests of consumers. This gap between what evidence-based practice promotes and what consumers want raises this question: To what end? This question may indeed hold the essential seed of controversy that is fueled by the evidence-based initiative.

Proponents of evidence-based nursing practice contend that the initiative is consistent with practices that are patient focused and with qualitative research methods. I respectfully disagree. The ultimate goal of evidence-based practice is control. No matter what patient-friendly words are picked up along the way and no matter what research methods are employed, the values and assumptions embedded in evidence-based practice lead to a particular place—prescriptive interventions aimed at managing patients. Nurses and other professionals have been trying to manage people for many decades, and people have indicated that the management approach is not wanted. It is folly to think that people will embrace professionals who judge them and who do not recognize their knowledge and their investment in the healthcare process.

It is my hope that nurses will seriously consider the complex issues surrounding the evidence-based initiative. Debate will continue to shed light on how nursing is evolving as a human science. There are alternative views and different roads that lie in nursing's path. The call issued here is for nurses to choose a path that ensures a value-specific, theory-guided knowledge base that clearly places the client as the expert about health and change—a path that places nurses as accountable to clients for the quality of nursing care.

References

DiCenso, A., Cullum, N., & Ciliska, D. (1998). Implementing evidence-based nursing: Some misconceptions. *Evidence-Based Nursing, 1*(2), 38–40.

Gerteis, M., Edgman-Levitan, S., Daley, J., & Delbancho, T. L. (Eds.). (1993). *Through the patient's eyes.* San Francisco: Jossey-Bass.

Macurdy, A. H. (1997). Mastery of life. In J. Young-Mason (Ed.), *The patient's voice: Experiences of illness* (pp. 9–15). Philadelphia: F. A. Davis.

Parse, R. R. (1998). *The human becoming school of thought.* Thousand Oaks, CA: Sage.

White, S. J. (1997). Evidence-based practice and nursing: The new panacea? *British Journal of Nursing, 6*(3), 175–178.

Chapter 29

Critical Thinking and Theory-Based Practice

Ellen Clark Birx,
PhD, RN

Critical thinking is an essential and ongoing process in using theory to guide nursing practice. Theory involves seeing patterns that bring order to chaos. Chinn and Kramer define theory as "a systematic abstraction of reality that serves some purpose."[1(p. 20)] This definition emphasizes the idea that theory is an abstraction and not reality itself. From a different perspective or for a different purpose an alternate theory might be developed and found to be useful. The purpose of nursing theory is the description, explanation, and prediction of phenomena within the domain of nursing with the ultimate aim of guiding nursing practice.

A key question in using theory to guide nursing practice is, "What theories are useful in particular nursing situations?" Critical thinking on the part of each nurse is required to select or develop theories to guide practice in diverse clinical settings. Although theories can be useful in organizing and guiding our practice, they can also be blinders that limit us from seeing things as they are. Critical thinking helps us gain awareness of how we are viewing and creating our world of practice.

There is a large body of literature in the fields of psychology, education, and nursing about critical thinking, what it is, how it is learned, and how it is applied in practice. The National League for Nursing (NLN)[2] mandates that nursing programs emphasize the development of critical thinking and independent decision making. However, there is a lack of clarity about just what critical thinking entails. In a national survey of 470 deans or directors of NLN-accredited nursing programs, 51% of whom responded, Jones and Brown[3] found that most of the respondents conceptualized critical thinking as an objective, rational, linear problem-solving process similar to the nursing process. They concluded that most of the sample defined critical thinking in a rather narrow way, excluding aspects of critical thinking like imaginative speculation.

Experts have defined critical thinking in various ways. Ennis defines critical thinking as "reasonable reflective thinking that is focused on deciding what to believe or do."[4(p. 10)] Although this definition includes reasoning and decision-making processes, it is not limited to these. It also incorporates reflective thought and creative thinking processes.

Smith[5] views critical thinking within the context of thinking in general. Smith describes thinking as "a single, continual, all-embracing

Source: Birx, E.C., (1993). Critical thinking and theory-based practice. *Holistic Nursing Practice.* 7(3):21–27. Reprinted with permission from and copyright ©1993 Springer Publishing Company.

operation of the mind, powered by an imagination that never rests, not a collection of disparate skills . . ."[5(p. 124)] Smith's holistic view of critical thinking as inseparable and overlapping with other natural thinking processes resonates with nursing's holistic world view. It is also consistent with the current trend in nursing toward integrating multiple types of thinking or patterns of knowledge—empirical, ethical, aesthetic, and personal—to guide clinical decision making.[6]

Smith's[5] emphasis on the role of imagination in our thinking processes is also especially pertinent. Critical thinking not only involves rational, linear thinking processes, but also intuitive, imaginative thinking processes. The ability to imagine an alternative leads us to question the current system and move toward more humanistic health care environments and relationships.

Viewing or defining critical thinking in a broad way, rather than limiting it to linear problem-solving processes encompasses the many aspects of critical thinking that are needed to select or develop theories to guide nursing practice. Increasing our awareness of various critical thinking processes facilitates our ability to use these processes in the complex world of practice.

Attitude of Inquiry and Openness

Smith[5] suggests that critical thinking is facilitated by an attitude of doubt. An attitude of doubt involves questioning what is happening within and around us and a comfort with uncertainty or not knowing. According to Smith, "Thought flourishes as questions are asked, not as answers are found."[5(p. 129)] An open and inquiring mind is needed to question the way things are in our clinical practice and to be open to new possibilities.

Through research and theory development, the profession is engaged in developing knowledge on which to base our clinical practice. The knowledge on which we base our practice is not just an accumulation of facts and theories, but also a dynamic, ongoing process of awareness, inquiry, investigation, integration, imagination, and openness to realities and possibilities. Our knowledge base is not static; it is constantly evolving.

Knowledge of the Discipline of Nursing

Critical thinking involves both process and content. We must have something to think about. In a practice discipline like nursing, we have a body of knowledge gleaned from our literature and the direct experience of clinical realities from our everyday practice to think critically about. While the undergraduate student and beginning nurse are able to think critically at a beginning level with freshness of vision, the graduate student and experienced nurses are able to think critically at an advanced level due to an expanded familiarity with nursing literature and a rich background of clinical experience.

Most of the nurses in the graduate course in nursing theory that the author teaches are currently practicing nurses from diverse clinical settings. Two major objectives of the course are to familiarize the students with a broad range of nursing theories in as interesting a manner as possible and to encourage critical thinking about the relevance of these theories to their own clinical practice. Students often comment that they were not looking forward to taking a course in nursing theory and expected it to be dry and tedious. However, by the end of the semester, they express much enthusiasm for the course and find it to be a real eye opener. They state that they have become more aware of the theories that, whether they realized it or not, have been guiding their clinical practice; they are able to critique and select useful theories to improve their practice; and they are inspired to imagine what new theories are needed to guide practice in their specialty area.

Metacognition and Metatheory

Another type of critical thinking process used in selecting or developing theories to guide clinical practice includes metacognition and metatheory. These terms refer to the processes of thinking about thinking and thinking about theory, respectively. Metacognition involves the awareness of the thought processes we are using and the ability to select appropriate thinking strategies to accomplish our task.[7] Metatheory focuses on philosophical and methodological issues related to nursing theory, such as questioning the type of theory needed in nursing, critiquing nursing theories, and analyzing nursing theories to identify recurring themes and trends.[8] Both of these critical thinking processes require that we step back from our clinical practice and reflect about the theories we need to guide our practice and the thought processes we need to use to select or develop these theories.

Metatheory involves asking questions such as
- "What are the values of the nursing profession?"
- "What are the assumptions we are making when we approach nursing situations in a particular way?"
- "What are characteristics of nursing's world view?"

The ability to identify underlying values, assumptions, and perspectives is an essential critical thinking skill.

Integrating Multiple Levels of Theory

Selection of theory to guide nursing practice involves multiple levels of theory, including metatheory, grand theory, and midrange theory. Grand theory "deals with broad goals and concepts representing the total range of phenomena of concern within a discipline."[1(p. 199)] Midrange theory is more specific and limited in scope, dealing with a single phenomenon or a limited number of phenomena within the domain of nursing.

The use of theory to guide clinical practice involves selecting, adapting, or developing a grand-level nursing theory or conceptual framework. This conceptual framework then guides the selection, adaptation, or development of midrange theories that are specific enough to guide nursing actions. The conceptual framework is like the two-by-fours that frame in a house, outlining where walls, windows, and doors will go. The midrange theories complete the house with various wall finishings and varieties of windows and doors. We first select the overall house plan, and then we select fixtures, colors, flooring, and so forth. Even when the house is finished, we are open to the possibility of remodeling to update or improve the house in various ways.

An example of this process is the use of Levine's[9] grand nursing theory to guide clinical practice in a neonatal intensive care unit. Levine's Conservation Principles provide a useful conceptual framework for organizing nursing care in this complex setting. The four conservation principles, (1) conservation of energy, (2) conservation of structural integrity, (3) conservation of personal integrity, and (4) conservation of social integrity, guide the nurse in providing holistic and comprehensive care for the neonate and family.

In addition to selecting this broad nursing conceptual framework, additional midrange theories must be selected to provide the specific knowledge to guide nursing action. Levine's conservation of energy principle guides the nurse in selecting or developing physiological theories and nursing theories related to temperature regulation, oxygenation, nutrition, fluids and electrolytes, and rest and activity aimed at conserving the energy of the neonate for growth and healing. The principle of conservation of structural integrity guides the nurse in selecting or developing theories related to immune response, positioning, range of motion, wound healing, and skin care. The principle of conservation of personal integrity guides the nurse in the selection of nursing theories and the adaptation of theories from related disciplines dealing with early psychological development. The principle of conservation of social integrity guides the nurse in the selection or development of nursing theories and the adaptation of theories from related disciplines, such as sociology and anthropology, to guide nursing care for neonates within the context of their family, community, and culture. Examples of mid-range theories that are useful in neonatal intensive care that can be integrated within Levine's broad nursing conceptual framework are the synactive theory of infant development,[10] crisis intervention theory,[11] attachment theory,[12] and maternal role attainment theory.[13] A wide range of theories from nursing and related disciplines are organized within Levine's conceptual framework to provide theory-based care that is congruent with nursing's holistic, caring world view.

Cromwell proposes a definition of critical thinking as "the ability to apply disciplinary frameworks in personal, academic, and professional settings and to monitor and evaluate that activity."[14(p. 40)] As the nurse engages in metatheoretical inquiry and in the evaluation of nursing conceptual frameworks and midrange theories for use in clinical practice, he or she is engaged in critical thinking. Critical thinking is an ongoing process in clinical practice as the nurse monitors and evaluates the usefulness of the theories he or she has applied. Critical thinking is a creative process as nurses identify areas within their clinical practice where new theories need to be developed.

In that critical thinking is both a rational and a creative process, the selection and application of theory to guide clinical practice is not performed in a mechanical way. It is a reflective, creative process. Johnston and Baumann[15] dis-

cuss a process for selecting and tailoring nursing models to meet the needs of particular clinical settings. Among the steps in the process they outline are reflection on the nurse's own values and ideas about person, environment, health, and nursing; categorizing the attributes of the client population served; and identifying effective intervention used on the unit. This is followed by the selection or development of a nursing conceptual framework that fits well with these considerations and that allows for collaboration with other disciplines practicing on the unit. Johnston and Baumann suggest selecting conceptual frameworks to guide practice at the unit level rather than at the level of an agency or institution as a whole. This allows the selection and development of theory that is most useful in guiding nursing practice in particular clinical settings.

Perspective Taking

A critical thinking process that is especially pertinent to the development of theory-based practice is the ability to view a situation from multiple perspectives. The discipline of nursing has a rich tradition of valuing not only the nurse's perception of a situation, but also the client's perception of the situation; of valuing subjective realities; and of valuing multicultural perspectives.[16–18] In addition, nursing practice requires consideration of multiple historical, philosophical, economic, and political viewpoints. Engaging in dialogue with nursing colleagues, colleagues from other disciplines, health care consumers, and families enhances perspective-taking ability.[19] Through critical dialogue, nurses can move toward a synthesis of multiple perspectives.[20]

Gebser[21] describes and predicts the evolution of human consciousness beyond the synthesis of multiple perspectives to an integral or aperspectival consciousness. According to Gebser, humankind has evolved through archaic, magical, mythical, and mental stages and is now on the verge of evolving to a stage of integral or aperspectival consciousness. He describes the awareness of a person in aperspectival consciousness in the following way: "For him them is no longer heaven or hell, this world or the other, ego or world, immanence or transcendence; rather beyond the magic unity, the mythical complementarity, the mental division and synthesis is the perceptible whole."[21(p543)] Aperspectival consciousness is characterized by integration rather than synthesis.

Lassalle emphasizes that in integral or aperspectival consciousness, "thinking is not determined solely by reason; in it intelligence, feeling, will, spirit, and the body play equally important roles."[22(p. 63)] In this new thinking, previous stages are not eliminated, rather they are integrated and brought into balance in an awareness of the whole. Ultimately, this level of holistic thinking is desirable to guide nursing practice.

Empowerment

A further consideration regarding critical thinking and theory-based nursing practice is empowerment. Smith[5] encourages examination of the extent to which individuals are allowed to be critical thinking in hierarchical, bureaucratic systems. He contends that a necessary ingredient in critical thinking is that people be given the authority to be independent thinkers. This he refers to as empowerment.

Empowerment that fosters critical thinking in nursing practice involves communicating to nurses that they have the authority, ability, and responsibility to think critically about their practice. The authority to think critically is conveyed by eliciting, listening to, and valuing the views and experiences of nurses engaged in clinical practice. Authority, is conveyed through an atmosphere of collaboration and equality with other disciplines. The ability to think critically

is cultivated through role-modeling. Nurses grow in their ability to think critically when they work with and observe other nurses engaged in inquiry, critical reflection, exploration of creative alternatives, and articulation of what they are seeing.

Theory-based practice is not just a matter of latching onto the latest theory. It goes far deeper than this. We must critically reflect on the theories, whether implicit or explicit, we are using to guide our practice. As nurses, we have not only the authority and ability, but also the responsibility to question and work toward better health care systems.

While the present emphasis on critical thinking as the use of problem-solving skills in nursing practice is necessary, it is not sufficient or representative of the broad range of critical thinking processes required for theory-based clinical practice. An attitude of openness and inquiry, knowledge and clinical experience in nursing, metacognition and metatheoretical reflection, the integration of multiple levels of theory, perspective taking, and empowerment are all important critical thinking processes.

In addition to taking a holistic approach to critical thinking, it is important to view critical thinking as an ongoing process in using theory to guide clinical practice. As the nurse engages in clinical practice, there is the need to continually question, "What is going on here?" "Are the theories I am using to guide my practice really helpful or are they limiting my authenticity, creativity, and compassion in helping this person?" "What new theories need to be developed in this practice setting?" Through critical thinking, we continually become more open, more inquiring, more knowledgeable, more experienced, more reflective, more integrated, more sensitive to multiple perspectives, and more empowered to refine and develop theory to improve clinical practice. Critical thinking creates theory-based practice that is nursing at its best.

References

1. Chinn PL, Kramer MK. *Theory and Nursing: A Systematic Approach,* 3rd ed. St. Louis: Mosby; 1991.

2. National League for Nursing. *NLN Self-Study Manual.* New York: NLN; 1989.

3. Jones SA, Brown LN. Critical thinking: Impact on nursing education. *Journal of Advanced Nursing.* 1991;16:529–533.

4. Ennis RH. A taxonomy of critical thinking dispositions and abilities. In: Baron JB, Sternberg RJ, eds. *Teaching Thinking Skills: Theory and Practice.* New York: W.H. Freemonk; 1987.

5. Smith F. *To Think.* New York: Teachers College Press; 1990.

6. Carper BA. Fundamental patterns of knowing in nursing. *Advances in Nursing Science.* 1978;1(1):13–23.

7. Beyer BK. *Practical Strategies for the Teaching of Thinking.* Boston: Allyn & Bacon; 1987.

8. Walker LO, Avant KC. *Strategies for Theory Construction in Nursing.* Norwalk, CT: Appleton-Century-Crofts; 1983.

9. Levine ME. The conversation principles: Twenty-years later. In: Riehl-Sisca J, ed. *Conceptual Models for Nursing Practice,* 3rd ed. Norwalk, CT: Appleton & Lange; 1989.

10. Als H. Neurobehavioral development of the premature infant. In: Avery ME, First LR, eds. *Pediatric Medicine.* Baltimore: Williams & Wilkins; 1989.

11. Aguilera DC, Messick JM. *Crisis Intervention: Theory and Methodology,* 5th ed. St. Louis: Mosby; 1986.

12. Klaus MH, Kennel JH. *Parent-Infant Bonding,* 2nd ed. St. Louis: Mosby; 1982.

13. Mercer RT. *First-Time Motherhood: Experiences from Teens to Forties.* New York: Springer; 1986.

14. Cromwell LS. Assessing critical thinking. In: Barnes CA, ed. *Critical Thinking: Educational Imperative.* San Francisco: Jossey-Bass; 1992.

15. Johnston N, Baumann A. Selecting a nursing model for psychiatric nursing. *Journal of Psychosocial Nursing.* 1992;30(4):7–12.

16. Orlando I. *The Dynamic Nurse–Patient Relationship.* New York: Putnam; 1961.

17. Watson J. *Nursing: Human Science and Human Care: A Theory of Nursing.* New York: National League for Nursing; 1988.

18. Leininger M. *Transcultural Nursing: Concepts, Theories, and Practices.* New York: Wiley; 1978.

19. Chaffee J. Teaching critical thinking across the curriculum. In: Barnes CA, ed. *Critical Thinking: Educational Imperative.* San Francisco: Jossey-Bass; 1992.

20. Lorensen M. Response to "Critical theory: A foundation for the development of nursing theories." *Scholarly Inquiry for Nursing Practice.* 1988;2(3):233–236.

21. Gebser J. *The Ever-Present Origin.* Athens, OH: Ohio University Press; 1985.

22. Lassalle HE. *Living in the New Consciousness.* Boston: Shambhala; 1988.

Chapter 30

The Circle of Caring: A Transformative Model of Advanced Practice Nursing

Lynne M. Dunphy, PhD, FNP, CNS

Jill E. Winland-Brown, EdD, MSN, FNP-c

This article presents a new and original approach to advanced practice nursing. A transformative model, the Circle of Caring, is described. Using a template that builds on both nursing and medicine, this model provides a synthesized approach to practice. The traditional medical model is reviewed, as well as the evolution of the nursing process. In response to changing societal need, the scope of nursing practice is constantly challenged and expanded. New elements of practice emerge. In an effort to clarify and elaborate the current realities of advanced practice nursing, the Circle of Caring was conceptualized. Components of traditional medical practice are combined with elements of traditional nursing practice; both are situated in an elemental nursing model of caring. Although a linear representation, the Circle of Caring encompasses process pieces taken in part from a theory of caring (Boykin & Schoenhofer, 1993; Mayerhoff, 1971). An underlying purpose of this model is to highlight in a concrete way the inclusion of nursing's voice in the new and emerging—and rapidly changing—healthcare system. It is theorized that this approach to practice will yield more positive outcomes for patients, families, and communities. Keywords: caring, advanced practice nursing, Circle of Caring.

As APNs, we do differ from other health care providers. . . . We take it into the lived experience [of the patient]. (B. Armstrong, personal communication, 1997)

The North American healthcare system is built on the traditional medical model of care and, as such, emphasizes organ pathology, inter-

ventionist acute care, and technological solutions (Venegoni, 1996; Watson, 1995). Currently, the healthcare needs of individuals, families, and communities are not adequately met; costs of healthcare continue to skyrocket; and social problems such as violence and environmental pollution are an ever-present backdrop (Buerhaus, 1996; Shalala, 1993; Smith, 1995). Chronic diseases abound and behavioral interventions oriented toward lifestyle changes often receive limited attention. Additionally, macro-level approaches that might impact the healthful or

Source: Dunphy, L. M., and Winland-Brown, J. E. The circle of caring: A transformative model of advanced practice nursing. *Clinical Excellence for Nurse Practitioners.* 2(4), 1998. Copyright © 1998 by Churchill Livingstone.

unhealthful structures in which people live out their lives often fall short (Brush & Capezuti, 1997; Roach, 1995).

It is the premise of this article that a more active addition of nursing-based knowledge is missing from today's healthcare system. Increasing numbers of nurses have traversed practitioner programs and now have their own advanced nursing practices in the day-to-day workplaces of primary and acute care (Division of Nursing, 1996). Frequently, these advanced practice nurses (APNs) struggle to articulate what it is as nursing-based care providers that they uniquely bring to their patients. This question has plagued nursing as a discipline and has gained new urgency in an age that necessitates collaboration (Brush & Capezuti, 1996; Cody, 1994; Huch, 1995; Rogers, 1972).

At present, an essential task is creating a clearer vision of disciplinary identity. A more lucid articulation of the uniquely nursing-based perspective used by APNs will make nursing's contribution more visible and effect meaningful change for patients, families, and communities as well as our current healthcare system. Both physicians, practicing medical science, and APNs, practicing nursing, are needed to fix our healthcare system. There is a need to collaborate, but this collaboration needs to include a more active addition of nursing to the current dominant medical mode of practice. The Circle of Caring offers a step in this direction.

The Traditional Medical Model: Based in Reductionist Science

Figure 30–1 is a representation of the traditional medical model. It is largely a reductionist model, a decontextualized view of the person. The assessment phase is built on subjective aspects of the patient's story, liberally prioritized and rationalized through the diagnostic

lens of hypothesis formation and hypothesis testing. The objective phase of the assessment includes the physical exam and data from diagnostic lab tests. These ideally validate the diagnostic hunches, or hypotheses. They are then correlated to the lexicon of diagnostic medical terminology, the International Classification of Diseases codes (ICD-o-CM, 1997). Reimbursement is predicated on this labeling.

Next, therapeutic interventions are prescribed for the identified malady, often pharmacologic and/or surgical. This generates a different set of codes for billing purposes, the Current Procedural Terminology (CPT) (American Medical Association, 1997). Some interventions are geared toward firming up the diagnosis

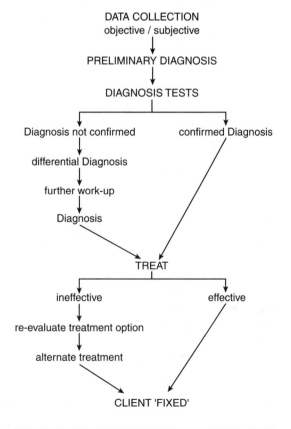

Figure 30–1 THE MEDICAL MODEL

DATA COLLECTION
objective / subjective

PRELIMINARY DIAGNOSIS

DIAGNOSIS TESTS

Diagnosis not confirmed   confirmed Diagnosis

differential Diagnosis

further work-up

Diagnosis

TREAT

ineffective   effective

re-evaluate treatment option

alternate treatment

CLIENT 'FIXED'

Figure 30-2 THE NURSING PROCESS: AS EASY AS PIE

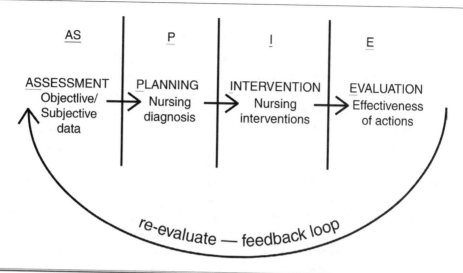

(i.e., referral and/or more diagnostic tests). Some are known to be merely palliative, and others are believed to be curative. Outcomes are traditionally measured in mortality and morbidity rates, with an occasional reference to quality of life in a way that may be objectified and defined.

The Traditional Nursing Model: A Nursing Process Approach

Nursing, in its need and desire to differentiate itself from medicine while nonetheless continuing its pursuit of a rationalized and scientific meaning for its existence, evolved the nursing process approach. This is frequently linked to the taxonomy of nursing diagnoses (**Figure 30–2**). These developments occurred explicitly and self-consciously in the late 1960s and early 1970s, spawning a spate of changes in nurse practice acts, which legally define nursing as the treatment of actual and potential human responses to illness.

The nursing process takes the form of assessment, analysis (or the labeling of the human response), planning, implementation, and evaluation. Nursing diagnosis, or the naming of the patient's subjective responses to the illness experience, is based on data gathering that includes the same subjective and objective database of medical science but with more emphasis on psychosocial and environmental factors.

The analysis of the subjective and objective cues displayed by the patient and/or family system are evaluated in light of nursing diagnostic hypotheses and are named accordingly. An example is *alteration in skin integrity,* meaning a break in the integrity of the skin. Often the goals dictated are a reflection of the underlying medical diagnosis, such as laceration or wound, recast in the cumbersome language of nursing diagnosis as *alteration in skin integrity.* In this sense, nursing diagnosis may be viewed as reactive stance, rooted in an attempt to differentiate nursing from medicine as opposed to a proactive conceptualization (Orlando, 1990).

The planning phase of the nursing process is conceptualized as mutual goal setting by the nurse and the patient/family (King, 1970). These goals are achieved through a combination of medical treatment, nursing interventions, and self-care. Some of these goals call for interventions uniquely suited to the nursing domain of knowledge, referred to as *independent nursing actions,* whereas many goals call for collaborative planning with the medical orders, termed *dependent nursing actions.*

The development of the Nursing Intervention Classification system (NIC) (McCloskey & Bulechek, 1996), the objectification of nursing-based knowledge into a taxonomy of unique nursing interventions, is an attempt at standardization of treatment, again mirroring the structuring of medically based diagnosis and treatment. However, neither nursing diagnosis, in the form of the North American Nursing Diagnosis Association (NANDA) (Gordon, 1987), nor nursing interventions, in the form of NIC, are currently accorded the status and privilege of being factored into the current healthcare system in any meaningful way. The external structure and processes of reimbursement and billing remain unenlightened as to what nurses, in this case APNs, are doing in their day-to-day practice and the positive healthcare outcomes that result.

The evaluation phase of the nursing process is traditionally a circular one, assessing the extent to which the goals have been achieved, complete with prescriptive remedies and room for modification. In this sense, the evaluation phase is partially related to the goals mutually set by nurse and patient/family, but in reality, more often dominated by the goals of medical science (Carpenito, 1993; Gordon, 1987). Nursing process is often criticized as being a linear, problem-solving approach to holistic phenomena (Mitchell, 1995).

A New Transformative Template: The Circle of Caring

A multiparadigmatic perspective has been selected to structure the Circle of Caring (Engebretson, 1997). Caring is suggested as one way to bridge the gulf between holistic nursing theories and biomedical nursing praxis.

The Circle of Caring (**Figure 30–3**) is a nursing-based template superimposed on a traditional medical model. The Circle of Caring is a synthesized view of the problem-solving method used in primary and acute care. Both the traditional medical model as well as traditional nursing process (**Figures 30–1 and 30–2**) are predicated on (1) a subjective and objective database, (2) a labeling of the patient problem/response, (3) a therapeutic plan, and (4) an evaluation of the outcome. Building on these features, the Circle of Caring also includes (1) a broadened and contextualized database, (2) a labeling of the patient's concern that more actively incorporates the patient's responses to the meaning of illness in their day-to-day lives, (3) a holistic approach to therapeutics that includes nursing-based interventions as well as complementary therapies, as appropriate, and (4) a view of outcomes based on the patient's/family's perceptions of improvement as well as the more traditional, quantified outcome measures such as mortality and morbidity data.

A Contextualized Database

Although the patient's subjective perception of experience is captured in the history portion of the assessment database, the Circle of Caring is predicated on hearing the patient's story in all

Figure 30–3 CIRCLE OF CARING

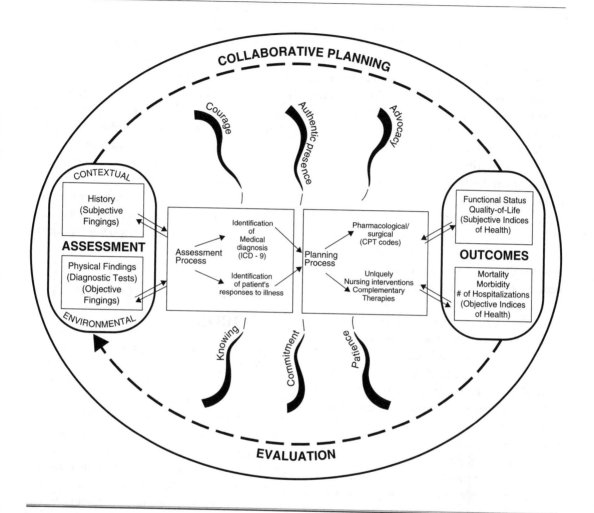

The Nature of Patient Responses
its complexity, as well as eliciting the meaning of health to the patient/family. Additionally, increased attention is focused on the interplay of perceptual, psychodynamic, that have impact on the patients health status. This contextualized approach—the lived experience of the patient/family—is central to this model and is one that nurses are educated about in their undergraduate programs.

The Nature of Patient Responses

The American Nurses Association's Social Policy Statement (1995) defines nursing as the diagnosis and treatment of human responses to actual and potential health problems. This statement provides continued support for the development and use of nursing diagnosis, formalized in the

NANDA. The language of nursing diagnosis is often rejected as (1) not reflective of a holistic perspective and (2) cumbersome and reactive. Nursing diagnoses, however, do provide for concrete labeling, in the form of a taxonomy, of patient responses. Boykin and Schoenhofer (1993) conceptualized the phenomenon of human responses as calls for nursing. As such, these responses remain unique and interactional, not amenable to generic labeling.

Medical texts have fastened onto the delineation between illness and disease, as elaborated by Kleinman, Einberg, and Good (1978). Rakel (1995), for example, described illness as "all the sensations of a patient and all the ramifications of a disorder" (p. 305). Disease is a taxonomic and theoretical concept, a useful tool that enables the caregiver to make inferences and predictions concerning phenomena. Illness and disease belong to two different universes of discourse: one of the world of theory; the other of the lived experience of the patient. For example, Mishler (1984), in studying physician–patient conversations, distinguished between the world of medicine and the voice of the "lifeworld," which represented a common-sense attitude, and the interpretation of events with reference to one's own experience.

The family physician, in particular, experiences the limitations and frustrations of the medical taxonomic classification system. *Medical diagnosis,* in the strict sense of the term, is possible in only approximately 50% of patients seen in primary care (Rakel, 1995)! Other literature (Howie, 1973) supports this. In the reality of practice, caregivers often make management decisions based on the absence and/or presence of certain clinical features, as opposed to clear congruence with a taxonomic set of disease criteria.

As collaborative practice increases, a more generic labeling of clinical phenomena may well emerge. One example is the Agency for Health Care Policy and Research (AHCPR) guidelines, generated around clinical conditions often labeled in a more generic fashion—for example, low back pain, heart failure, post-stroke rehabilitation. The democratization of information and databases used by increasingly informed consumers all necessitate such a transition.

The importance of the labeling of the patient's problem, be it in medical and/or nursing diagnostic terminology or a more generic format, is that it helps the patients' responses to be better addressed. This labeling involves the acknowledgment and knowledge of the complex interplay of perceptual, psychodynamic, socioeconomic, cultural, and environmental factors that contribute to health. APNs are especially skilled at eliciting and understanding this human phenomenon, and fashioning nursing-based responses uniquely suited to the individual.

A Broadened Approach to Therapeutics

Another hallmark of the proposed model is a broadened approach to therapeutics. In reality, this is actualized in day-to-day practice, yet it remains an especially invisible piece of nursing work (Wolf, 1989; Zerwekh, 1993). This nursing-based approach entails working with the individual patient to tailor interventions geared to the meaning of health to that unique patient/family. Building on current standards of medical and nursing practice, interventions are fine tuned. This requires a flexible approach to therapeutics that includes holistic approaches to healing. Research in this area is proliferating as patients and their families are calling for alternative and complementary approaches (Achterberg, 1996; Dossey, 1996).

Additionally, to quote Donna Shalala (1993) from her keynote address at the National League for Nursing's Centennial Conference, patients and families are calling for the appearance of the "good fairy" in the managed care experience—someone who really hears them and their concerns, the nitty-gritty of their day-to-day experiences and struggles. They need someone to hear why they did not take the medication that their healthcare provider was so quick to prescribe but that they just could not tolerate, or could not afford, or could not get to the pharmacy to pick up, or could not understand the directions for administration; why they did not have the mammogram because they were afraid; why the baby was not immunized because food on the table was more important. This is the iceberg that our healthcare system, traditionally focused on the easily visible peaks above the water, has plowed into. Nurses understand the whole of the iceberg: we are educated to see below the water, as well as above.

Outcomes: Who Decides? According to Whom?

The Circle of Caring also predicates a broadened view of outcomes. Outcome-based research of today demonstrates the need to incorporate patients' perceptions as measured objectively (functional assessments and the like) and subjectively (Cody, 1994). Quality-of-life measures, and most importantly the meaning of health and illness to the patient/family, must be taken more fully into consideration. Plans must be assessed by their ability to assist patients and families to meet their goals in ways that are meaningful to them, not just to improve mortality and morbidity measures. The voice of an increasingly informed, information-savvy consumer demands no less.

Environmental science and the interplay of environmental factors on health and the experience of a healthful life are recognized pieces of the healthcare puzzle, although often they are underdeveloped in the traditional medial model. Labeled *community-oriented primary care* in current medical textbooks (Rakel, 1995), these approaches along with preventive aspects of care were largely abandoned by medical science in the earlier parts of this century in favor of science, technology, and specialization. Medicine has awakened to the renewed need for such approaches to deal with current healthcare realities such as violence and AIDS. Likewise, nursing has renewed its emphasis on community-based approaches, reaffirming its historic roots (Zerwikh, 1993).

Encircled by Caring

A broadened, although essentially linear, approach to problem solving is necessitated in practice. A linear representation of the problem-solving approach was also chosen for ease of communication; it is embedded in the middle of the schemata (Figure 30-3). This process is encircled by *caring,* a visual representation of the interpersonal process occurring between caregiver and patient/family. The ability to provide effective and meaningful care for the patient is predicated on the processes of care, as exemplified in the Circle of Caring. This is what enables the nurse to adequately hear the patient's call and fashion appropriate nursing responses (Boykin & Schoenhofer, 1993). This process of care is actualized through caring processes drawn from Mayerhoff (1971) and Boykin and Schoenhofer (1993). These are described as patience, courage, advocacy, authentic presence, commitment, and knowing.

The Return of the Good Fairy

The frustration of patients and families in dealing with today's healthcare system is heard daily in practice. Although the technology of medical care continues unabated (Locsin, 1995), the interactional and collaborative aspects of care are often underdeveloped. The Circle of Caring is needed for patients and families to document and describe the practice of APNs, who respond to calls from patients and who imaginatively, creatively, and powerfully foster responses. These may be fashioned on a micro level—the one-to-one nurse-patient relationship in primary or acute care—or on a macro level, as uniquely nursing-based knowledge is applied to the care of communities and/or populations. This transformative model, the Circle of Caring, incorporates the individual strengths of both nursing and medicine but reformulates them in a new model of care. APNs are the appropriate providers to demonstrate the efficacy of an integrated model of caregiving, rooted in the lived experience of the patient.

The following is an example that uses the Circle of Caring in clinical practice.

Mary, aged 54, presented to the ambulatory care setting with fatigue. Her chief complaint was inability to sleep, and she requested a prescription for sleeping pills. I ran a complete blood count (CBC) to rule out anemia and a thyroid profile to rule out hypothyroidism, then pulled out my prescription pad to write a prescription for a soporific. Following the traditional medical model, I would have spent a few more minutes exploring the reason for her insomnia and made a diagnosis of fatigue, rule-out (R/O) anemia, and R/O hypothyroidism. I sensed, however, the need to explore further. I discovered that Mary was caring for her husband, who had recently suffered a stroke, and that she also cared for her elderly mother, who lived with her. Her inability to sleep was only the tip of the iceberg. In reality, Mary was experiencing "caregiver strain." What she needed was time to care for herself. What was really called for were some concrete nursing interventions, such as home-maintenance assistance and respite care, as well as coping enhancement. We discussed a caregiver support group that met Thursday evenings at a nearby hospital and provided volunteers to sit with family members to allow principal caregivers to attend. Ability to care for oneself was also addressed. Suggestions included resuming her weekly canasta club and going to movies with her friends. I also prescribed a hot bath with aromatic oils at bedtime. When she left, she stated that she had never felt so cared for. She called me a week later with an update, stating that she was feeling less strained, was sleeping better, and that she had not needed the sleeping medication.

References

Achterberg, J. (1996). What is medicine? *Alternative Therapies, 2*(3), 58–61.

American Medical Association. (1997). *Physicians' current procedural terminology—CPT 97.* Chicago: Author.

American Nurses Association, (1995). *Nursing: A social policy statement.* Washington, DC: Author.

Boykin, A., & Schoenhofer, S. (1993). *Nursing as caring: A model for transforming practice.* New York: National League for Nursing Press.

Brush, B. L., & Capezuti, E. A. (1996). Revisiting "A nurse for all settings: The nurse practitioner movement, 1965–1995." *Journal of the American Academy of Nurse Practitioners, 8*(1), 5–11.

Brush, B. L., & Capezuti, E. A. (1997). Professional autonomy: Essential for NP survival in the 21st century. *Journal of the American Academy of Nurse Practitioners, 9*(6), 265–269.

Buerhaus, P. L. (1996). Economics and health care financing. In J. V. Hickey, R. M. Ouimette, & S. L. Venegoni (Eds.), *Advanced practice nursing* (pp. 188–205). Philadelphia: Lippincott.

Carpenito, L. J. (1993). *Nursing diagnosis: Application to clinical practice.* Philadelphia: Lippincott.

Cody, W. K. (1994). Nursing theory-guided practice: What it is and what it is not. *Nursing Science Quarterly, 7*(4), 144–145.

Division of Nursing. (1996). *1996 Report to Congress.* Division of Nursing, Health Resources & Services Administration, Public Health Services. Rockville, MD: Division of Nursing.

Dossey, B. (1996). *Holistic nursing.* Frederick, MD: Aspen Publishing Co.

Engebretson, J. (1997). A multiparadigm approach to nursing. *Advances in Nursing Science, 20*(1), 21–33.

Gordon, M. (1987), *Nursing diagnosis: Process and application* (2nd ed.) New York: McGraw-Hill.

Howie, J. R. R. (1973). A new look at respiratory illness in general practice: A reclassification of respiratory illness based on antibiotic prescribing, cited in Rakel, R. (1995). *Textbook of family practice.* Philadelphia: W. B. Saunders.

Huch, M. H. (1995). Nursing science as basis for advanced practice. *Nursing Science Quarterly, 8*(1), 6–7.

King, I. (1970). *Toward a theory of nursing.* Philadelphia: E. A. Davis.

Kleinman, A., Einberg, L., & Good, B. (1978). Culture, illness, and care: Clinical lessons from anthropological and cross-cultural research. *Annals of Internal Medicine, 88,* 251.

Locsin, R. C. (1995). Technology and caring. In A. Boykin (Ed.) *Power, politics and public policy* (pp. 24–36). New York: NLN Press.

Mayerhoff, M. (1971). *On caring.* New York: Harper & Row.

McCloskey, J. C., & Bulechek, F. M. (Eds.). (1996). *Nursing intervention classifications* (2nd ed.). St. Louis: Mosby.

Mishler, E. G. (1984). *The discourse of medicine: dialectics of medical interviews.* Norwood, NJ: Ablex Publishing.

Mitchell, G. (1995). Nursing diagnosis: An obstacle to caring ways. In A. Boykin (Ed.), *Power, politics and public policy* (pp. 11–23). New York: NLN Press.

Orlando, I. (1990). Nursing in the 21st century: Alternative paths. In C. A. Linderman, & M. McAthie (Eds.), *Nursing trends and issues* (pp. 13–21). Springhouse, PA: Springhouse Corp.

Rakel, R. (1995). *Textbook of family practice.* Philadelphia: W.B. Saunders.

Roach, S. M. (1995). The dominant paradigm of the modern world. In A. Boykin (Ed.), *Power, politics and public policy* (pp. 3–10), New York: NLN Press.

Rogers, M. E. (1972). Nursing: To be or not to be? *Nursing Outlook, 20,* 42–46.

Shalala, D. E. (1993). Nursing and society: The unfinished agenda for the 21st century. *Nursing and Health Care, 14*(6), 289–291.

Smith, M. C. (1995). The con of advanced nursing practice. *Nursing Science Quarterly, 8*(1), 2–3.

St. Anthony's. (1997). *ICD-9-CM: Code book for physician payment,* Vol. 1 & 2, Cincinnati, OH: St. Anthony Publishing.

Venegoni, S. L. (1996). Changing environment in health care. In J. V. Hickey, R. M. Oulmette, & S. L. Venegoni (Eds.), *Advanced practice nursing* (pp. 77–90). Philadelphia: Lippincott.

Watson, J. (1995). Advanced nursing practice: and what might be. *Nursing and Health Care, 10,* 463–467.

Zerwekh, J. (1993). Commentary: Going to the people— public health nursing today and tomorrow. *American Journal of Public Health, 83*(12), 1676–1678.

Chapter 31

Theory-Based Advanced Nursing Practice

Janet W. Kenney, RN, PhD

All professional disciplines are based on their unique knowledge, which is expressed in models and theories that are applied in practice. The focus of nursing knowledge is on humans' health experiences within the context of their environment and the nurse–client relationship. Theory-based nursing practice is the application of various models, theories, and principles from nursing science and the biological, behavioral, medical, and sociocultural disciplines to clinical nursing practice. Conceptual models and theories provide a broad knowledge base to assist nurses in understanding and interpreting the client's complex health situation and in planning nursing actions to achieved desired client outcomes. "Explicit use of conceptual models of nursing and nursing theories to guide nursing practice is the hallmark of professional nursing"; it distinguishes nursing as an autonomous health profession (Fawcett, 1997, p. 212).

This chapter describes the value and relevance of theory-based nursing for advanced practice nurses and discusses some underlying concerns about applying theories in nursing practice. The structure of nursing knowledge and the transformative process for theory-based practice are explained, along with the importance of critical thinking. An overview of various models and theories of nursing, family, and other disciplines is provided. Finally, the process for selecting and applying appropriate models and theories in nursing practice is thoroughly described.

Relevance of Theory-Based Practice in Nursing

The value of theory-based nursing practice is well documented in numerous books and journal articles. Although many articles illustrate the application of a nursing model or theory to clients with a specific health problem, Alligood (1997b) recently reviewed the nursing literature and found that about 68% of the articles reflect a medical approach to nursing. She also noted that most nurses described their practice in terms of a specialty area, types of care or health problems, and nursing interventions.

All nurses use knowledge they acquired during their formal education and clinical experience to guide their practice. Some nurse practitioners consistently use models and theories to guide their practice, but most nurses are unaware of existing theories and models or do not know how to apply them. Many nurses are not aware of what knowledge they use or where they learned it; thus, their implicit knowledge tends to be fragmented, diffused, incomplete, and greatly influenced by the medical model (Fawcett, 1997). Although graduate nurse practitioner students learn about nursing models and theories, their education often emphasizes application of medical knowledge as the base for their nursing practice. Thus, the use of medical knowledge and policies of health care delivery systems has replaced nursing knowledge and influenced some nurses to become "junior doctors," instead of "senior nurses" (Meleis, 1993).

Theories and models from nursing and behavioral disciplines are used by advanced practice nurses to provide effective, high quality nursing care. Many nurses believe that use of nursing theories would improve the quality of nursing care but that they do not have sufficient information about them or the opportunity to use them (McKenna, 1997b). According to Meleis (1997), theories improve quality of care by clearly defining the boundaries and goals of nursing assessment, diagnosis, and interventions and by providing continuity and congruency of care. Theory also contributes to more efficient and effective nursing practice and enhances nurses' professional autonomy and accountability. Aggleton and Chalmers (1986) claim that providing nursing care without a theory base is like "practicing in the dark." Kenney (1996) reported that professional nurses can effectively use theories and models from nursing and behavioral disciplines to:

- collect, organize, and classify client data
- understand, analyze, and interpret client's health situations
- guide formulation of nursing diagnoses
- plan, implement, and evaluate nursing care
- explain nursing actions and interactions with clients
- describe, explain, and sometimes predict clients' responses

- demonstrate responsibility and accountability for nursing actions
- achieve desired outcomes for clients (p. 9)

As we enter the next millennium, the health care revolution requires that nurses demonstrate efficient, cost-effective, high-quality care within organized delivery systems. "Nursing theory-based practice offers an alternative to the dehumanizing, fragmented, and paternalistic approaches that plague current delivery systems" (Smith, 1994, p. 7). With changes in the current third-party reimbursement systems, nurses will be paid for effective theory-based practice that enhances clients' health and their quality of life. To accomplish this, nurse practitioners must use critical thinking skills combined with theory-based knowledge and clinical expertise to achieve desired client outcomes.

Issues Related to Theory-Based Nursing Practice

In recent years, the enthusiasm for using nursing models and theories in practice has waned due to criticisms about the "theory–practice gap" and the lack of relevance to clinical practice. Also, there are philosophical concerns about whether only nursing models should guide practice and whether models and theories of nursing and other disciplines may be integrated in practice. This section discusses some of these issues.

The "theory–practice gap" refers to the lack of use or inability of nurses to use nursing and other theories in clinical practice. McKenna (1997b) claims that theories are not being used in a systematic way to guide nursing practice, although using theories may improve the quality of care. He believes nurses do not use nursing theories because they do not know about them, understand them, believe in them, know how to apply them, or are not allowed to use them. Professional nursing practice more often reflects the medical or organizational model of care than application of relevant nursing models or theories.

According to Rogers (1989, p. 114), "Nursing knowledge . . . is often seen as being unscientific, intuitive, and highly subjective." Some nurses believe that conceptual models and theories are too abstract to apply in nursing practice: they do not provide sufficient information to guide nursing judgments, are subject to different interpretations, are incomplete, and lack adequate testing and refinement (Field, 1987; Firlet, 1985). Others argue that some nursing theories were never meant to be directly applied in nursing practice but were intentionally abstract to stimulate thinking, provide new insights, and develop creative ways of viewing nursing (McKenna, 1997b).

As a practice discipline, nursing models and theories should be useful in practice, or their value is questionable. When models and theories are logical and consistent with other validated theories, they may provide the rationale and consequences of nursing actions and lead to predictable client outcomes. There are numerous articles and chapters describing application of various models to clinical nursing practice. However, rigorous research studies on how nursing models and theories contribute to desirable nursing actions and client outcomes are lacking.

Another issue is whether only nursing models and theories are appropriate for the discipline, as nursing is an applied science. Most professional nurses are familiar with theories from other disciplines, such as systems theory, family theories, developmental theories, and others; in clinical practice, nurses often combine their nursing and medical knowledge with theories from other disciplines. Some nurse scholars argue that nursing practice must be based on nursing models and theories, as they are consistent with nursing's view of human science and provide the structure for explaining nursings'

unique contribution to health care (Cody, 1996; Mitchell, 1992). Because nursing models or theories represent the theorist's unique beliefs about persons, health, and nursing and guide how nurses interact with clients, McKenna (1997b) believes that an eclectic approach, combining theories from nursing and other disciplines, may compromise nursing theories if the concepts are removed from their original context and interwoven with other theories.

In contrast, Meleis (1997) argues that because nurses study other disciplines, nursing theory tends to reflect a broad range of perspectives and premises. Many nursing theorists have incorporated or "borrowed" theories from other disciplines and then transmuted them to fit within the context of nursing so that their nursing theories comprise shared knowledge used in a distinctive way (Timpson, 1996).

A related issue is whether professional nurses should consistently use only one nursing model, or use various models and theories from nursing and other disciplines in their practice. Most professions, like nursing, have multiple theories that represent divergent and unique perspectives about the phenomena of concern to their practice. Within nursing, conceptual models and theories range from broad conceptual models, or grand theories, to specific practice theories. There are advantages and disadvantages to using one or more theories in clinical practice. Depending on the nurse's knowledge and clinical practice area, some nursing models and theories may be more appropriate than others. However, some would argue that use of only one nursing theory limits the nurse's assessment to only those things addressed by the theory, and the nurse may be forced to "fit" the client situation to the theory.

Others believe that nurses should consider a variety of nursing theories and select the model or theory that best "fits" the client's health problems. The majority of early nursing theories were based on traditional scientific methods and reflect a reductionistic perspective of humans as passive beings, consisting of elementary parts that respond to external stimuli in a linear, causal, and predictive way (Benner & Wrubel, 1989). Nursing models based on this perspective ultimately dehumanize individuals into disparate parts and systems and lead to fragmented, non-holistic nursing care (Aggleton & Chalmers, 1986). More contemporary nursing models view humans as continuously changing during reciprocal interactions with their environment, thus individual reactions to nursing care are not predictable, nor can they be controlled. However, these newer nursing models are more abstract than earlier models and are less likely to offer specific guidelines for nursing actions. Professional nurses are expected to develop unique, creative nursing actions suitable for each client's health problem and lifestyle, and theories from other disciplines may be integrated to complement and strengthen some limitations in both early and contemporary nursing models.

Cody (1996) contends that eclecticism, or selecting the best theory from other sources, is not necessarily wrong, but constantly borrowing theories from other disciplines does not contribute to the science of nursing or differentiate nursing from other professions. He believes that nursing practice ought to reflect a coherent, nursing theoretical base to guide practice in specific ways and contribute to the quality of care.

Since professional nurses provide health care for a variety of clients, each of whom is unique yet may have similar health concerns, nurses must use a broad knowledge base from nursing and other disciplines to select and apply relevant models and/or theories that are congruent with the client's situation. Health care, based on appropriate nursing models and theories, that integrates appropriate family, behavioral, and developmental theories, is most likely to achieve desired client health outcomes.

Structure of Nursing Knowledge and Perspective Transformation

Advanced practice nurses must first understand the structure of nursing knowledge and the process of transforming nursing models and theories into useful perspectives prior to implementing theory-based practice. In her recent book, Fawcett (1995) described the structural hierarchy of nursing knowledge, or nursing science. Nursing's metaparadigm, which includes the major concepts of person, health, environment, and nursing, provides the foundation from which nursing philosophies, conceptual models, and theories are derived. Each nurse theorist developed unique definitions of her major concepts, based on her education, practice, and personal philosophy (values, beliefs, and assumptions) about humans, health, nursing, and environment. The theorist's philosophy also influenced her conceptual model, which describes how the concepts are linked: the model explains the relationships among client-health-nursing situations (Sorrentino, 1991). Conceptual nursing models are usually called "grand theories" because they are broad and abstract and may not provide specific directions for nursing actions. Some nurse theorists have developed midrange or practice theories from their models that describe specific relationships among the concepts and suggest hypotheses to be tested.

According to Rogers (1989), an individual's personal "meaning" perspective or conceptual model provides a frame of reference or lens that influences how one perceives, thinks, and behaves in the world, yet most people are not aware of how their perspective influences and affects their view of themselves, others, and their world because underlying beliefs are held in the unconscious mind. In practice, nurses' perceptions, thoughts, feelings, and actions are guided by their personal framework or perspective of nursing, which provides a cognitive structure based on their assumptions, beliefs, and values about nursing (Fawcett, 1995). Many nurses unconsciously use a medical or institutional model as their perspective for organizing care. The prevalent values of such models or perspectives are efficiency, standardized care, rules, and regulations, such as "critical care pathways" (Rogers, 1989). As nurses become aware of the differences between the present and potential possibilities of nursing practice, they experience a cognitive dissonance or discomfort from an awareness of "what is" versus "what could be" (Rogers, 1989). Thus, only when nurses experience cognitive dissonance in practice will they change their frame of reference and use nursing models and theories.

For professional nurses to apply conceptual nursing models and theories, a dramatic change, or "perspective transformation," must occur (Fawcett, 1995; Rogers, 1989). Perspective transformation is the process of moving from one frame of reference or perspective to another, when unresolved dilemmas arise and creat dissonance in one's current perspective (Mezirow, 1979). It is a process of critical reflection and analysis of other explanations or perspectives that might resolve the dilemma and explain or guide one's understanding and actions. The process involves gradually acquiring a new perspective that leads to fundamental changes in the way nurses experience, interpret, and understand their world and their relationships with others (Fawcett, 1995).

Fawcett (1995) describes nine phases leading to "perspective transformation." Initially, the prevailing *stability* of the current nursing practice is disrupted when use of a nursing conceptual model or theory-based practice is introduced. *Dissonance* occurs as nurses consider their own perspective for practice and the challenge of changing to a new conceptual model or theory.

Some nurses identify discrepancies between their current practice and how the new model or theory could affect their practice. *Confusion* may follow as nurses struggle to learn about the model or theory and how to apply it in practice. Nurses often feel anxious, angry, and unable to think during these phases and may grieve the loss of familiar perspectives of nursing. Their former perspective no longer seems useful, yet they have not internalized the new model or theory well enough to use it effectively. While *dwelling with uncertainty,* nurses acknowledge that their confusion is not due to personal inadequacy, and as their anxiety diminishes, they begin to critically examine former practice methods and explore the possibilities of implementing a new model or theory (Fawcett, 1995; Rogers, 1989).

With the discovery that a new model or theory is coherent and meaningful, *synthesis* occurs. As ways to apply the new model become clearer, new insights assist nurses to understand the usefulness of the conceptual model or theory in nursing practice (Fawcett, 1995). *Resolution* occurs as nurses become comfortable using the new model; they may feel a sense of empowerment and view their practice differently. Gradually, nurses consciously change their practice during *reconceptualization;* they shift from their former patterns to new ways of thinking and acting within the new model or theory. The final phase, *return to stability,* occurs when nursing practice is clearly based on the new nursing model or theory. Acceptance of a new perspective or paradigm, along with the corresponding assumptions, values, and beliefs concludes the transformation process.

Models and theories from nursing and other disciplines provide the cognitive structures that guide professional nursing practice. This body of knowledge helps nurses explain "what they know" and the rationale for their nursing actions that facilitate the client's health (Fawcett, 1997). Theory-based nursing practice depends on the depth of nurses' knowledge of models and theories and their understanding about how to apply them in practice (Alligood, 1997a). Nursing models and theories represent ideal, logical, unique perspectives or "maps" of the person and health. They provide a structure and systematic approach to examine clients' situations, identify relevant information, interpret data for nursing diagnoses, and plan effective nursing care through critical thinking, reasoning, and decision making (Alligood, 1997a; Mayberry, 1991; Timpson, 1996).

Nurses must use *critical thinking* skills to apply models and theories to their clients' health concerns. Paul and Nosich's (1991) definition of critical thinking is a commonly accepted one:

> *Critical thinking is the intellectually disciplined process of actively and skillfully conceptualizing, applying, analyzing, synthesizing, or evaluating information gathered from, or generated by, observation, experience, reflection, reasoning, or communication, as a guide to belief and action. (p. 4)*

According to Cradock (1996), *it is not what they know* that makes nurses advanced practitioners, but *how they use what they know.* They must make expert clinical decisions based on reflection, complex reasoning, and critical thinking to apply theoretically based knowledge to diverse client situations (Spiracino, 1991). Critical thinking incorporates ideas from both models or theories with clinical experience and provides the structure for unique, creative nursing practice with each client (Alligood, 1997a; Field, 1987; Mayberry, 1991; Sorrentino, 1991). Several nurse authors believe that nursing theories will become the stimuli for reflection and critical thinking, leading to realms for creative expressions in nursing practice (Chinn, 1997; Marks-Moran & Rose, 1997). Theory-based nursing and critical thinking are the foundations of advanced nursing practice

(Mitchell, 1992). Specific critical thinking skills for each component of the nursing process are identified in **Table 31–1.**

Models and Theories Applicable in Advanced Nursing Practice

Theory-based nursing practice is the creative application of various models, theories, and principles from nursing, medical, behavioral, and humanistic sciences. Models and theories from relevant disciplines provide the knowledge base to understand various aspects of the client's health concerns and guide appropriate nursing management. In advanced nursing practice, the client may be an individual, families or an aggregate, such as a community or special population. Knowledge of relevant models and theories from nursing and other disciplines enables the nurse to select those that "best fit" each client. This section provides a brief overview of some nursing, family, community, and other models and theories that may be relevant and useful to nurse practitioners.

Nursing Models and Theories

Numerous nursing models and theories have been reported in the literature since the 1950s. Some well-known nurse theorists' works are cited: readers are encouraged to seek other sources for more information about their models and theories. The early nurse theorists' conceptual models focused on individual clients and described nursing goals and activities. Peplau's "Interpersonal Model" described a goal-directed, nurse–client interpersonal process to promote the client's personality and living. Orlando's model explained a deliberative nursing approach to understand nurse–patient relationships and the communication process. Hall's "Core-care-cure Model" expanded and clarified nursing

Table 31–1 APPLICATION OF CRITICAL THINKING SKILLS TO THE
NURSING PROCESS

Components & Definitions	Critical Thinking Skills & Activities
Assessment An ongoing process of data collection to determine the client's strengths and health concerns	Collect relevant client data by observation, examination, interview and history, and reviewing the records Distinguish relevant data from irrelevant Distinguish important data from unimportant Validate data with others
Diagnosis The analysis/synthesis of data to identify patterns and compare with norms and models A clear, concise statement of the client's health status and concerns appropriate for nursing intervention	Organize and categorize data into patterns Identify data gaps Recognize patterns and relationships in data Compare patterns with norms and theories Examine own assumptions regarding client's situation Make inferences and judgments of client's health concerns Define the health concern and validate with the client and health team members Describe actual and potential concerns and the etiology of each diagnosis Propose alternative explanations of concerns
Planning Determination of how to assist the client in resolving concerns related to restoration, maintenance, or promotion of health	Identify priority of client's concerns Determine client's desired health outcomes Select appropriate nursing interventions by generalizing principles and theories Transfer knowledge from other sciences Design plan of care with scientific rationale
Implementation Carrying out the plan of care by the client and nurse	Apply knowledge to perform interventions Compare baseline data with changing status Test hypotheses of nursing interventions Update and revise the care plan Collaborate with health team members
Evaluation A systematic, continuous process of comparing the client's response with the desired health outcomes	Compare client's responses with desired health outcomes Use criterion-based tools to evaluate Determine the client's level of progress Revise the plan of care

actions to promote clients' health. Levine's model identified four principles of human conservation to guide nursing activities.

More contemporary nursing theories have been published since 1970, when Rogers introduced her "Science of Unitary Man." She described mutually evolving relationships between humans and their environment that are expressed as changing energy fields, patterns, and organization. Orem's "Self-care Model" identified requisites for an individual's self-care, and specific nursing systems to deliver care according to the client's self-care needs. King designed a systems model that included the individual, family, and society, then developed her "Theory of Goal Attainment," which described nurse–patient transactions to achieve the client's goals. Roy's "Adaptation Model" identified three types of stimuli that affect a patient's four modes of functioning. She described how the nurse identifies maladaptive behaviors and alters stimuli to enhance the client's adaptation. Paterson and Zderad developed a model of "Humanistic Nursing." Leininger's "Transcultural Nursing Model" explained differences between universal and cultural specific views of health and healing, and how nurses can provide culturally congruent health care. According to Watson, nursing is the art and science of human care: nurses engage in transpersonal caring transactions to assist persons achieve mind–body–soul harmony. Johnson's "Behavioral Systems Model" focused on nurturing, protecting, and stimulating the individual's seven subsystems to maintain balance and stability. Neuman designed a complex "Health Care Systems" model that identified different types of stressors and levels of defense: nursing actions were based on three levels of prevention. Parse developed a "Man–living–health Theory" in which nurses assist individuals to explore their past–present–future life experiences and illuminate possible lifestyle choices to enhance their health and lives. Newman's theory of "Health as expanding consciousness" considers disease as part of health, and explores time and rhythm pattern recognition with changes in life and health.

Family Models

Although most nursing models were originally designed to focus on individual clients, a few are applicable to families. King views the family as a social system or group of interacting individuals, and family health as dynamic life experiences. Roy views the family as part of the client's immediate social environment, whereas Neuman's concept of family is harmonious relationships among family members. These nurse theorists focused on the individual client with the family seen as context. If the family is viewed as the client, the nurse must decide what the model should focus on—family development, interactions and stress, family systems, structure and function, or a combination of these models, such as the Calgary Family Model.

Family development models are based on the premise that the life cycle of families follows a common sequence of events from marriage through childrearing, retirement, and bereavement. Most are based on the typical nuclear two-parent family and emphasize the stages and adult's responsibilities to accomplish desired goals. Duvall's (1977) model is well-known, and Stevenson (1977), a nurse theorist, also designed a family model.

Family interactional models view family members as a unit of interacting personalities within a dynamic life process. These models focus on how members' perceptions and interpretations of themselves and other family members determine their behaviors and actions. Also, these models consider how members' roles affect their interaction with others. Satir's "Family Interaction Model" is an example. Family stress and coping models, based on the work of Lazarus and Folkman, were developed by Moos and Billings (1982) to identify how the family appraised the situation, dealt with their problems, and handled the resulting emotions. McCubbin and McCubbin (1993) designed the "Double ABCX Model," which examines family life stressors and resources, along with changes that affect their adaptation to health problems, and ability to manage family crises. Curran's (1985) "Healthy Family Model" identified characteristics of healthy families and common stressors affecting families.

Family systems models view the whole family as greater than and different from the sum of its parts or members. These models focus on the family with a hierarchy of subsystems (mother–father, parent–child) and supersystems in the community (social, occupational, recreational, and religious networks) that interact with the family system. Olson, Russell, and Sprenkle's (1983) model identifies 16 types of family systems based on the premise that a balance must be maintained in family *cohesion,* so that members do not become too enmeshed or too distant, and *adaptability,* wherein too much change creates chaos and too little change leads to rigidity. *Communication* between family members is the third dimension. The "Beaver's System Model" (Beavers & Voeller, 1983) examines the *structure, flexibility,* and *competence* of a family and its members. Centripetal families enjoy close family relationships, while centrifugal families seek satisfaction outside the family.

Family structural–functional models view the family as a social system composed of nuclear and extended family members, and their social–communicative interactions to achieve family functions. According to Friedman (1992), the structural components include family composition, values, communication patterns, members' roles, and the power structure. Functional components of this model include physical necessities and care, economic, affec-

tive, and reproductive behaviors, socialization and placement of family members, and family coping abilities. The structural and functional components are interrelated, and each part is affected by changes in other parts.

A model that combines many of the above models is the Calgary Family Model, developed by Wright and Leahey (1994). The major components include the internal and external family structure, similar to Friedman's (1992) model, along with family context, such as race, ethnicity, social class, religion, and environment. Family functions are viewed as "instrumental" or daily living activities, and "expressive" activities, including communication (emotional, verbal, and behavioral), problem-solving, roles, influences, beliefs, and alliances or coalitions. Family developmental stages and tasks, similar to Duvall's (1977), are also part of this comprehensive model.

Any family model may be combined with and complement a nursing model because nursing practice may involve individual clients or families. Nurses with knowledge of various family models are more likely to select the most appropriate and relevant one to meet the family's health concerns.

Community Models

There are many community models that are useful to nurses, but they differ according to whether "community" is considered a target population or aggregate or a geographical area. McKay and Segall (1983) described an aggregate model, in which the focus is on a group of individuals who share common characteristics, but may not interact with each other. Shamansky and Pesznecker (1981) identified three interdependent factors that constitute a geographical community: (1) *persons* who reside in an area; (2) *space and time,* which includes the community's history and environmental features; and (3) *purpose* factors that explain functional processes such as government policies, educational services, and forms of communication. The "Community-as-Client Model," designed by Anderson, McFarlane, and Helton (1986) combines both the aggregate and geographical community. It addresses the following eight subsystems of the aggregate in the community: physical environment, education, safety and transportation, politics and government, health and social services, communication, economics, and recreation. A community nursing process model was developed by Goeppinger, Lassiter, and Wilcox (1982) that examines the following eight processes in a community: commitment of members, awareness of others' views, articulation of community needs, effective communication within and among members, conflict containment and accommodation, participation in organizations, management of relations with the larger society, and mechanisms to facilitate participant interactions and decision making. Knowledge of several community models facilitates selection of the most appropriate one.

Other Useful Models and Theories

Nurses, and theorists in other disciplines, have developed many relevant models and theories that are useful in advanced nursing practice. Some of these models include Maslow's Hierarchy of Needs, Erikson's "Stages of Development," Piaget's "Cognitive Development of Children," Pender's (1987) "Health Promotion/Disease Prevention" model, and Loveland-Cherry's (1989) "Family health promotion" model. In addition, there are numerous theories of stress, crises, coping, grief, bereavement, death, and dying developed in psychology and behavioral disciplines. Nurses have transformed some of these theories to encompass a health–illness context. Nurses who

are cognizant of a variety of nursing, family, community, and behavioral models and theories are more likely to select the "best fitting" model for their clients.

Selection of Relevant Models and Theories

This section provides an overview of several nurse scholar's criteria and guidelines for selecting models and theories. Meleis (1997) identified six criteria to guide selection of suitable models and theories for practice. McKenna (1997a) described seven selection criteria based on a review of the literature. Kim (1994) constructed a framework for practice theories with four dimensions to consider in selecting nursing models and theories. Fawcett and associates (1992) suggested that nurses consider three questions to determine the best "fit" between the client's health concerns and various models and theories. Relevant criteria from the above scholars' work were integrated with the author's prior work to delineate five guidelines for selecting appropriate models and theories (Christensen & Kenney, 1996).

Meleis (1997) wrote that selecting models and theories for nursing practice is both a subjective and objective process. She identified six criteria for nurses to consider in the selection process.

- Personal—the nurse's comfort with the theory and congruency with the nurse's own philosophical views of life
- Mentor—the model or theory learned from a nurse mentor or educator
- Theorist—their reputation in the discipline and degree of recognition
- Literature—support the amount of literature available about the theory and the theory's significance for one's specialty
- Sociopolitical congruency—the model or theory's acceptability within the nurse's

workplace and whether major structural or practice changes are required

- Utility—the ease in which nurses can understand and apply the model or theory in practice settings

McKenna (1997a) reviewed the literature and identified the following seven criteria for selecting models and theories.

- The type of client—the client's needs should direct the choice because the theory provides guidelines to achieve the client's goals.
- Health care setting—the type of clinical setting and nursing practice are contextual factors that affect selection of theories.
- Parsimony/simplicity—simple and realistic theories are more likely to be understood and applied in practice.
- Understandability—nurses must understand a theory if they expected to use it.
- Origins of the theory—the credibility, prior use, and testing of the theory should also be considered.
- Paradigms as a basis for choice—nurses must decide between the totality or simultaneity paradigm, as each provides a different view of clients and nursing actions.
- Personal values and beliefs—the theory must be congruent with the nurse's own views about humans, health, and nursing.

In her article on practice theories, Kim (1994) defined two dimensions of theories, which include four "sets of practice theories" relevant to selecting models and theories. One dimension is the "target," which addresses both the philosophy of care for the person and the philosophy of therapy for the client's problems. The other dimension is the "nurse–agent," which includes two phases, deliberation, and enactment. The four "sets of practice theories" serve to guide nurses in choosing theories that

will (1) explain the patient's problems and ideas about therapy for the problems; (2) provide ideas about how the nurse should approach the patient, such as through communication, caring, or empowerment; (3) explain how to make decisions about appropriate nursing actions for the patient; and (4) explain what happens during enactment of nursing actions. Kim proposed that a science of nursing practice could be developed from this framework.

Fawcett and associates (1992) identified questions to guide nurses' selection of appropriate theories and models. The nurse must understand the differences among various models and theories in nursing and other disciplines to answer these questions. The following three questions will help the nurse identify the most appropriate model:

1. Does the theory or model address the client's problems and health concerns?
2. Are the nursing interventions suggested by the model consistent with the client's expectations for nursing care?
3. Are the goals of nursing actions, based on the model or theory, congruent with the client's desired health outcomes?

These questions help nurses decide which models and theories will assist them to organize the data into patterns, identify other health concerns, and determine congruency of the client's and nurse's view of nursing and health.

The first step toward theory-based nursing practice is the *conscious decision to use theories in practice* (Fawcett, 1997). The second step is recognizing that use of conceptual nursing models and theories requires a major change in how the nurse thinks about and interacts with clients to alleviate their health concerns. This change, referred to earlier as a "perspective transformation," occurs gradually as the nurse discards one framework of practice and learns another perspective. Adopting and applying new models and theories in practice depends on nurses having knowledge of various models and theories and understanding how these models and theories relate to each other (Alligood, 1997a).

Guidelines for Selecting Models and Theories for Nursing Practice

After deciding to implement theory-based nursing practice, the author believes that each nurse must engage in the five steps described here:

1. *Consider your personal values and beliefs about nursing, clients, health, and environment.* Each nurse has a personal frame of reference or perspective of nursing practice, based on his/her conscious or unconscious assumptions, beliefs, and values about nursing. One's perspective of nursing provides a cognitive structure that guides one's perceptions, thoughts, feelings, and nursing actions (Fawcett, 1995). Clarifying one's own values and beliefs about clients, health, and nursing practice is necessary before a "perspective transformation" can occur.

2. *Examine the underlying assumptions, values, and beliefs of various nursing models, and how the major concepts are defined.* After clarifying one's own values and beliefs, the nurse examines the definitions of major concepts in various models and theories to determine whether they are congruent with one's own beliefs (Alligood, 1997a). Nursing models and theories are based on different values and beliefs about the nature of the client's behaviors and abilities, what is health and environment, and what nursing actions facilitate clients' health. Each nursing model and theory provides a unique view for specific nursing practice. Some nursing models reflect a "totality"

paradigm, and view humans as having separate biological, social, psychological, and spiritual parts that respond to environmental stimuli or change, and the nurse's role is to facilitate adaptation or equilibrium to maintain health. Other nursing models reflect a "simultaneity" paradigm, and believe humans are intelligent beings, capable of making informed decisions about their lives, and that they continuously engage in a dynamic, mutual interaction with their environment. In this paradigm, the nurse's role is to guide clients in choosing lifestyles and/or therapies that are acceptable to them and facilitate their growth and life–health process.

3. *Identify several models that are congruent with your own values and beliefs about nursing, clients, and health.* Each nurse must consider whether the theorist's underlying values are congruent with one's own personal values and beliefs about clients, health, and nursing because the theorist's values guide the nurse's critical thinking and reasoning processes (Alligood, 1997a). Models and theories reflect the theorist's views about people and nursing. They directly effect how nurses approach their clients, what information they gather, how that information is processed, what nursing activities are appropriate, and, what client outcomes are expected based on the model. For example, some traditional nursing models define the person as a bio–psycho–social being who responds to environmental stimuli, and health results from nursing actions that lead to predictable changes. These models would be incongruent for contemporary nurses who believe that people are free agents, dynamically interacting with their environment as a whole, and capable of making rational decisions, and that the

nurse's role is to assist clients to explore various options and choose ones that are acceptable with their values and lifestyle.

4. *Identify the similarities and differences in client focus, nursing actions, and client outcomes of these models.* Nursing models and theories consist of concepts with specific definitions, and statements that describe how the concepts are interrelated. Some propose specific nursing actions and expected client outcomes. The major concepts guide what data is collected during the assessment and how the data is organized to identify and interpret bio–behavioral patterns and determine nursing diagnoses. Nursing models also guide development of the nursing care plans and designate desired outcomes to evaluate. By comparing various models, nurses recognize which ones are congruent with their values and beliefs about nursing and offer the best "fit" with the client's health concerns.

5. *Practice applying the models and theories to clients with different health concerns to determine which ones best "fit" specific situations and guide nursing actions that will achieve desired client outcomes.* The nurse explores specific models in depth, and may analyze their usefulness before implementing them. By comparing several models and examining the attributes of the client, the focus of nursing actions, and the proposed outcomes, the nurse will acquire a more in-depth understanding of different models. Each nursing model describes different areas for assessment, unique nursing diagnoses, and specific nursing interventions to assist the client toward health. The nurse must decide which models and theories are most appropriate for each client. Which one offers the best "fit" for the client's health concerns? Selecting appropriate models and theories for each unique client health situation requires

nurses to use their broad knowledge base from various disciplines, critical thinking skills, clinical expertise, and intuition to identify the best 'fit' between the client's health concerns and nursing models (Fawcett, et al., 1992).

Application of Theory-Based Nursing Practice

The choice of theories and models suitable to the client's health concerns occurs during the initial data assessment process. The initial data focus on the client's primary expressed concerns and how they are related to or affect the client's lifestyle and patterns of living. These data assist the nurse to identify and understand the client's common and unique patterns. The client's view of health, along with past and present "lived experiences," and future lifestyle and health concerns, are also considered. Using this information, the nurse considers various models and theories from nursing and other disciplines that are relevant to the client's unique health concerns, and congruent with the nurse's own beliefs. Then, the nurse selects those models and other theories that best "fit" the client's situation and health concerns and will systematically direct nursing practice.

The major concepts of the chosen models and theories guide each component of the nursing process, as shown in **Table 31–2**. The concepts serve as categories to guide additional data collection. They suggest, either directly or indirectly, *what* information is relevant and should be collected. The models and theories assist the nurse to organize, categorize, and interpret pertinent data that illustrate the client's bio–behavioral patterns and identify appropriate nursing diagnoses that are linked to relevant etiological factors.

Nursing and other models and theories guide development of a care plan by suggesting appropriate types of nursing interventions and specific

Table 31-2 THEORY-BASED NURSING PRACTICE

Component	Nursing Process Use	Nursing Model Use
Assessment	Describes how to collect data	Guides what data to collect
Diagnosis	Describes how to process data	Guides organizing, categorizing, and interpreting data
	Provides format for nursing diagnosis	Provides concepts for nursing diagnosis
	Describes *how* to plan	Guides *what* to plan
	Facilitates development of care plan unique to client	Designates appropriate types of nursing interventions
Implementation	Describes phases of implementation	Directs model-specific nursing actions
Evaluation	Identifies *how* to evaluate	Guides *what* to evaluate
General	Requires accountability through use of systematic approach to nursing practice	Enhances accountability of theory-based practice
	Process enhances continuity of care	Provides a comprehensive, coherent approach to care of client

nursing actions. Desired client outcomes are derived from the models and theories and define what changes in the client should be evaluated. For example, if Roy's model is chosen, data about the client's physiological needs, self-concept, role mastery, and interdependence, along with related stimuli would be collected, and used to identify adaptive and maladaptive behavioral patterns. The nurse who uses Orem's Self-Care Model would assess and judge clients' ability to meet their universal and developmental self-care requisites and whether they had any health deviations. From analysis of this data, the nurse would diagnose self-care deficits and determine appropriate nursing plans for partial, compensatory, or health education nursing care. Nursing care plans are based on the model and describe the client's desired outcomes, along with nursing actions to achieve the client's outcomes. Nurses who use Johnson's Behavioral Systems Model would consider ways to nurture, protect, or stimulate the client to facilitate health, whereas the Neuman's Health Care System's model assists the nurse to explore ways to reduce stressors within the three levels of disease prevention.

Some nurses believe that family models complement nursing models and provide a more holistic and comprehensive perspective of clients and their health concerns. Selection of a family model occurs after the nurse gathers preliminary data about the family and identifies its unique and common patterns. Then the nurse decides whether the "family as context" or "family as client" would be more appropriate and best "fit" the client's situation. Also, the nurse's perception and definition of family and health guide the selection of a family model. For example, a pediatric nurse who works in an outpatient clinic may choose Orem's Self-Care Model to guide care of a nine-year-old child with an ear infection and the mother's treatment of the child. Friedman's Family System model may complement Orem's model and enhance understanding of the family's structure and functions. The nurse may also use Erikson's Developmental Framework to help the mother recognize and encourage her child's normal developmental behaviors. Pain management theories may also be applied to reduce the child's earache.

This example illustrates how nurses examine and judge the value of various models and theories and select those that are most congruent and useful and best "fit" the client's health concerns and the nurse's perspective of practice. Gradually, nurse practitioners develop an expertise in selecting theories and models that are appropriate and relevant to their client's health concerns and congruent with their own views of advanced practice.

Summary

This chapter described the importance and value of applying models and theories from nursing and other disciplines in advanced nursing practice. Issues related to the nursing theory-practice gap were discussed, along with concerns about using only one nursing model in practice and about integrating models and theories from other disciplines with nursing models and theories. The structure of nursing knowledge was explained and the need for a "perspective transformation" to occur prior to implementing theory-based nursing practice. Critical thinking, logical reasoning, and creatively applying nursing models and theories were emphasized. Different types of nursing, family, community, and other models and theories were discussed. Finally, the process of selecting and applying models and theories was thoroughly described.

In the last few decades, the emergence of nursing models and theories has illuminated several nursing paradigms and explicated their underlying assumptions, beliefs, and values that guide nursing practice. The science of nursing and empirical patterns of knowing is represented by these nursing models and their theories. Application of models and theories from nursing and other disciplines depends on nurses having a broad knowledge base and understanding how models and theories are interrelated. Empowerment of nurses through "perspective transformation" and the use of nursing models and theories is essential. They provide the framework for critical thinking within the context of nursing and guide the reasoning that professional nurses need to survive in an era of cost containment and evidence-based practice. Use of models and theories from nursing and related health disciplines enables nurses to demonstrate accountability for their decisions and actions through scientific explanation and provides a coherent approach to theory-based nursing practice.

References

Aggleton, P. J., & Chalmers, H. (1986). *Nursing models and the nursing process.* Basingstoke: Macmillan.

Alligood, M. R. (1997a). Models and theories: Critical thinking structures. In M. R. Alligood and A. Marriner-Tomey. *Nursing Theory: Utilization & Application,* St. Louis: C. V. Mosby, pp. 31–45.

Alligood, M. R. (1997b). Models and theories in nursing practice. In M. R. Alligood and A, Marriner-Tomey. *Nursing Theory: Utilization & Application,* St. Louis: C. V. Mosby, pp. 15–30.

Anderson, E. T., McFarlane, J. M., & Helton, A. (1986). Community as client: A model for practice. *Nursing Outlook, 3*(5), 220.

Beavers, W. R., & Voeller, M. N. (1983). Family models: Comparing and contrasting the Olson circumplex models with the Beaver's systems model. *Family Process, 22,* 85–98.

Benner, P., & Wrubel, J. (1989). *The primacy of caring.* Menlo Park, CA: Addison-Wesley.

Chinn, P. L. (1997). Why middle-range theory? *ANS, 19*(3), viii.

Christensen, P. J., & Kenney, J. W. (1996). *Nursing process: Application of conceptual models,* 4th ed. St. Louis: C.V. Mosby.

Cody, W. K. (1996). Drowning in eclecticism. *Nursing Science Quarterly, 9*(3), 86–88.

Cradock, S. (1996). The expert nurse: Clinical specialist or advanced practitioner? In Gary Rolfe (Ed.). *Closing the theory-practice gap: A new paradigm for nursing.* Oxford, UK: Butterworth-Heinemann Ltd.

Curran, D. (1985). *Stress and the healthy family.* Minneapolis, MN: Winston Press.

Duvall, E. M. (1997). *Marriage and family development,* 5th ed. Philadelphia: Lippincott.

Fawcett, J. (1995). Implementing conceptual models in nursing practice. In J. Fawcett (Ed.). *Analysis and evaluation of conceptual models of nursing,* 3rd ed. Philadelphia: F. A. Davis.

Fawcett, J. (1997). Conceptual models of nursing, nursing theories, and nursing practice: Focus on the future. In M. R. Alligood and A. Marriner-Tomey (Eds.). *Nursing Theory: Utilization & Application.* St. Louis: C. V. Mosby, pp. 211–221.

Fawcett, J., Archer, C. L., Becker, D., et al. (1992). Guidelines for selecting a conceptual model of nursing: Focus on the individual client. *Dimen Critical Care Nursing, 11*(5), 268–277.

Field, P. A. (1987). The impact of nursing theory on the clinical decision making process, *Journal of Advanced Nursing, 12,* 563–571.

Firlet, S. I. (1985). Nursing theory and nursing practice: Separate or linked? In J. McCloskey & H. K. Grace (Eds.). *Current issues in nursing.* Boston: Blackwell Scientific Publications, pp. 6–19.

Friedman, M. M. (1992). *Family nursing: Theory and practice,* 3rd ed. New York: Appleton & Lange.

Goeppinger, J., Lassiter, P. G., & Wilcox, B. (1982). Community health is community competence. *Nursing Outlook, 30*(8), 464.

Kenney, J. W. (1996). Relevance of theory-based nursing practice. In P. J. Christensen & J. W. Kenney (Eds.). *Nursing Process: Application of Conceptual Models,* 4th ed. St. Louis: C. V. Mosby, pp. 1–23.

Kim, H. S. (1994). Practice theories in nursing and a science of nursing practice. *Scholarly Inquiry for Nursing Practice: An International Journal, 8*(2), 145–158.

Loveland-Cherry, C. J. (1989). Family health promotion and health protection. In P. Bomar (Ed.). *Nurses and family health promotion: Concepts, assessment, and interventions.* Baltimore, MD: Williams & Wilkins.

Marks-Moran, D., & Rose, P. (Eds.). (1997). *Reconstructing nursing: Beyond art and science.* Philadelphia: Bailliere Tindall.

Mayberry, A. (1991). Merging nursing theories, models, and nursing practice: More than an administrative challenge. *ANS, 15,* 44.

McCubbin, M. A., & McCubbin, H. I. (1993). Families coping with illness: The resiliency model of family stress, adjustment and adaptation. In C. B. Danielson, B. Hamel-Bissell, & P. Winstead-Fry (Eds.). *Families, health and illness: Perspectives on coping and intervention.* St. Louis: Mosby, pp. 21–65.

McKay, R., & Segall, M. (1983). Methods and models for the aggregate. *Nursing Outlook, 31*(6), 328.

McKenna, H. (1997a). Choosing a theory for practice. In Hugh McKenna (Ed.). *Nursing theories and models.* New York: Rutledge, pp. 127–157.

McKenna, H. (1997b). Applying theories in practice. In Hugh McKenna (Ed.). *Nursing theories and models.* New York: Rutledge, pp. 158–189.

Meleis, A. I. (1993). *Nursing research and the Neuman model: Directions for the future.* Panel discussion conducted at the Fourth Biennial International Neuman Systems Model Symposium, Rochester, NY.

Meleis, A. I. (1997). *Theoretical nursing: Development and progress,* 3rd ed. Philadelphia: Lippincott.

Mezirow, J. (1979). Perspective transformation. *Adult Education, 28*(3), 100–110.

Mitchell, G. (1992). Specifying the knowledge base of theory in practice. *Nursing Science Quarterly, 5*(1), 6–7.

Moos, R. H., & Billings, A. G. (1982). Conceptualizing and measuring coping resources and processes. In L. Goldberger & S. Breznitz (Eds.). *Handbook of stress.* New York: Free Press.

Olson, D. H., Russell, C. S., & Sprenkle, D. H. (1983). Circumplex models of marital and family systems: VI. Theoretical update. *Family Processes, 22,* 69–83.

Paul, R. W., & Nosich, G. M. (1991). Proposal for the national assessment of higher-order thinking (revised version). The United States Department of Education Office of Educational Research and Improvement, National Center for Education Statistics.

Pender, N. J. (1987). *Health promotion in nursing practice.* New York: Doubleday.

Rogers, M. E. (1989). Creating a climate for the implementation of a nursing conceptual framework. *Journal of Continuing Education in Nursing, 20*(3), 112–116.

Shamansky, S. L., & Pesznecker, B. (1981). A community is. . . . *Nursing Outlook, 29*(3), 182–185.

Smith, M. C. (1994). Beyond the threshold: Nursing practice in the next millennium. *Nursing Science Quarterly, 7*(1), 6–7.

Sorrentino, E. A. (1991). Making theories work for you. *Nursing Administration Quarterly, 15*(3), 54–59.

Spiracino, P. (1991). The reciprocal relationship between practice and theory. *Clinical Nurse Specialist, 5*(3), 138.

Stevenson, J. (1977). *Issues and crises during middlescence.* New York: Appleton-Century-Crofts.

Timpson, J. (1996). Nursing theory: Everything the artist spits is art? *Journal of Advanced Nursing, 23,* 1030–1036.

Wright, L. M., & Leahey, M. (1994). *Nurses and families: A guide to family assessment and intervention,* 2nd ed. Philadelphia: F. A. Davis.

Index

A

accomplishment, as expression of health, 148, 151–152
accreditation and licensing, 92
action, principles for, 217–218
activity, as expression of health, 148, 150
adaptation, 20
advanced nursing practice. *See* practice of nursing
affect, as expression of health, 147–149
ANA Code for Nurses, 102–103
ANA Social Policy Statement, 184, 289–290
antipositivism. *See* interpretative paradigms
aperspectival consciousness, 283
APN. *See* practice of nursing
appreciating wholeness, healing as, 155–169
    appreciating context, 155–157
    appreciating process, 158–161
    case study, 161–168
apprenticeship system of nursing, 88
approaches (nursing), knowledge of, 16
art of nursing (esthetics), 32. *See also* interpretative paradigms
    ability to learn, 137
    conceptualizations of, 133–140
    humanistic nursing model, 233–238
    morality of, 139–140
    patterns of knowing, 259
    science vs., 21–22
aspiration, as expression of health, 148, 150–151
attending nurses, 56
attitude

as expression of health, 148–149
of openness and inquiry, 77, 280
perspective taking, 282–283
authentic consciousness, 211–213
authenticity of patient relationship, 23, 136
autonomy, 210–211
avoiding bias, 7
    American value system, 102–104
    critical multiplism, 226
    critical multiplism for, 224
    misrepresentation of evidence, 276–277
awareness
    authentic, 211–213
    integral (aperspectival), 283

B

behavioral ability, nursing art as, 136–137
bias, 7
    American, in value system, 102–104
    critical multiplism, 226
    misrepresentation of evidence, 276–277
    reducing with critical multiplism, 224
blending nursing and other sciences, 62
Board of Medical Research, Sweden (MFR), 111
body of nursing knowledge, 43
Buber, Martin, 135
Bunch, Haugen, 103

311

W